T0134719

Anatomy for Urologic Surgeons in the Digital Era

Emre Huri • Domenico Veneziano

Editors

Anatomy for Urologic Surgeons in the Digital Era

Scanning, Modelling and 3D Printing

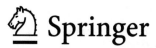 Springer

Editors
Emre Huri
Department of Urology
Hacettepe University
Ankara, Turkey

Domenico Veneziano
Grande Ospedale Metropolitano
Reggio Calabria
Italy

ISBN 978-3-030-59481-7   ISBN 978-3-030-59479-4   (eBook)
https://doi.org/10.1007/978-3-030-59479-4

This Springer imprint is published by the registered company Springer Nature Switzerland AG
The registered company address is: Gewerbestrasse 11, 6330 Cham, Switzerland

I dedicate this book to my daughter Melya and my wife Meral.

—Emre Huri

Preface

Enterprises with social or economic value are considered innovations. Considering a historically important concept such as anatomy together with innovative methods in urology is important for finding new surgical methods and teaching surgery better. We are in the era of widespread use of digital in the medical field. Research, education and patient care, which are the three basic requirements of a medical academy, are developing in parallel with the developments in health technologies. For this reason, it is known that "anatomy", which is the basis of urological surgery, also keeps up with this change, and new methods used in surgical training and surgical planning are popular in the digital era. This book, *Anatomy for Urologic Surgery in Digital Era,* consist of 25 chapters; however, we aimed to include important topics such as anatomical standards of 3D models used in urology, innovations in imaging, surgical planning and visualization tools, use of 3D medical printing in urology and anatomical classification in urological surgery. Thanks to the contribution of some of the most relevant names in the field, we hope that this volume will help the reader to increase awareness of being in a digital era for urologic surgery; we hope that every urologist can find a visional perspective in this book.

During the preparation phase of this book, my aim was to describe urological surgery in the digital era in a single book. However, in a period when digital transformation is experienced intensively in urology, when you consider the anatomy and future surgical modalities, we felt the need to prepare two separate books in this field. We did these studies with my esteemed colleague Domenico Veneziano. In addition, we have received the contributions of academics of international importance in their fields. Two separate books have emerged, describing the use of 10 years' technologies in urology and reinforced with anatomy.

As a urologist who has been working on urological anatomy for more than 10 years, I would like to thank my family for their support throughout this process.

Ankara, Turkey   Emre Huri

Foreword

Emre Huri and Domenico Veneziano gave me the pleasure to comment on their book "Anatomy for the urologic surgeons in the digital era." The book is timely and comprehensive of all present advancements in the field. Surgical anatomy is the alphabet of any surgeon and the digital era, thanks to tremendous innovations in imaging, 3D reconstruction, virtual reality, and real-time virtual navigation, provides marvelous tools to be used by novices and experts. I can imagine the astonishment of Leonardo da Vinci, if he had the opportunity to experience a glimpse of all this. Easy to say that we are witnessing just the beginning of a process and soon more than later, anatomic surgical navigation will match what we have seen in modern science fiction movies. It is my hope that the outstanding value of anatomic surgical navigation will be understood by those big companies that are involved in creating and marketing digital games. Many of the readers know the level of reality and interaction achieved by these games and I believe that the underlying technology could be easily employed in producing "surgical anatomy games." It is just a matter of financial commitment.

All this is transforming surgical teaching and training: interactive anatomic navigation will provide the opportunity to simulate simple and complex surgical procedures, measuring accurately the progress, and the performance of the trainee.

All Authors should be commended for their contributions to such a great work.

Verona, Italy   Walter Artibani

Contents

Chapter 1
History of Urological Anatomy

José María Gil-Vernet Sedó and José María Gil-Vernet Vila

1.1 The History of the Urinary Tract Anatomy

The Greek physician Galen (129 AD-*ca.* 210), when studying the urinary tract in his *De Anatomicis administrationibus* [1] erroneously described that the right kidney was higher than the left one, as these were findings from dissections on animals, mainly the Barbary macaque (*Macacus inuus*). He assumed that inside the kidney there was a membrane filter separating urine from blood. He demonstrated the existence of the renal sinus and the intrasinusal space, while the pelvis was defined as a "membranous body" where the ureter was born. At bladder neck level, he described the existence of a muscle he called sphincter. In *De uso partium* (Hakkert 1968) Galen observed, by means of the ligation of ureters in dogs, that urine was produced in kidneys and not in the bladder, and accurately describes the layout of the ureter and its intravesical oblique path, a layout considered key for preventing vesicoureteral reflux. He believed that the bladder only has three muscle layers, i.e. a longitudinal outer layer an oblique intermediate layer and a circular inner layer. Galen's anatomical concepts remain valid and unwavering until the sixteenth century.

In the fourteenth century, the Italian anatomist Mondino da Luzzi (*ca.* 1270–1336), a professor at the university of Bologna and one of the leading proponents and restorers of anatomy, tapped into the ancient Hellenistic tradition of Herophilos and Erasistratus, and all its unique character. He performed dissections on human corpses and in his *Anatomia* (1316) he described the bladder with its

J. M. Gil-Vernet Sedó (✉)
Teknon Medical Center, Barcelona, Spain

Complutense University of Madrid Research Group 920547, Madrid, Spain

Gil-Vernet Urology Center, Barcelona, Spain

J. M. Gil-Vernet Vila
University of Barcelona, Barcelona, Spain

© Springer Nature Switzerland AG 2021
E. Huri, D. Veneziano (eds.), *Anatomy for Urologic Surgeons in the Digital Era*,
https://doi.org/10.1007/978-3-030-59479-4_1

ureters and, with great detail, the vessels of the penis and the venous system of the cavernous bodies.

The Bologna tradition reaches the University of Montpelier through Henri de Mondeville (*ca.* 1260–1320), Professor of Anatomy and Surgery. Mondeville used in his classes a skull he could dismantle, with thirteen tables. In a reduced and simplified form, these tables were used to illustrate the French translation of his *Chirurgia* (1312). In this work, Mondeville describes, without naming them, the renal pelvis and the renal calyces [2]. The urinary system illustration (Fig. 1.1) departs from traditional Medieval representation and approaches the artistic anatomy later found in Vesalius.

Berengario da Carpi (*ca.* 1460–1530), Professor of Anatomy and Surgery in Bologna, was one of the most important pre-Vesalius anatomists. In the chapter titled *De renibus* of his *Carpi commentaria cum amplissimis aditionibus super anatomiam Mundini* (1521), he describes that the injection of warm water in the renal vein of a pig does not reach the renal pelvis, but is instead accumulated in the kidney substance and that, when cutting the kidney along its convex side, the injected water oozes out and its exit is observed through the papillae, which he defines as "female nipples". In this way, the old Galen concept of a filtering membrane that serves to separate urine from the blood coming from the renal vein is refuted [3].

Further on, the Venetian physician Niccolò Massa (1485–1569), when describing kidneys in his *Liber introductorius anatomiae* (1536), he demonstrates by blowing air through a rod into the renal veins, that these do not continue on to the renal pelvis [4].

Fig. 1.1 Front view of a male body opened from the xiphoid process to the pubis, showing the urinary system. Mondeville, H. Chirurgia, 1314

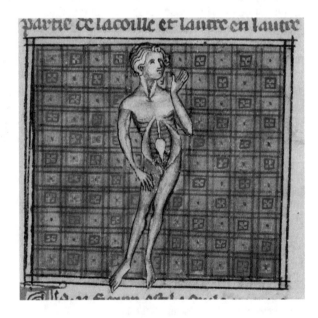

Andreas Vesalius (1514–1564), Professor of Anatomy and Surgery at the University of Padua (Italy), in his monumental work *De humani corporis fabrica libri septem* (1543) breaks with the false opinion that the right kidney is higher than the left one. Although this error appears in the illustration of book V (Fig. 1.2), the text asserts that the opposite is true. In his dissections, using the uni-papilla kidney of a dog, he mistakes the projection of the papilla for a dividing septum and does not describe the area cribrosa.

Vesalius also rejects Galen's theory according to which urine passes through the kidney via a filtering membrane. Berengario da Carpi and Niccolò Massa had already rejected the filter theory, but Vesalius went a step further by confirming that the "serum blood" was deliberately selected or directed towards the kidney's membranous body (pelvis) and its "branches" in order to release its "serous humour" and the excreted matter was later taken to the bladder by the ureters. He believed that the bladder was made up of a mucosal layer and a muscular tunic, comprising three fibre groups, several transversal external fibres, some intermediate oblique fibres, and other, internal ones. Vesalius thought that the intramural layout of the ureter prevented the vesicoureteral reflux based on the fact that, when the bladder was filled with air, the air did not escape through the ureters [5].

The Cremonese Realdo Colombo (*ca.* 1515–1558), a discipline and assistant of Vesalius in Padua, questions some of his master's descriptions. In the chapter *De*

Fig. 1.2 Plate 25. Female urinary system. The bladder (β) has been reflected downward to the left side, showing the right ureter sectioned (**b**). Vesalius, A. De humani corporis fabrica libri septem. V Book, 1543

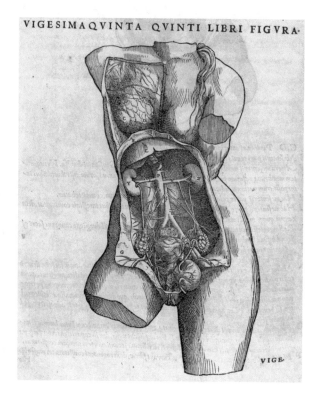

VIGESIMAQVINTA QVINTI LIBRI FIGVRA·

renibus from the work *De re anatomica libri XV* (1559), he contends that the right kidney is lower than the left [6].

Grabiele Fallopio (*ca.* 1523–1562), an anatomist from Modena, taught at the universities of Pisa and Padua. In his work *Observationes anatomicae* (1562), he intended to discuss the illustrations of *Fabrica* and to rationally correct the inaccuracies of Vesalius; he provides a detailed description of the papillae and the renal calyces [7].

Bartolomeo Eustacchio (1510–1574), Professor of Anatomy at the medical school of the Archigimnasio della Sapienza in Rome, wrote between 1562 and 1563 a series of treaties published under the name *Opuscula anatomica* (1563–1564). In this work, in the *Tractatio de renibus* and specifically in the chapter *De renum structura* [8], he shows that the right kidney is located below the left one, and describes the adrenal glands for the first time (Fig. 1.3a). He depicts the layout of the calyces, the uriniferous tubule in the renal medulla and the papillae with their area cribrosa and, using vascular injection and corrosion techniques, he describes the kidney's vasculature with its terminal arches (Fig. 1.3b). He is also the first to describe the kidney's anatomical variations (Fig. 1.3c). Eustacchio provided the illustrations himself, and his drawings are more detailed and accurate than those in Vesalius' *Fabrica*.

In the seventeenth century, the English surgeon Nathaniel Highmore (1613–1685) in his work *Corporis humani disquitio anatomica; in qua sanguinis circulationem in quavis corporis particula plurimis typis novis* (1651), describes for the first time the interlobular vessels and the arcuate arteries and veins [9], located between the cortex and the renal medulla (Fig. 1.4a and b).

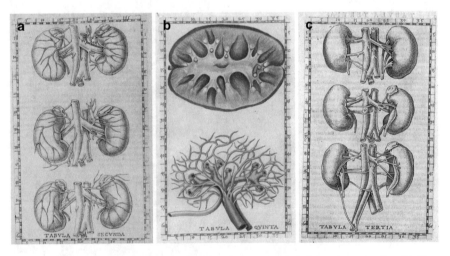

Fig. 1.3 (**a**) Plate II. The kidneys and the adrenal glands, with their arteries and veins. (**b**) Plate V. Calyces and renal pelvis. Papillae and cribrosa areas. (**c**) Plate III. Renal anatomical variations. Eustaccchio, B. Opuscula anatomica, 1564

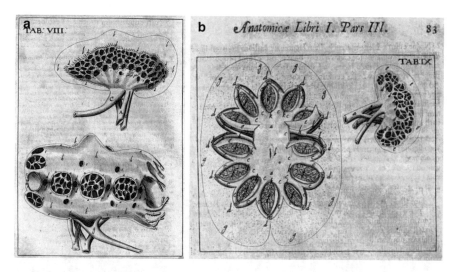

Fig. 1.4 (**a**) Plate VIII. Renal interlobular arteries and veins (**b**) Plate IX. Arcuate renal vessels. Highmore, N. Corporis humani disquisitio anatomica, 1651

In 1662, the Florentine Lorenzo Bellini (1643–1704), Professor of Anatomy at Padua, published *Exercitatio anatomica duae de structura et usu renum*. In the chapter *De structura renum* [10] he demonstrates, by injecting dye injections in the renal veins of lamb and deer, that blood reaches the cortex and implying that urine is filtered at this level (Fig. 1.5a). Also, using loupes or microscopes, he demonstrates for the first time the existence of "filaments" that reach the kidney surface from the renal papillae. These are the collecting tubules and they are called Bellini ducts in his honour (Fig. 1.5b).

The Italian Marcello Malpighi (1628–1694), Professor of Medicine at the University of Bologna and the founder of microscopic anatomy, published in 1687 his enormous *Opera omnia, seu, thesaurus locupletissimus botanico-medico-anatomicus*. This work includes the treaty *Exercitationes anatomicae de structura viscerum* with the chapter *De renibus*, where through the use of a mixture of Indian ink and alcohol injected in the renal artery, he finds some tiny corpuscles hanging, like apples, from the blood vessels. These are the renal glomeruli [11], although Malpighi believed they were small glands responsible for urine secretion.

Later on, the Dutch Anatomist Frederik Ruysch (1638–1731), an unrivalled master at preparing vascular trees through melted wax injections, in his work *Thesaurus anatomicus primus* (1701) rejected the glandular theory of the kidney as he observed that the glomeruli were formed of capillary skeins [12].

In 1774, the French Anatomist Exupère Joseph Bertin (1712–1781), Professor of Anatomy at the University of Paris, in his essay *Mémoirs pour servir à l'histoire des reins*, divides the renal parenchyma into two portions, i.e. a cortical and a medullary section. He discovers some formations of the renal cortex which descend among the

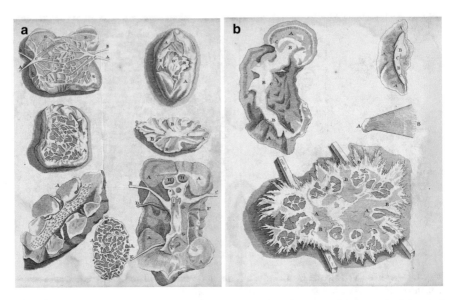

Fig. 1.5 (**a**) Dissections of sheep kidneys. Microscopic view of the superficial vessels of the renal cortex after the injection of dye in the renal blood vessels (6) (**b**) Dissections of human and deer kidneys. Isolated papilla with its collector tubules (10). Bellini, L. De structura renum, 1662

Fig. 1.6 Intrarenal vascularization. Intrusions of cortical tissue between the renal pyramids (Bertin's columns). Bertin, EJ. Mémoirs pour servir à l'histoire des reins, 1744

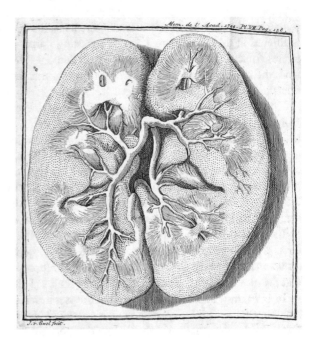

pyramids and will become known as Bertin's columns (Fig. 1.6). He also discovered, for the first time, the nephron loop, a century before Henle's description [13].

The Italian physician Giovanni Battista Morgagni (1682–1771), Professor of Anatomy at the University of Bologna, in his work *Adversaria anatomica omnia:quorum tria posteriora nunc primum prodeunt* (1723) describes the navicular fossa of the urethra, the penile suspensory ligament and the urethral glands [14].

The Venetian Anatomist, Giovanni Domenico Santorini (1681–1737), in his works *Observationes anatomicas* (1774) and *Septemdecim tabulae quas nunc primum edit* (1775), offers a detailed description of the different layers of the vesical musculature, the pubovesical ligaments coming down from the external longitudinal layer of the detrusor, the external urethral sphincter and the *plexus pubicus impar* or venous plexus of Santorini (Fig. 1.7) and the male perineal musculature [15].

The Italian anatomist Paolo Mascagni (1725–1815), using the mercury injections technique through capillary tubes, performed the most accurate and detailed description of the lymphatic system of the human body. In 1787, he published his work *Vasorum linfaticorum corporis humani historia et ichnographia* [16], where he described the lymphatic vessels and nodes of the urogenital tract (Fig. 1.8a and b).

In the nineteenth century, Anatomy would complete its descriptive stage and focus on the study of the human body from a regional or topographic concept, with the aim of building bridges between anatomy and surgery.

Fig. 1.7 Plate 15. Bladder musculature and pubovesical ligaments sectioned (I and II) In Santorini's venous plexus (III). External urethral sphincter (IV). Santorini, GD. Septemdecim tabulae quas nunc primum edit, 1775

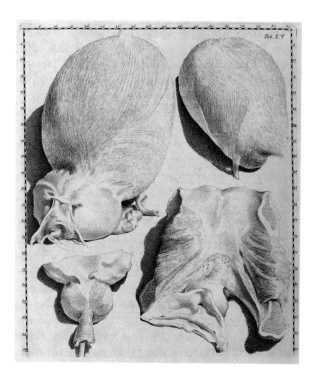

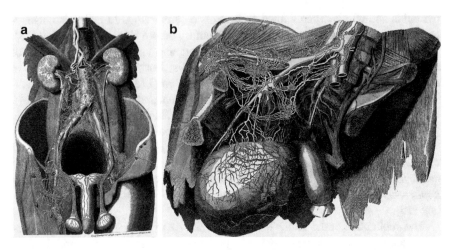

Fig. 1.8 (**a**) Lymph nodes and lymph vessels of the kidneys, ureters, testicles and penis. (**b**) Lymph nodes and lymph vessels of the bladder, prostate and seminal vesicles. Mascagni, P. Vasorum linfaticorum corporis humani historia et ichnografia, 1787

The German Anatomist, Friedrich Gustav Jacob Henle (1809–1885) in his work *Zur Anatomie der Niere* (1862) observed that there were two types of tubules in the renal medulla. One was the Bellini ducts, while the others smaller in diameter, run in parallel to the collector ducts and return in a loop towards the medulla, thus forming the loop bearing his name [17].

The French surgeon, Charles-Pierre Denonvilliers (1808–1872) in his doctoral thesis *Propositions et Observations d'Anatomie, de Physiologie et de Pathologie* (1837) studied the male pelvic and perineal region and described the prostato-peritoneal aponeurosis, now also known as Denonvilliers' aponeurosis [18].

The anatomist Jean Cruveilhier (1791–1874) through his work *Traite d'anatomie descriptive* (1871), sets forth a detailed study of the anatomy both macroscopic and microscopic of the urinary tract [19].

The anatomist Jean Baptiste Marc Bourgery (1797–1849) with his monumental work *Traité complet de l'anatomie de l'homme* (1831–1854) where descriptive anatomy successively leads to the comparative anatomy and the urogenital topographic anatomy (Fig. 1.9a and b) with the subsequent projection to surgical technique [20].

In the early twentieth century, the German anatomist Otto Kalischer (1869–1492) in his work *Die Urogenitalmuskulatur des Dammes mit besonderer Berücksichtigung des Harnblasenverschlusses* (1900) using serial anatomical cutting techniques of 20–50 microns sections, describes the internal vesical sphincter and the layout of the perineal musculature in men [21]. This method enables highly accurate "dissection" and avoids the notorious artefacts of macroscopic dissection in a region as complex as the male perineum.

Half way through the century, the Spanish anatomist and urologist Salvador Gil Vernet (1892–1987) in *Patología Urogenital: Biología y Patología de la Próstata*

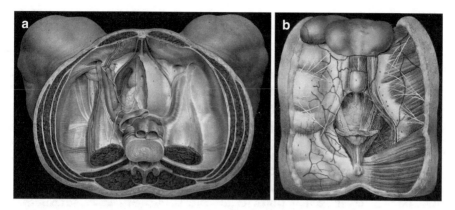

Fig. 1.9 (**a**) Plate 9. Volume VI. Surgical anatomy. Male pelvis. Ureter, bladder, prostate, seminal vesicles and vas deferens. (**b**) Plate 4. Volume VI. Surgical anatomy. Male perineum. Bulbospongiosus muscle, external urethral sphincter and levator ani muscles. Bourgery, JB. Traité complet de l'anatomie de l'homme, 1866

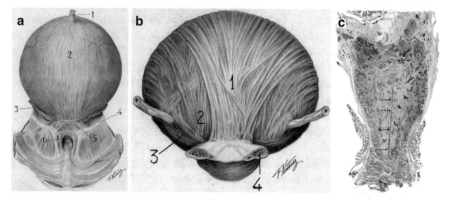

Fig. 1.10 (**a**) Transverse pre-cervical arch. (**b**) Posterior longitudinal bundle of the detrusor. (**c**) Coronal prostate section. Posterior prostato-urethral muscular bundle of the urethral crest (arrows). Gil Vernet, S. Morphology and function of vesico-prostato-urethral musculature, 1968

[*Urogenital Pathology: Biology and Pathology of the Prostate*] (1953) and *Morphology and function of vesico-prostato-urethral musculature* (1968), in his dissection works, after exhausting the macroscopic description and by using the Kalischer method, completes the vesical musculature study and describes, for the first time, the pre-cervical transverse arch of the detrusor (Fig. 1.10a), the posterior longitudinal muscular bundle of the detrusor or *musculus vesicoprostaticus* (Fig. 1.10b) and the posterior prostate-urethral muscular bundle or *musculus ejaculatorius* [22], the muscle making up the relief of the urethral crest (Fig. 1.10c). In 1953, the American urologist, Eduard Uhlenhuth (1885–1961) publishes *"Problems in the anatomy of the pelvis: an atlas"*, where he conducts an exhaustive and impressive study of the topographic anatomy of the pelvis and the perineum [23].

1.2   The History of the Male Genital Anatomy

In the fourth century BC, Aristotle, in his work *Historia Animalium* examines the anatomy of the testicle, the spermatic cord, the vas deferens and describes the epididymis [24]. In *De Generatione Animalium*, he attempts to explain the role of semen in reproduction and reaches the erroneous conclusion that testicles are not necessary for fertilization and that their main function is to extend the copulation time [25].

In the third century BC, the Greek physician from the School of Alexandria, Herophilos of Chalcedon (335–280 BC) was the first to practice public dissections on human corpses. In his work *De Anatomia* which unfortunately perished in the Alexandria library fire and for which references exist through the Galenic texts, uses the words "*adenoidis parastatai*" (glandular assistants) also defining what we now call the prostate gland and seminal vesicles and "*kirsoidis parastatai*" (varicose assistants) which we now know as the ampullae of vasa deferentia [26]. Herophilos also describes the vas deferens, which he calls "*spermatikos poros*" (spermatic vessel).

In the second century AD, Galen (129- ca. 210) in his works *De uso partium* and *De musculorum dissectione* describes the bulbospongiosus muscle, although he believes this comprises two muscles with the function of dilating the urethra to enable semen to pass through. He also describes the cremaster muscle, which he believed was the muscle suspending the testicle [27]. In *De semine*, he describes the testicle, the epididymis, the vas deferens and the ampulla of the vas deferens.

In the sixteenth century, the Italian Jacopo Berengario da Carpi (*ca.* 1460–1530), used the term vas deferens for the first time and described the seminal vesicles in the chapter *De Vasis Seminaris* of his work *Isagogae breves* (1525) which he believed to be a sperm reservoir [28]. Soon after, the Venetian physician Niccolò Massa (1485–1569), in his *Liber introductorius anatomiae* (1536) describes the prostate gland that he called "*glandular flesh*" and believes its function is to provide a secretion that neutralises urine acidity [4].

The first illustration of the prostate [29] is found in the *Tabulae anatomicae sex* (Fig. 1.11) (1538) by the Belgian Andreas Vesalius (1514–1569), and in the chapter on the organs of men serving generation in Book V of *De Humanis Corporis Fabrica Libri Septem* (1543) where he describes the prostate, calling it "*corpus glandulosum*" (glandular body) (Fig. 1.12a and b). He writes that: "The glandular body into which the vessels carrying semen are inserted after they join, and which Herophilus calls "*adenoidis parastatai*" placed at the lowest part of the bladder, about halfway between the body of the bladder and its neck. This is a single body, and hence larger than the testicles themselves but not exactly round, being depressed in front and behind and round like a globe on the sides."

Vesalius confirms, in the dissection of a hanged man who ejaculated during the execution, the presence of a secretion when cutting the prostate and confused this with sperm. He describes the vas deferens, which he calls a "vessel which guides the sperm" and indicates that it widens at its distal end. He does not describe the

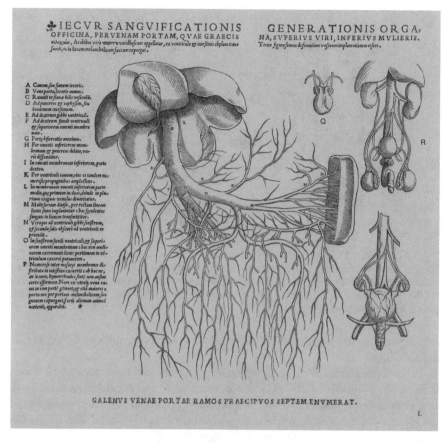

Fig. 1.11 Plate 1. Bladder, ureters, prostate and ampulla vas deferens (Q). Urogenital apparatus in the male (R). Vesalius, A. Tabulae anatomicae sex, 1538

seminal vesicles and believes that both deferens join, distally, to go through the prostate and discharge in the urethra through a single duct [5].

In the gonads study, he describes the pampiniform plexus, the tunica vaginalis, the head and tail of the epididymis, the tunica albuginea of testis, the efferent ductules and the septa (Fig. 1.12b). He shows the external urethral sphincter, in its vertical layout and which is made up of transversal fibres, the penis with the *corpora cavernosa* and the *bulbospongiosus* muscle which he thought, repeating Galen's error, were two separate muscles, and the *ischiocavernosus* muscles (Fig. 1.13).

Later, Bartolomeo Eustacchio (1510–1574), in an illustration prepared for his *Opuscula anatomica* (1563–1564) but unused, and that did not appear until the eighteenth century when recovered and published by Giovanni Maria Lancisi in the work *Tabulae Anatomicae clarissimi vir Bartholomaei Eustachii quas é tenebris tandem vindicatas* (1714), we find several illustrations of the seminal vesicles, the prostate and the ejaculatory ducts flowing into the *veru montanum* [30]. The

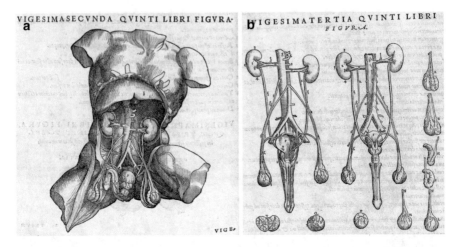

Fig. 1.12 (**a**) Plate 22. The male urogenital system. Bladder (ν). Glandular body (prostate) (ξ). External urethral sphincter (ρ). Corpora cavernosa (ς,τ). (**b**) Plate 23. Right testis from the front and along the left side (**a**, **b**). Vas deferens and epididymis (H, I). Ductuli efferentes (Q). Bladder (ν). Prostatic urethra (o). Prostate (ξ). External urethral sphincter (ρ). Vesalius, A. De humani corporis fabrica libri septem. V Book, 1543

vesicoprostatic vascular pedicles and the arteries and dorsal veins of the penis also appear (Fig. 1.14).

In the seventeenth century, the English surgeon Nathaniel Highmore (1613–1685) in his work *Corporis humani disquitio anatomica; in qua sanguinis circulationem in quavis corporis particula plurimis typis novis* (1651) shows a detailed study of the testicle and describes the mediastinum testis, which he calls "*ductiu novus testiculi*" and that will become known as Higmore's body.

Later, the Dutch anatomist Reignier de Graaf (1641–1673), a pioneer in the vascular injection of solidifiable and coloured substances, will publish his work *De virorum organis generationi inservientibus* (1668). With great accuracy, he describes the seminiferous tubules, the efferent ducts, the perforating arteries of the testicle's tunica albuginea and the intratesticular vascularization (Fig. 1.15a). The glandular and muscular nature of the prostate is highlighted and, through injection techniques, he makes painstaking observations of the prostate collecting ducts and describes the trajectory and the end of the ejaculatory ducts into the veru montanum, which he calls "*caput gallinagum*", and the slope that the urethral crest forms (Fig. 1.15b). By injecting air into the vas deferens, he observes that the seminal vesicules fill up before reaching the urethra, which leads him to believe that these act as a sperm reservoir. Furthermore, using intravascular injection techniques, he describes the intracavernous artery and its branches, the septum pectiniforme and the spongious body of the penis (Fig. 1.15c) [31].

The French surgeon Jean Mery (1645–1722) describes, for the first time, the bulbourethral gland in the *Journal des Sçavans* (1684). He confirms that these are

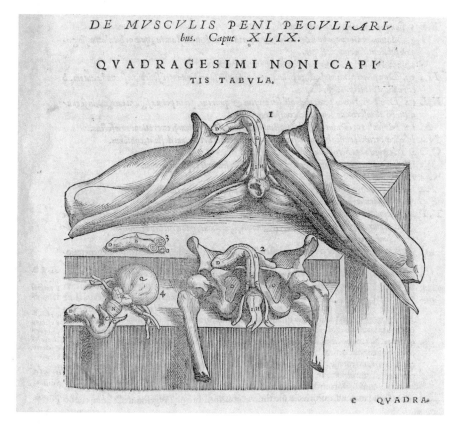

DE MVSCVLIS PENI PECVLIARI-
bus. Caput XLIX.

QVADRAGESIMI NONI CAPI-
TIS TABVLA.

e   QVADRA-

Fig. 1.13 Plate of the 49 chapter. On the muscles intrinsic to the penis. Corpora cavernosa (AB). Crura penis (CC). Urethra (G). Bulbospongiosus muscles (HI). KL Ischiocavernosus muscles (KL). External urethral sphincter (N). Bladder (Q). Glandular body (prostate) (R). Vesalius, A. De humani corporis fabrica libri septem. II Book, 1543

two small glands as thick as a pea and located below the bulbospongiosus muscle an inch away from the prostate [32].

Soon after, the English physician William Cowper (1666–1709) will describe them far more accurately and comprehensively in *An Account of Two Glands and Their Excretory Ducts Lately Discover'd in Human Bodies* (1699), both in humans and in other mammals [33].

In the eighteenth century, the Italian anatomist Giacomo Lorenzo Terraneo (1666–1714), in his work *De glandulis universum et speciatim ad urethram virilem novis* (1721), correctly locates the bulbourethral glands in the heart of an external urethral sphincter [34], illustrates the periurethral glands of the posterior urethra and very accurately describes the external urethral sphincter with a cylindrical form and surrounding the membranous urethra (Fig. 1.16).

In the early nineteenth century, the German physician, Johannes Peter Müller (1801–1858), Professor of Anatomy and Physiology at the University of Berlin, in

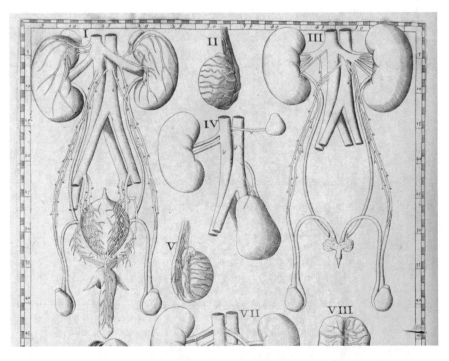

Fig. 1.14 Plate 12 (detail). Bladder and prostate vascular pedicles and dorsal penile vessels (I). Seminal vesicles, ampulla vas deferens and prostate with the opening of the ejaculatory ducts (III). Lancisi, G. Tabulae Anatomicae clarissimi vir Bartholomaei Eustachii quas é tenebris tandem vindicatas, 1714

his work *Über die organischen Nerven der erectilen männlichen Geschlechtsorgane des Menschen und der Säugethiere* (1835), studies the male perineal musculature and observes the layout of the pubovesical ligaments and of the detrusor fibres covering the front face of the prostate. He shows an accurate and detailed description of the external urethral sphincter and its relationship with the prostate. However, his most important discovery and published in the aforementioned work, was the detailed, accurate description of the pelvic *plexus* and its origin, and the trajectory of the cavernous nerves and their relationship with the prostate and the seminal vesicle, both in humans and in stallion [35].°

In 1858, the English urologist Henry Thompson (1820–1904) in his work "*The enlarged prostate: its pathology and treatment*" (1858) offers a detailed description of the dimensions and weight of the gland, noting its muscular-glandular nature and rejecting the existence of a" third lobe" or subcervical lobe which he considered pathological [36].

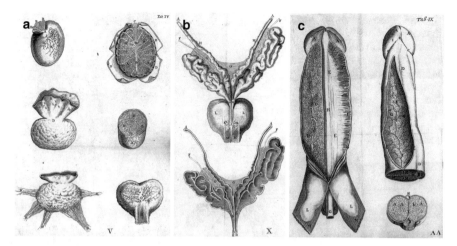

Fig. 1.15 (**a**) Plate IV. Testis and epididymis, seminiferous tubules, efferent ductules (I, II, III, IV and V). Prostate with the collecting ducts and their openings (VI). (**b**) Plate VI. Vas deferens, ampulas vas deferens, ejaculatory ducts, prostate, collecting ducts and veru montanum (I and II). (**c**) Plate IX. Corpora cavernosa, septum pectiniforme, intracavernosal arteries, and bulb of the penis (I and II). De Graaf, R. De virorum organis generationi inservientibus, 1668

At the beginning of the twentieth century, the Cuban urologist Joaquín María Albarrán (1860–1912) in his research on the microscopic anatomy of the prostate *Exposé des travaux scientifiques* (1906) divides the prostatic glands into a "central group", made up of inframontanal glands and some small submucosal glands in subcervical situation, the Albarrán glands, and a "peripheral group" of glands surrounding the prostatic urethra like a half moon [37].

In 1912, the North American urologist Oswald Lowsley (1884–1955), through the study of embryo and foetuses, confirms that the prostate is made up five lobes, two sides one, one front, another rear and another in the middle [38].

In 1953, Salvador Gil Vernet, through embryonic and microscopic anatomy studies, describes the first regional model of the prostate. In his *Patología Urogenital: Biología y patología de la prostata* (1953), he demonstrated that the gland consisted of three regions: the craneal, the caudal and the intermediate glands [39]. This model was urethrocentric, with areas defined according to the location of their collecting ducts opening into the urethra and was later used by North American pathologist John McNeal (1931–2006), as the foundation of the zonal anatomy model [40].

Fig. 1.16 Plate
II. External urethral
sphincter (I) with the
bulbourethral glands (M)
and their excretory ducts.
Urethral crest (g).
Terraneo, L. De glandulis
universum et speciatim ad
urethram virilem
novis, 1721

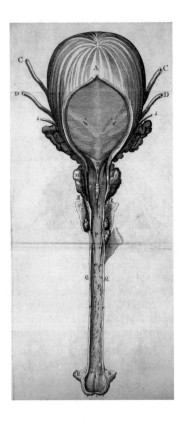

References

1. Singer C. Galen on anatomical procedures: de Anatomicis administrationibus. London: Oxford University Press for the Wellcome Historical Medical Museum; 1956. p. 67–171.
2. Mondeville H. Chirurgia. Bibliothèque nationale de France. Département des Manuscrits. Français 2030; 1312 1301–1400. p. 29.
3. Berengario da Carpi J. Commentaria cum amplissimis aditionibus super anatomiam Mundini. Bologna; 1521. p. 178–180.
4. Massa N. Liber Introductorius anatomiae. Venice: Francisci Bindoni; 1536. p. 29–34.
5. Garrison DH, Hast MH. A. Vesalius. The Fabric of the Human Body. An Annotated Traslation of the 1543 and 1555 Editions of De Humani corporis fabrica libri septem. Basel: S. Karger; 2014. p. 1037–1064.
6. Colombo R. De re Anatomica libri XV. Paris: Andream Wechelum; 1572. p. 427.
7. Fallopio G. Observationes anatomicae. Paris: Apud Bernardum Turrisanum, via Iacobea in Aldina bibliotheca; 1562. p. 108–110.
8. Eustachio B. Opuscula anatomica. Venice: Vincentinus Luchinus;1564. p. 20–147.
9. Highmore N. Corporis humani disquitio anatomica; in qua sanguinis circulationem in quavis corporis particula plurimis typis novis, ac aengymatum medicorum succinta dilucidationen ornatam prosequutus est. Ex officina Samuelis Broun bibliopolae anglici; 1651. p. 74–93.
10. Bellini L. Exercitationes anatomicae duae de structura et usu renum ut et de gustus organo novissime deprehenso. 9th ed. Lugduni Batavorum, apud Joannem à Kerkhem; 1726. p. 1–40.
11. Malpighi M. Opera omnia, seu, thesaurus locupletissimus botanico-medico-anatomicus. Lugduni Batavorum: Apud Petrum Vander Aa. Leiden; 1687. p. 278–89.
12. Ruysch F. Thesaurus anatomicus sextus. Amsterdam: J. Wolters; 1701. p. 11–5.

13. Bertin EJ. Mémoire pour servir a l'histoire des reins. Histoire de L'Académie Royales des Sciences. Paris: J. Boudot; 1744. p. 77–116.
14. Morgagni JB. Adversaria anatomica omnia:quorum tria posteriora nunc primum prodeunt, novis pluribus aeris tabulis. Lugduni Batavorum: Apud Johannem Arnoldum Langerak; 1723. p. 52–3.
15. Santorini GD. Septemdecim tabulae quas nunc primum edit atque explicat iisque alias addit de structura mamarum et de tunica testis vaginali Michael Girardi. Parmae: Ex regia typographia; 1775. p. 165–203.
16. Mascagni P. Vasorum lymphaticorum corporis humani historia ichnografia. Ex Typographia Pazzini Carli; 1787. p. 88–92.
17. Henle J. Zur Anatomie der Niere. Göttingen: Verlag der Dieterichschen Buchandlung; 1862. p. 15–23.
18. Denonvilliers CP. Propositions et Observations d'Anatomie, de Physiologie et de Pathologie. Paris: Impr. Et fonderie de Rignoux et Ce; 1837. p. 23.
19. Cruveilhier J. Traite d'anatomie descriptive. Paris: P. Asselin; 1871. p. 307–47.
20. Bourgery J, Bernard C. Traité complet de l'anatomie de l'homme comprenant l'anatomie chirurgicale et la médicine opératoire. Volume 6. Paris: L. Guérin editeur; 1866–1871. Planche IV.
21. Kalischer O. Die Urogenitalmuskulatur des Dammes mit besonderer Berücksichtigung des Harnblasenverschlusses. Berlin: S. Karger; 1900.
22. Gil Vernet S. Morphology and function of vesico-prostato-urethral musculature. Treviso: Canova; 1968. p. 32–234.
23. Uhlenhuth E. Problems in the anatomy of the pelvis. An atlas. J.B. Philadelphia: Lippincott; 1953. p. 8–65.
24. Pallí Bonet J. Aristóteles. Investigación sobre los animales. Madrid: Gredos; 1992. p. 132–133.
25. Aristóteles SE. La reproducción de los animales. Madrid: Gredos; 1994.
26. Barcia Goyanes JJ. El mito de Vesalio. Valencia: Real Academia de Medicina de la comunidad valenciana. Universitat de València; 1994. p. 117.
27. Galen. On the usefulness of the parts of the body, vol. II. Ithaca: Cornell University Press; 1968.
28. Berengario da Carpi J. Isagogae breves. Venice; 1525. p. 61–64.
29. Vesalius A. Tabulae Anatomicae Sex. Venice: Imprimebat B. Vitalis; 1538. Plate I.
30. Lancisius GM. Tabulae Anatomicae clarissimi vir Bartholomaei Eustachii quas é tenebris tandem vindicatas. Roma: Ex officina typographica Francisci Gonzagae; 1714. p. 33.
31. De Graaf R. Virorum organis generationi inservientibus, de clÿsteribus et de usu siphonis in anatomia. Ex Officina Hackiana. Lugd Batav. et Roterod; 1668. p. 1–160.
32. Méry J. Observations anatomiques faites per M. Mery. Journal des Sçavans, vol. XVII. Paris: Chez Florentin Lamber et Chez Jean Cusson; 1684. p. 301.
33. Cowper W. An Account of Two Glands and Their Excretory Ducts Lately Discover'd in Human Bodies. Philosophical Transactions (1683–1775), vol. 21; 1699. p. 364–369.
34. Terraneo L. De glandulis universim, et speciatimad urethram virilem novis. Ex Officina Boutesteniana. Lugduni Batavorum; 1721. p. 49–78.
35. Müller JP. Über die organischen Nerven der erectilen männlichen Geschlechtsorgane des Menschen und der Säugethiere. Berlin: F. Dúmmler; 1836. p. 117–34.
36. Thompson H. The enlarged prostate: its pathology and treatment: with observations on the ralation of this complaint to stone in bladder. London: J. Churchill; 1858. p. 1–8.
37. Albarrán JM. Exposé des travaux scientifiques. Paris: Masson; 1906. p. 2–3.
38. Lowsley O. The development of the human prostate with reference to the development of other structures at the neck of the urinary bladder. Am J Anat. 1912;13:299–349.
39. Gil-Vernet JM, Arango O, Álvarez-Vijande R. Topographic anatomy and its development in urology in the 20th century. The work of Salvador Gil Vernet. Eur J Anat. 2016;20:231–47.
40. McNeal JE. Regional morphology and pathology of the prostate. Am J Clin Pathol. 1968;49:347–57.

Part I
Standards in Anatomical Representation

Chapter 2
3D Reconstruction and CAD Models

Andrew Shea Afyouni, Aurus Dourado, and Zhamshid Okhunov

2.1   Introduction

Human beings have been gifted the ability to interact with the world around them in three dimensions. When studying anatomy, planning for a surgical case, or learning about physiological processes of different organ systems, students and medical professionals, alike, truly understand and appreciate anatomical relationships when they are given tools to visualize structures, such as cadavers, printed models, and interactive visual representations.

Until only three decades ago, medical imaging technology was limited to simple 2D renderings of anatomical structures, such as with ultrasonography (US), computerized tomography (CT), and magnetic resonance imaging (MRI). A physician's ability to prepare for a complex case preoperatively was confined to solely reviewing a patient's scans and consulting with colleagues who may have encountered similar cases in the past. Patients with little-to-no practical knowledge of their disease or treatment plan often went into a surgical operation with only a vague understanding of what they could hope to expect intraoperatively and/or postoperatively.

Since the early 1990s, however, advances in cross-sectional imaging technology combined with an exponential increase in processing power have allowed medical professionals to portray and interact with human anatomy in 3D space. Specifically, within the field of urology, this rise of computational power has coincided with beginning of an era of "precision surgery" [1] where laparoscopic and robot-assisted surgical techniques have allowed for a minimally-invasive approach for the treatment of many genitourinary malignancies. As surgical techniques to treat a myriad

A. S. Afyouni · Z. Okhunov (✉)
Department of Urology, University of California, Irvine, California, USA
e-mail: aafyouni@uci.edu; zokhunov@uci.edu

A. Dourado
Department of Urology, Sao Marcos Hospital, Teresina, Brazil

© Springer Nature Switzerland AG 2021
E. Huri, D. Veneziano (eds.), *Anatomy for Urologic Surgeons in the Digital Era*,
https://doi.org/10.1007/978-3-030-59479-4_2

of different urological diseases have evolved over the years, so has the 3D imaging technology physicians have used to optimally prepare for a case and better understand a patient's unique anatomy [2].

2.1.1 Basic Methodologies of 3D Reconstruction

Broadly speaking, the process of constructing a 3D image involves first acquiring raw data points from a 2D image, then using a computer algorithm to estimate and extrapolate new data points (interpolation), subsequently rendering those data points into a rough image, and finally visualizing that image in 3D space. (Fig. 2.1).

2.1.1.1 Data Acquisition

For every step in the stepwise sequence of constructing a 3D image, data regarding the spatial orientation of elements within an image as components of three spatial planes (i.e. x, y, and z) must be registered. In more advanced imaging modalities, such as CT and MRI, this process is not difficult to achieve. With these imaging types, the scanning table, which captures cross-sectional images of target areas, is able to automatically identify the position of every segment of an image in 3D space as the patient moves through the scanner [3].

However, an imaging modality like US lacks the ability to map an image in 3D space (i.e. register images in the z axis), making the process of 3D reconstruction far more difficult. US is unable to register the positional orientation of images in 3D space in the same manner CT and MRI are able to achieve using the scanning table. Rather, US relies on acoustic, electromagnetic, and/or optical positional devices, such as the US transducer, to register the coordinates of each US image recorded.

Ultrasonography, in nature, is a non-mechanized imaging modality that relies on mostly "freehand" scanning techniques, unlike CT and MRI [3, 4]. With a non-mechanized image scanning system, there are no imposed restrictions on the movement of the imaging probe (or transducer) as a human being, rather than a computer, is tasked with determining where he or she wishes to select as a region of interest to image. In the case of US, physicians are given full control over both where they wish to position the ultrasound transducer and how they want to position the probe in order to get an image they feel best represents the region of interest they are examining.

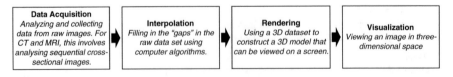

Fig. 2.1 Schematic representation of the stepwise processes required when creating a 3D reconstruction of a 2D image

2.1.1.2   Interpolation

After sequential images and raw positional data are collected, they are subsequently processed and edited in a process known as interpolation. Interpolation of data points effectively involves using several computer algorithms to fill gaps present in the raw data set in order to produce a data set that can be used to produce a 3D image [4]. Due to the non-mechanized nature of US imaging, images collected by US often contain far more "gaps" and artifacts than CT and MRI-based images, making the process of interpolation more difficult and less precise. For this reason, US images often contain more porous 3D datasets, resulting in the final 3D reconstructed image not being a true representation of the imaged anatomy [3]. Although 3D technology has advanced quite significantly over time and has partially addressed this issue, the gaps present in US-based datasets are a major reason why 3D US reconstruction is used less frequently than 3D CT and 3D MRI reconstruction.

2.1.1.3   Rendering

Once the final 3D dataset is obtained through interpolation algorithms, computer-generated 3D images can be rendered in several different ways. The term "rendering" refers to the process of mapping a 3D dataset onto a 2D screen for purposes of visualization. While rendered images do not present more information than typical axial images, they do, however, offer viewers a significantly better understanding of spatial information and anatomical relationships [3].

There are four major rendering methodologies that are important to note: (1) maximum intensity projection (MIP), (2) multi-planar reformatting (MPR), (3) surface rendering (or shaded surface display, SSD), and (4) volume rendering.

The MIP rendering method is a method for visualizing 3D data that presents only the brightest voxels (i.e. a value on a 3D grid, similar to what a "pixel" represents in 2D space) [3]. MIP is best utilized when the target objects are the brightest objects in the image and is often used to evaluate structures that are injected with contrast material, such as in CT angiography and CT urography [5, 6]. In addition, MIP is also a great rendering modality to expose high attenuation arteries or calculi because of these properties [3, 7, 8]. However, because this technique only draws from data with the highest values, MIP images usually contain 10% or less of the original dataset, thus limiting the fidelity of the produced images [7]. For this reason, the MIP rendering technique was commonly used when computer processing power limited accessibility to advanced imaging techniques.

Multi-planar reformation (MPR) is a rendering technique that pulls data from axially-oriented CT images to create non-axial 2D images [9]. MPR images can be described to be either coronal, sagittal, oblique, or curved plane images that are generated from a plane only 1 voxel in thickness transecting a stack of axial images [10–13]. This technique is particularly useful for evaluating 3D representations of transrectal ultrasounds (3D TRUS), since some regions of interest may not be easily apparent solely on axial sections [3].

Shaded surface display (SSD) (i.e. surface rendering) provides a 3D view of the surface of an object and shades various apparent surfaces with different densities (or opacities), giving an element of depth to the image. SSD shades each apparent surface in an image with varying degrees of gray-scale depending on the amount of observed light intensity and shadowing that is present [14–16]. This technique is particularly useful in reconstructing images from CT/MR cystoscopy [3]. However, just as MIP discards any lower valued data, SSD discards all data but the surface-defining data, which typically only consists of less than 10% of the acquired data [17].

Volume rendering is a technique that can produce higher fidelity images that use all available volume in a 3D image [9]. Using technology originally developed for motion picture computer animation [17, 18], volume rendering assigns opacity values on a complete spectrum from 0 to 100% (complete transparency to total opacity) using a variety of computational techniques [19, 20]. Volume rendering uses information on the opacity and lighting of structures to expose spatial relationships between structures. In addition, volume rendering involves applying various colors for different tissue classifications while reserving gray-scale hues for solely lighting effects. In this way, the volume rendering process can rapidly process a 3D dataset and create/shade an image in such a way that appears more natural to human optical capabilities and intuitive for the perception of depth [21, 22]. Because all acquired data may be used with this rendering modality, volume rendering requires much more processing power than MIP, MPR, or SSD.

2.1.2   History of 3D Reconstruction Modalities in Clinical Urological Practice

2.1.2.1   First Iteration of 3D Reconstruction in Clinical Urology

The first mention of 3D reconstruction in clinical urological practice came in 1990 when Kaneto and colleagues aimed to map the 3D muscular architecture of the ureteropelvic junction (UPJ) in patients with congenital hydronephrosis [23]. In this study, serial UPJ histological sections from patients with congenital hydronephrosis were taken longitudinally along the ureteral axis, fixed in formalin, and embedded in celloidin-paraffin. Each histological section was subsequently subjected to stereo-morphometric analysis (i.e. quantitative analysis of size and shape) to determine any architectural changes of the smooth muscle layer. In order to visualize 3D muscular architecture of the UPJ from these sequential histological sections, Kaneto and colleagues used computer-aided reconstructive techniques that simplified sections into a series of vector bundles so that the arrangement of slices may be expressed as a vector distribution. From the final vector distribution, information regarding each UPJ's anatomy and its variation from the norm UPJ architecture could be collected and analyzed.

2.1.2.2   Computerized Tomography and Ultrasonography

Several years following Kaneto and colleagues' feat of creating a 3D representation of the UPJ from a series of histological sections, Hubert and colleagues demonstrated the capability of using helicoidal CT acquisition technology to make 3D reconstructions of various renal vessels, calices, and parenchymal surfaces. Not only was this study influential in documenting the first instance of using CT technology to create 3D renal reconstructions but it also demonstrated the feasibility of making 3D reconstructions of various urological phenomena, including congenital malformations (i.e. horseshoe kidney, megaureter, ectopic organs), acquired malformations (i.e. diverticulum and trabeculated bladder), renal stones (including staghorn calculi), and renal transplantations [24, 25].

While Hubert and colleagues were publishing their preliminary data on CT-based 3D reconstruction, Crivianu-Gaita and colleagues wished to repurpose 3D reconstruction technology at their small county hospital in Romania to assist in calculating the volume of the prostate as a means of better evaluating patients with suspected prostate adenoma. However, unlike Hubert's team, this team did not have access to either a CT machine or endorectal ultrasonography (the most suitable imaging modality for studying prostatic tumors), forcing Crivianu-Gaita and colleagues to come up with a novel means of modeling the prostate.

Urologists at the county hospital were trained in using echographic estimation through transabdominal examination, a far less precise method of determining prostatic tumor volumes. However, precise calculation of prostatic volume is especially important in choosing a surgical method to treat prostate adenomas and Crivianu-Gaita noted that, within their institution, there was a tendency of overestimating prostate volumes in cases of small and medium adenomas. Thus, Crivianu and colleagues created a software tool that synthesized realistic 3D prostate models from 2D ultrasound images and minimized errors made in calculating prostatic volume. In comparing 29 patients' true prostate volumes to those calculated by both echographic equipment and the 3D US software, Crivianu-Gaita found that their application yielded an average error of 9.4% compared to 20.9% when using conventional US echographic estimation methods [26].

After Crivianu-Gaita's study examining prostatic tumor volumes, 3D US technology was quickly adapted for a number of other urological purposes, including examining the endoluminal tract of the ureter [27] and creating models for core biopsy simulations [28–30]. Bagley and colleagues first published preliminary data demonstrating the efficacy of 3D endoluminal ultrasonography of the ureter in examining ureteral strictures, obstructed ureteropelvic junction, ureteral neoplasms, and ureterovesical junctions. In their study, they utilized 6.2F endoluminal ultrasound catheter connected to a dedicated ultrasound unit to take serial cross-sectional images of the endoluminal tract of the ureter. Subsequently, Bagley and colleagues were able to use volume rendering techniques to generate high-fidelity 3D models of the ureter that were able to expose irregular structures and internal characteristics of the lumen. Bagley noted that the use of 3D US technology for imaging the ureter can give important information regarding the longitudinal appearance of various ureteral segments without the need for developing novel ultrasound transducers in addition to revealing anatomic features that would not otherwise be evident on 2D images alone [27].

Egevad and colleagues utilized 3D reconstruction for purposes of modeling prostate lesions from transrectal ultrasound-guided biopsies. In their study, they compared the cancer detection rate and correlative tumor volume of a simulated 10-biopsy protocol to a conventional sextant preoperative biopsy protocol. Transrectal ultrasound-guided core biopsies were taken from 81 patients and these same patients underwent radical prostatectomy and had their specimens step-sectioned and whole-mounted. Using these sections, a 3D volume of each prostate was reconstructed, virtual core biopsy needles imitating the positions of the real biopsies were inserted into the prostate, and cancer yield was calculated. Egevad and colleagues found that, of the cancers detected with 10 standard virtual biopsies, 24% would have remained undetected with sextant biopsies. In addition, the cancer yield of these 10 virtual biopsies correlated closely with preoperative biopsies and were similar in calculated tumor volume [28]. Egevad and colleagues gave support to the notion that 3D simulation of prostate biopsies could improve biopsy protocols, a fact that was further corroborated in subsequent studies [29, 30].

2.1.2.3 Magnetic Resonance and Fluoroscopy

By the mid-2000s, contrast-enhanced magnetic resonance angiography (MRA) and imaging (MRI) had become more commonplace as laparoscopy and minimally invasive surgery became standard practice in the field of urology. MRA (and MRI) became increasingly popular as it has a distinct advantage over CT imaging in that it does not require nephrotoxic and allergenic contrast material and avoids ionizing radiation. For many years, the use of non-contrast MRA in the abdomen was limited by long imaging times, motion artifacts, and a lack of standardization in techniques. However, novel advances in MR hardware, software, and scanning at the beginning of the century contributed to decreases in imaging times and significant improvements in overall image quality [31–33]. Wang and colleagues published one of the first studies that utilized preoperative 3D MRA techniques to create renal reconstructions prior to laparoscopic renal surgeries. In comparing their 3D MRA image reconstructions to actual intraoperative findings, Wang and colleagues found that their 3D models closely correlated (96%) with true renal anatomy, especially with regards to aberrant vasculature (i.e. duplicated renal arties or veins, accessory vessels, and crossing vessels). These findings were some of the first to demonstrate the value of 3D MRA in providing highly accurate and detailed recreations of renal vasculature [34].

Traditionally, renal vascular anatomy and functional patterns had been examined with the aid of radiological imaging, such as angiography, contrast CT, or MRI, and computerized into 3D reconstructive models. However, one issue that remained with these radiological methods was the 3D image quality was insufficient to view renal micro-vascularity. As surgical and radiological practices continued to develop towards highly selective nephron-sparing techniques, examining microvasculature and understanding intricate renal anatomy became of vital importance prior to treatment. Following in the footsteps of a prior study that showed that vessels as small as 40 µm in diameter in a goat heart could be clearly exposed using fluorescent imaging cryomicrotomy [35], Lagerveld and colleagues assessed whether the combined use of fluorescent casting, cryomicrotome imaging, and 3D computer reconstruction could provide a novel means of visualizing the renal vascular tree in a porcine renal model. Lagerveld and his team were able to create a 3D reconstruction of the arterial vascular tree that showed the complete porcine renal arterial anatomy up to a resolution of 50 µm [36]. (Fig. 2.2).

2.1.3   Modern Applications of 3D Reconstruction

2.1.3.1   3D Printing

While 3D printing has been commonplace with manufacturers for many years, the application of 3D printing and models has been a relatively novel development in the field of urological medicine. One of the first studies to examine the usefulness of 3D printing in clinical urological practice came at the hands of Priester and colleagues in 2014 as a means of evaluating MR imaging of prostate cancer using patient-specific 3D printed molds [37]. Since then, many studies have published

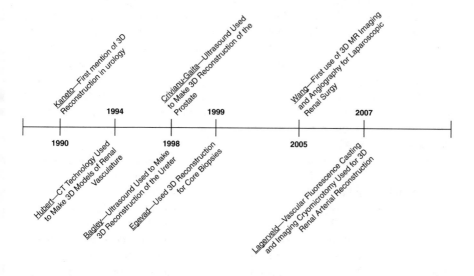

Fig. 2.2 Chronological timeline of important and innovative studies in the evolution of 3D reconstruction technology

data that have underlined the importance and value of 3D printing technology in aiding with the comprehension of renal and prostatic vascular and structural anatomy, particularly in instances of cancer.

With regards to prostatic cancers, 3D printing technology has proven to be a valuable clinical and educational tool. Physical 3D printed models have aided physicians with gaining a stronger understanding of the location of tumors with respect to surrounding vasculature [38]. In addition, a close examination of 3D printed prostate models preoperatively have helped bolster physicians' confidence preoperatively and perceived surgical precision intraoperatively, according to Porpiglia and colleagues [39]. Others have also shown that 3D printed models showing suspected prostatic lesions have helped influence the course of surgical management and encourage surgeons to favor nerve-sparing techniques with higher frequency [40].

Regarding the surgical treatment of various renal cortical neoplasms, Silberstein and colleagues have shown that 3D models of renal malignancies have served as a useful diagnostic reference tool for physicians when planning nephron-sparing surgeries, especially in cases when conventional 2D imaging is suboptimal [41]. 3D printed models have been shown to encourage surgeons to adopt more complex and precise surgical treatment options, as surgeons gain a more profound understanding of patients' unique tumor morphology and volume preoperative after consulting physical models [42–44].

2.1.3.2 Augmented Reality (AR)

Augmented Reality (AR) refers to the superimposition or alignment of 3D virtual images onto a patient's actual diagnostic images or videos preoperatively or intraoperatively [45]. In order to implement AR into surgical procedures, several key steps are necessary. First, reconstruction of 3D surgical models from standard 2D images is required. Second, these 3D models must be integrated into imaging softwares so that they can be superimposed onto a patient's diagnostic images or live videos. Finally, intraoperatively, surgeons must use a head-mounted wearable device, such as Sony's head-mounted 3D viewer or Google Glass™, to be able to track both the motion of surgical instruments relative to the target organs in the operative field [46, 47].

Several studies have examined the value and efficacy of utilizing AR and head-mounted displays to visualize endoscopic images in real time. In these cases, the head-mounted displays were wired physically to surgical endoscopes, cameras, and AR software so that the display could superimpose 3D model renderings onto live intraoperative video. To date, AR has been demonstrated to be effective in helping surgeons better understanding patient's anatomy and malignancies during radical nephrectomies [48, 49], partial nephrectomies [50, 51], nephroureterectomies [52], placement of urethral stents [53], and treatment of various neoplasms, such as urothelial prostate, and renal carcinomas [54, 55].

2.1.3.3 Immersive Virtual Reality (iVR)

A physician's ability to visualize 3D models has far transcended simply examining static images on a flat computer screen. Fortunately, the advent of various virtual reality headsets, such as Oculus™, Sony VR™, and Google Glass™, has given physicians the ability to both visually and cognitively process 3D images. Immersive Virtual Reality, or iVR, is one visualization modality that has given physicians the perception of being physically present with 3D models within interactive simulation. Recently, Parkhomenko and colleagues have demonstrated the value and potential of using CT-based iVR models to view patient's anatomy preoperatively in percutaneous nephrolithotomy (PCNL) procedures. (Fig. 2.3) Using iVR, surgeons were found to be able to manipulate, segregate, and visualize all relevant anatomic components of their patients in fine detail, including renal parenchyma, collecting system, calculi, and surrounding organs. Parkhomenko and colleagues found that iVR improved surgeons' understanding of the optimal calyx of entry along with the

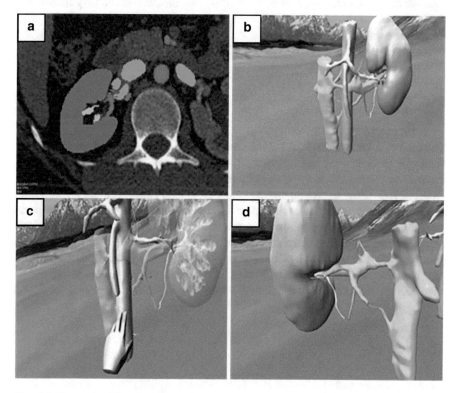

Fig. 2.3 Immersive Virtual Reality (iVR) technology. (**a**) Sequential cross-sectional images (2–3 mm thickness) of patients' non-contrast CT scans are closely examined and renal vasculature and parenchyma are shaded in 3D Slicer (National Institute of Health, Bethesda, MA) (**b-d**) Patients' renal anatomy can be visualized in 3D space and, using an Oculus Rift and Touch controllers (Facebook Inc., Menlo Park, CA), viewers can interact with renal vasculature and parenchyma

stone's size, location, and orientation in these PCNL cases. In cases where surgeons were able to view a patient's images using iVR, patients experienced a significant decrease in fluoroscopy time intraoperatively, in addition to a decrease in blood loss, fewer nephrostomy tracts, and overall higher stone-free rates [56].

2.1.3.4 Redefining Urological Physiology and Disease

3D reconstruction has demonstrated its value in furthering the scientific community's understanding of genitourinary physiology, specifically with regards to intrarenal and extrarenal nerves. Modern advances to 3D reconstruction technology have made it possible to better visualize and map the autonomic distribution of microscopic nerves in the renal artery, renal vein, segmental vessels and intrarenal vasculature [57], bladder [58], and ureter [59]. Information gathered from these virtual 3D models have provided a means of mapping connections between nervous tissue and various segments of the urinary tract, a field that was previously ill-defined. Furthermore, improved understanding of local neural anatomy could help improve targeted nerve-modulating therapies and prevent unwarranted tissue damage during invasive procedures.

2.2 Conclusions

Over the past three decades, 3D reconstruction technology has developed quite dramatically from its early stages, especially within the field of urology. This improvement is attributed not only to rapidly advancing technological advancements in imaging modalities and computer processing but also to a concerted effort within the urology community to better understand patients' unique anatomy preoperatively and minimize surgical invasiveness intraoperatively. Nowadays, 3D virtual/printing practices have entered daily practice for the treatment of many different urological diseases across hundreds of institutions internationally. 3D reconstruction has demonstrated its value as a useful clinical tool for surgical planning, physician education and training, and more comprehensive patient counseling.

References

1. Autorino R, Porpiglia F, Dasgupta P, et al. Precision surgery and genitourinary cancers. Eur J Surg Oncol. 2017;43:893–908.
2. Porpiglia F, Amparore D, Enrico C, et al. Current use of three-dimensional model technology in urology: a road map for personalized surgical planning. Eur Uro Focus. 2018;4:652–6.
3. Ghani KR, Pilcher J, Patel U, et al. Three-dimensional imaging in urology. BJU Int. 2004;94:769–73.
4. Udupa JK, Herman GT. 3D imaging in medicine. Philadelphia: CRC Press; 1999.

5. Calhoun PS, Kuszyk BS, Heath DG, et al. Three-dimensional volume rendering of spiral CT data: theory and method. Radiographics. 1999;19:745–64.
6. Napel S, Marks MP, Rubin GD, et al. CT angiography with spiral CT and maximum intensity projection. Radiology. 1992;185:607–10.
7. Heath DG, Soyer PA, Kuszyk BS, et al. Three-dimensional spiral CT during arterial portography: comparison of three rendering techniques. Radiographics. 1995;15:1001–11.
8. Keller PJ, Drayer BP, Fram EK, et al. MR angiography with two-dimensional acquisition and three-dimensional display: work in progress. Radiology. 1989;173:527–32.
9. Dalrymple NC, Prasad SR, Freckleton MW, et al. Introduction to the language of three-dimensional imaging with multidetector CT. Radio Graphics Info RAD. 2005;25:1409–29.
10. Rankin SC. Spiral CT: vascular applications. Eur J Radiol. 1998;28:18–29.
11. Rubin GD, Napel S, Leung AN. Volumetric analysis of volumetric data: achieving a paradigm shift [editorial]. Radiology. 1996;200:312–7.
12. Rubin GD. Multislice imaging for three-dimensional examinations. In: Silverman PM, editor. Multislice helical tomography: a practical approach to clinical protocols. Philadelphia, Pa: Lippincott Williams & Wilkins; 2002. p. 317–24.
13. Rubin GD, Silverman SG. Helical (spiral) CT of the retroperitoneum. Radiol Clin N Am. 1995;33:903–32.
14. Magnusson M, Lenz R, Danielsson PE. Evaluation of methods for shaded surface display of CT volumes. Comput Med Imaging Graph. 1991;15:247–56.
15. Rubin GD, Dake MD, Napel S, et al. Spiral CT of renal artery stenosis: comparison of three-dimensional rendering techniques. Radiology. 1994;190:181–9.
16. Rubin GD, Dake MD, Napel SA, et al. Three-dimensional spiral CT angiography of the abdomen: initial clinical experience. Radiology. 1993;186:147–52.
17. Fishman EK, Drebin B, Magid D, et al. Volumetric rendering techniques: applications for three-dimensional imaging of the hip. Radiology. 1987;163:737–8.
18. Drebin RA, Hanrahan P. Volume rendering. Comput Graph. 1988;22:65–74.
19. Rubin GD. 3-D imaging with MDCT. Eur J Radiol. 2003;45(suppl 1):S37–41.
20. Levoy M. Display of surfaces from volume data. IEEE Comput Graph Appl. 1988;8:29–37.
21. Vannier MW, Rickman D. Multispectral and color-aided displays. Investig Radiol. 1989;24:88–91.
22. Ward J, Magnotta V, Andreasen NC, et al. Color enhancement of multispectral MR images: improving the visualization of subcortical structures. J Comput Assist Tomogr. 2001;25:942–9.
23. Kaneto H, Orikasa S, Takahashi T. The muscular architecture at the ureteropelvic junction in congenital hydronephrosis—a stero-morphometric study. Nihon Hinyokika Gakkai Zasshi. 1990;81:268–74.
24. Hubert J, Blum A, Chassagne S, et al. Value of three-dimensional surface reconstruction scanning in urology—preliminary results. Prog Urol. 1994;4(6):937–50.
25. Hubert J, Blum A, Cormier L, et al. Three-dimensional CT-scan reconstruction of renal calculi. A new tool for mapping-out staghorn calculi and follow-up of radiolucent stones. Eur Urol. 1997;31(3):297–301.
26. Crivainu-Gaita D, Miclea F, Gaspar A, et al. 3D reconstruction of prostate from ultrasound images. Int J Med Inform. 1997;45(1–2):43–51.
27. Bagley DH, Liu JB. Three-dimensional endoluminal ultrasonography of the ureter. J Endourol. 1998;12(5):411–6.
28. Egevad L, Frimmel H, Norberg M, et al. Three-dimensional computer reconstruction of prostate cancer from radical prostatectomy specimens: an evaluation of the model by core biopsy simulation. Urology. 1999;53(1):192–8.
29. Bogers HA, Sedelaar JP, Beerlage HP, et al. Contrast-enhanced three-dimensional power Doppler angiography of the human prostate: correlation with biopsy outcome. Urology. 1999;54(1):97–104.
30. Egevad L, Frimmel H, Mattson S, et al. Biopsy protocol stability in a three-dimensional model of prostate cancer: changes in cancer yield after adjustment of biopsy positions. Urology. 1999;54(5):862–8.

31. Schoenberg SO, Essig M, Bock M, et al. Comprehensive MR evaluation of renovascular disease in five breath holds. J Magn Reson Imaging. 1999;10:347.
32. Prince MR, Chenevert TL, Foo TKF, et al. Contrast-enhanced abdominal MR angiography: optimization of imaging delay time by automating the detection of contrast material arrival in the aorta. Radiology. 1997;203:109.
33. Korosec FR, Frayne R, Grist TM, et al. Time-resolved contrast-enhanced 3D MR angiography. Magn Reson Med. 1996;36:345.
34. Wang DS, Stolpen AH, Bird VG, et al. Correlation of preoperative three-dimensional magnetic resonance angiography with intraoperative findings in laparoscopic renal surgery. J Endourol. 2005;19(2):193–9.
35. Spaan JA, ter Wee R, van Teeffelen JW, et al. Visualization of intramural coronary vasculature by an imaging cryomicrotome suggests compartmentalization of myocardial perfusion areas. Med Biol Eng Comput. 2005;43:1–4.
36. Lagerveld BW, ter Wee R, Rosette J. Vascular fluorescence casting and imaging cryomicrotomy for computerized three-dimensional renal arterial reconstruction. BJU Int. 2007;100:387–291.
37. Priester A, Natarajan S, Le JD, et al. A system for evaluating magnetic resonance imaging of prostate cancer using patient-specific 3D printed models. Am J Clin Exp Urol. 2014;2(2):127–35.
38. Schawalenberg T, Neuhaus K, Liatsikos E, et al. Neuroanatomy of the male pelvis in respect to radical prostatectomy including three dimensional visualization. BJU Int. 2010;105(1):21–7.
39. Porpiglia F, Bertolo R, Checcucci E, et al. Development and validation of 3D printed virtual models for robot-assisted radical prostatectomy and partial nephrectomy: urologists' and patients' perception. World J Urol. 2018;36(2):201–7.
40. Ukimura O, Aron M. Nakamoto, et al. three dimensional surgical navigation model with TilePro display during robot assisted radical prostatectomy. J Endourol. 2014;28(6):625–30.
41. Silberstein JL, Maddox MM, Dorsey P, et al. Physical models of renal malignancies using standard cross-sectional imaging and 3-dimensional printers: a pilot study. Urology. 2014;84(2):268–72.
42. von Rundstedt FC, Scovell JM, Agrawal S, et al. Utility of patient-specific silicone renal models for planning and rehearsal of complex tumor resections prior to robot-assisted laparoscopic partial nephrectomy. BJU Int. 2017;119(4):598–604.
43. Wake N, Chandarana H, Huang WC, et al. Application of anatomically accurate, patient-specific 3D printed models from MRI data in urological oncology. Clin Radiol. 2016;71(6):610–4.
44. Wake N, Rude T, Kang SK, et al. 3D printed renal cancer models derived from MRI data: application in pre-surgical planning. Abdom Radiol. 2017;42(5):1501–9.
45. Checcucci E, Amparore D, Fiori C, et al. 3D imaging applications for robotic urologic surgery: an ESUT YAUWP review. World J Urol. 2019;
46. Ukimura O, Gill IS. Augmented reality for computer-assisted image-guided minimally invasive urology. London: Springer; 2009. p. 179–84.
47. Yoon JW, Chen RE, Kim EJ, et al. Augmented reality for the surgeon: a systematic review. Int J Med Robot. 2018;14:e1914.
48. Matsuoka Y, Kihara K, Kawashima K, et al. Integrated image-navigation system using head-mounted display in "RoboSurgeon" endoscopic radical prostatectomy. Videosurg Other Miniinvasive Tech. 2014;9:613–8.
49. Kihara K, Fujii Y, Masuda H, et al. New three-dimensional head- mounted display system, TMDU-S-3D system, for minimally invasive surgery application: procedures for gasless single-port radical nephrectomy. Int J Urol. 2012;19(9):886–9.
50. Kihara K, Saito K, Komai Y, et al. Integrated image monitoring system using head-mounted display for gasless single-port clampless partial nephrectomy. Videosurg Other Miniinvasive Tech. 2014;9:634–7.
51. Yoshida S, Ito M, Tatokoro M, et al. Multitask imaging monitor for surgical navigation: combination of touchless interface and head-mounted display. Urologia Int. 2015;98:486–8.

52. Ishioka J, Kihara K, Higuchi S, et al. New head-mounted display system applied to endoscopic management of upper urinary tract carcinomas. Int Braz J Urol. 2014;40(6):842–5.
53. Yoshida S, Kihara K, Takeshita H, et al. Head-mounted display for a personal integrated image monitoring system: ureteral stent placement. Urol Int. 2014;94(1):117–20.
54. Yoshida S, Kihara K, Takeshita H, et al. A head-mounted display-based personal integrated-image monitoring system for transurethral resection of the prostate. Videosurg Miniinv. 2014;9:644–9.
55. Borgmann H, Socarrás MR, Salem J, et al. Feasibility and safety of augmented reality-assisted urological surgery using smartglass. World J Urol. 2016:1–6.
56. Parkhomenko E, O'Leary M, Safiullah S, et al. Pilot assessment of immersive virtual reality renal models as an educational and preoperative planning tool for percutaneous nephrolithotomy. J Endourol. 2019;33(4):283–8.
57. Lusch A, Leary R, Heidari E, et al. Intrarenal and extrarenal autonomic nervous system redefined. J Urol. 2014;191:1060–5.
58. Spradling K, Khoyilar C, Abedi G, et al. Redefining the autonomic nerve distribution of the bladder using 3-dimensional image reconstruction. J Urol. 2015;194:1661–7.
59. Vernez SL, Okhunov Z, Wikenheiser J, et al. Precise characterization and 3-dimensional reconstruction of the autonomic nerve distribution of the human ureter. J Urol. 2017;197:723–9.

Chapter 3
Physical Models

İlkan Tatar

3.1   Introduction

As well as improving technology effects many surgical fields, urological surgery is strengthened by new aspects of imaging and scanning, anatomical modelling and especially 3D printing in the digital millennium era. To universalize these affects for routine surgical procedures, standard anatomical representation is really important and crucial. It includes medical illustration and imaging, 3D reconstruction and printing, physical models, cadavers and lab animal models for human analogy. In this chapter; history, methodologies, benefits and limitation and the future of physical models in the urological surgery field will be reviewed. It is also beneficial for better understanding of the both normal and pathological anatomy and translating it to everyday surgical practice.

When we looking at a simple definition of the physical model term (most commonly referred to simply as a model but in this context distinguished from a conceptual model), it is a smaller or larger physical copy of an object. The object being modelled may be small (for example, an atomic compound) or large (for example, the Solar system).

The geometry of the model and the object represents often similar in the sense that one is a rescaling of the other. The scale is an important characteristic. However, in many cases the similarity is only approximate or even intentionally distorted. Sometimes the distortion is systematic (e.g., a fixed scale horizontally and a larger fixed scale vertically when modelling topography of a large area, as opposed to a model of a smaller mountain region, which may well use the same scale horizontally and vertically, showing the true slopes).

İ. Tatar (✉)
Department of Anatomy, Hacettepe University, Faculty of Medicine, Ankara, Turkey
e-mail: ilkan@hacettepe.edu.tr

© Springer Nature Switzerland AG 2021   35
E. Huri, D. Veneziano (eds.), *Anatomy for Urologic Surgeons in the Digital Era*,
https://doi.org/10.1007/978-3-030-59479-4_3

Physical models allow visualization, from examining the model, of information about the thing the model represents. A model can be a physical object such as an architectural model of an organ. Uses of an architectural model include visualization of internal relationships within the structure or external relationships of the structure to the environment. Other uses of models in this sense are as toys.

3.2   Brief History and Methodologies

In the past two decades, surgical education has been greatly influenced by industries such as aviation and defense, which heavily rely on simulation training before real-life exposure. Through the use of simulation, a large part of the procedural learning curve can be acquired using training models; thus, training in the simulation laboratory has been widely adopted to enhance performance in the operating room. As a result, surgical simulation has advanced at a rapid pace, becoming an established and valid method of training.

Technical skills can be acquired using a number of different simulation modalities including virtual reality (VR) and augmented reality (AR) simulators, benchtop or synthetic models, physical models (3D printed or not), animal tissue or live animals, and human cadavers (fresh-frozen or embalmed), each with their own advantages and disadvantages [1].

When we looking at the previous decade literature about physical models in the field of Urology, most of the models were created by 3D printing technology and methods. Several 3D printing methods have been developed for which a variety of applications have been found, including creating prototypes of new products, fabricating architectural models, and rapidly generating replacement parts and other products for consumers. The medical field in particular has been an early adopter of 3D modelling technology. 3D constructs are used in various specialties, including main surgical fields. Early adopters used computer-assisted milling machines to create computer- generated surgical models as early as 1980. The early constructs had to provide only structural support and, therefore, were the most easily modelled and produced. Implementation of 3D-printed objects in urology and other specialties that involve soft tissue has lagged, owing to the need for dynamic constructs with the ability to conform to multiple states. Additionally, urological bioengineering applications of 3D printing require solid and hollow viscous organs, such as the bladder, ureter, or kidney, and fabrication of such structures adds a further level of complexity [2].

The main three applications of 3D printing that are relevant to urology and have demonstrable or anticipated medical applications: 1-the use of 3D printing to generate inorganic models for surgical planning and education; 2-the use of 3D printing for the production of inorganic prostheses and devices; and 3-the current and future use of 3D printing for bio- engineering of organic structures.

All 3D printing processes start with the design of a virtual model regardless of the printing technique used. This step includes collecting size and tensile requirements for a construct and entering them into a 3D modelling software. For the generation of medical constructs, size requirements are often generated through medical imaging, such as CT and MRI. Modern imaging software generally saves files in the digital imaging and communications in medicine (DICOM) format and is the standard for most hospital information technology setups. Modern 3D modelling packages, such as Mimics (Materialise, Belgium) or OsiriX (Pixmeo, Switzerland), are able to convert these data into the stereolithography (.stl) format that is used by 3D printers. These files can be produced using DICOM data from both CT and MRI with equal efficacy. Once the model has been created, four different techniques can be used to create the construct: inkjet printing; extrusion printing; laser-assisted sintering; or stereolithography [2]. We can review the physical models in the field of Urology according to organs of urinary system.

3.3   Kidney/Ureter

There is a recent growing literature about physical modelling (mostly 3D printed) of the kidney and ureter pathologies because of they are main affected organs.

Silberstein et al. produced 5 physical models (all patients successfully underwent 4 robotic and one open partial nephrectomy) of renal units with suspected malignancies before surgery. Construction of models did not require any special or additional imaging. The physical models constructed using standard CT scans with 3- to 5-mm cuts have high fidelity to the actual malignancy and obviate any repeat or specialized imaging, which may expose the patient to excess risk or cost. Limitations from the third party additive manufacturing technique prevented constructing the lesion of interest, arteries, veins and collecting system, each in a unique color. They used firm resins that bear little resemblance to natural organic tissues; in the future, they anticipated having the ability to construct 3D models with materials that recapitulate the organ of interest. This will allow instructors and trainees to perform the operation on a model before the actual operation to improve surgical outcomes. Alternatively, the models may be used as a metric to assess trainee surgical acumen or as a tool for improvement by surgical simulation after the surgery [3].

Knoedler et al. evaluated the effect of 3-dimensionally (3D) printed physical renal models with enhancing masses on medical trainee characterization, localization, and understanding of renal malignancy. Six different models were printed from a transparent plastic resin; the normal parenchyma was printed in a clear, translucent plastic, with a red hue delineating the suspicious renal lesion. Twenty-three medical students, who had completed their first year of training, were given an overview and tasked with completion of renal nephrometry scores, separately using CT imaging and 3D models. Trainees were also asked to complete a questionnaire about their experience. Overall trainee nephrometry score accuracy was significantly improved with the 3D model vs CT scan. Furthermore, 3 of the 4 components of the nephrometry score (radius, nearness to collecting system, and location) showed significant improvement using the models. Qualitative evaluation with questionnaires filled out by the trainees further confirmed that the 3D models improved their ability to understand and conceptualize the renal mass [4].

Maddox et al. aimed to construct patient-specific physical 3D models of renal units with materials that approximates the properties of renal tissue to allow pre-operative and robotic training surgical simulation. Seven models of renal units with suspected malignancies were constructed using multi-jet 3D printers that selectively deposit photopolymer material that is cured immediately after deposition with an ultraviolet lamp. 3D printer materials are jetted through a print head in tiny droplets, and the process allows for multiple materials to be blended and deposited together creating a composite flexible structure. A firm but malleable renal capsule was created using this technique with a hollow cavity. Next, an agarose gel solution was prepared and injected into the cavity of the kidney shell creating an accurate model of the patient- specific pathology with texture that approximated normal anatomic tissue. Multiple contrasting materials and colors allowed delineation of the enhancing renal mass, collecting system and renal vasculature from the normal parenchyma. Partial nephrectomy was performed on each of the replicas. Subsequently all patients successfully underwent robotic partial nephrectomy. Patients with surgical models had larger tumors, higher nephrometry score, longer warm ischemic time, fewer positive surgical margins, shorter hospitalization, and fewer postoperative complications; however, the only significant finding was lower estimated blood loss. Pre-operative resectable physical 3D models can be constructed and used as patient-specific surgical simulation tools [5].

Libby and Silberstein produced physical model of clear cell renal carcinoma with inferior vena cava extension created from a 3D printer to aid in surgical resection. The 3D model of this patient's kidney tumor clearly shows the tumor's vascularity and thrombus extension into the IVC. The size and shape of the 3D printed model reflected the actual size of the kidney and thrombus. The 3D printed model provided advantages for all parties, including the patient, the patient's family, medical trainees, surgeons, surgical technicians, and anesthesiologists. The use of this model prior to surgery allowed residents and physicians to gain an appreciation for what to expect upon surgical entry and identify spatial relations in a novel manner. During the consenting process prior to surgery, the patient was given the opportunity to hold and manipulate the physical model of her anatomy. This allowed for a more informed discussion of the risks, benefits, and alternatives of the procedure and thus enhanced the informed consent process. The model demonstrated that the tumor thrombus was located below the hepatic venous drainage, which gave the surgeons more confidence that bypass was not necessary. The surgical technicians had a better understanding of the operative intervention because they were able to see from different angles this patient's unique anatomy prior to surgery and, potentially, were better assistants. Likewise, the anesthesia team also had a better understanding of the risks involved in the procedure and was abler to assess for thrombus with an intraoperative transesophageal echocardiogram [6].

Lee et al. studied on personalized 3D kidney model produced by rapid prototyping method and evaluation their usefulness in performing partial nephrectomy (PN) and also in the education of medical students. Models produced by using 3D-printing methods from preoperative computed tomography images in a total of 10 patients. Two different groups (3 urologists and 20 medical students) appraised the clinical usefulness of 3D-renal models by answering questionnaires. After application of 3D renal models, the urologist group gave highly positive responses in asking clinical usefulness of 3D-model among PN (understanding personal anatomy: 8.9/10, preoperative surgical planning: 8.2/10, intraoperative tumor localization: 8.4/10, plan for further utilization in future: 8.3/10, clinical usefulness in complete endophytic mass: 9.5/10). The student group located each renal tumor correctly in 47.3% when they solely interpreted the CT images. After the introduction of 3D-models, the rate of correct answers was significantly elevated to 70.0%. The subjective difficulty level in localizing renal tumor was also significantly low (52% versus 27%) when they utilized 3D-models [7].

Fan et al. published firstly their experiences about the data of five patients with completely endophytic renal tumors, who had undergone 3D kidney models-assistant laparoscopic PN by a single surgeon. The accuracy of 3D models was evaluated and discussed by surgeons and radiologists preoperatively. The postoperative results showed the deviations between the models and renal masses were acceptable, and the average deviation was 0.2 cm. During surgery, the entire kidney was fully dissociated from surrounding tissues to expose the renal anatomical landmarks. Intraoperative 3D printing models were found to be highly associated with the appearance of the tumor surface. The surgical assistant adjusted the 3D models to aid the surgeon for quickly and accurately locating the site of renal masses based on the dimensions and landmarks on the surface of the 3D kidney models. Thus, endophytic mass resection was successful as planned, and the depth of masses was achieved by the surgeons without any change in surgical modality. Postoperative review showed the navigation of 3D kidney models potentially help shorten the duration of warm ischemia time for LPN in endophytic tumors. Postoperatively, three participants, including one operating surgeon and two surgical assistants, were surveyed as part of the assessment for face and content validity. All participants advocated that 3D individual kidney models would be a beneficial advancement for helping to improve understanding of endophytic tumors and for performing laparoscopic PN [8].

Similar efforts can be seen in the field of Percutaneous Nephrolithotripsy (PCNL) Surgery, which focused more on the anatomy of pelvicalyceal system rather than renal parenchyma, which is important for the tumors. Adams et al. produced soft phantoms of the kidney with collecting system built by a novel fabrication process-combining 3D printing and polymer molding. The method is versatile since it replicates anatomical details with sub-millimeter resolution and permits a wide range of materials to be used, including biocompatible hydrogels. They validated anatomical details and material properties of the phantoms in detail by CT scan, ultrasound, and endoscopy. CT reconstruction, ultrasound examination, and endoscopy showed that the designed phantom mimics a real kidney's detailed anatomy and correctly corresponds to the targeted human cadaver's upper urinary tract. Soft materials with a tensile modulus of 0.8–1.5 MPa as well as biocompatible hydrogels were used to mimic human kidney tissues. They predicted a number of applications for the kidney phantom, including surgical planning, simulation and training of urological endoscopic procedures, and medical device testing [9].

Atalay et al. studied on the impact of 3DP kidney models on residents' understanding of pelvicalyceal system anatomy before PCNL surgery. Five patients' (with unilateral staghorn renal stones and clinical indications for PCNL) anatomically accurate models of the human renal collecting system were successfully generated. After presentation of the 3D models, 10 urology residents were 86% and 88% better at determining the number of anterior and posterior calyces, respectively, 60% better at understanding stone location, and 64% better at determining optimal entry calyx into the collecting system [10]. Same authors also studied the impact of personalized 3DP pelvicalyceal system models on patient information for PCNL surgery. After the 3D printed model presentation, patients demonstrated an improvement in their understanding of basic kidney anatomy by 60%, kidney stone position by 50%, the planned surgical procedure by 60%, and understanding the complications related to the surgery by 64%. In addition, overall satisfaction of conservation improvement was 50% [11].

More experimental studies related with the physical modelling of the kidney for PCNL procedure were also published in the literature. Akand et al. described a novel technique that uses mathematical calculation software, 3D modeling and augmented reality (AR) technology for access during PCNL in two different ex-vivo models. Novel software was created in order to calculate access point and angle by using pre-operative CT obtained in 50 patients. Two scans, 27 s and 10 min after injection of contrast agent, were taken in prone PCNL position. By using DICOM objects, mathematical and software functions were developed to measure distance of stone from reference electrodes. Vectoral 3D modeling was performed to calculate the access point, direction angle and access angle. With specific programs and AR, 3D modeling was placed virtually onto real object, and the calculated access point and an access needle according to the calculated direction angle and access angle were displayed virtually on the object on the screen of tablet. The system was tested on two different models—a stone placed in a gel cushion, and a stone inserted in a bovine kidney that was placed in a chicken—for twice, and correct access point and angle were achieved at every time. Accuracy of insertion of needle was checked by feeling crepitation on stone surface and observing tip of needle touching stone in a control CT scan [12].

Tatar et al. produced three physical models related with kidney and its vasculature during the MedTRain3DModsim Erasmus+ European union project, which started on October 2016 and completed on October 2018, was led by Hacettepe University in Ankara, Turkey, and partner organizations Chosun University, South Korea; Charles University, Czech Republic; and Rome 3 University, Italy and Hellenic Urological Association, Greece. The models were standard percutaneous nephrostomy, standard laparoscopic nephrectomy (partial/total) (available also as Virtual Reality/Augmented Reality formation) and standard percutaneous nephrolithotomy (C-arm depended) [13].

Tatar et al. also created 3D printed female anatomical model for the evaluation of hands on training of Trans-Obturator Tape (TOT) and Tension Free Vaginal Tape

(TVT) sling procedures from the same project. During two learning & teaching & training activities and a multiplier event of the project between 2016 and 2018; 41 medical students, 30 residents and 19 specialists of urology and gynecology were educated and performed TOT and TVT procedures with this model under the mentorship of 3 experts. All participants were assessed and scored for their achievement on both procedures with model according to 7 parameters including: identification anatomical landmarks in pelvic model, performing anterior vaginal wall dissection, right transobturator route of needle, left transobturator route of needle, right transvaginal route of needle, left transvaginal route of needle and good positioning and hand's position) by the experts. There was no any statistical difference between the student's and resident's category for each parameter. Since these activities are based on practical hand movements, while learning the initial steps of trans-obturator and trans-vaginal tape procedure; students and residents got similar scores. All the parameters for the student's and specialist's category were statistically different. The previous experience of specialists might be the most probable factor of this result [14].

3.4 Bladder/Urethra

More sophisticated projects were done in the field of Urological surgery especially for the bio-printing of urethra. Zhang et al. applied 3D bio-printing technology to fabricate cell-laden urethra in vitro with different polymer types and structural characteristics for the treatment of urethral stricture. They used polycaprolactone (PCL) and polylactidecocaprolactone (PLCL) polymers with a spiral scaffold design for mimicking structural and mechanical features of natural urethra of rabbits and cell-laden fibrin hydrogel for a better cell growth microenvironment. With using an integrated bio-printing system, tubular scaffold was formed with the bio-materials. Urothelial cells and smooth muscle cells were delivered evenly into inner and outer layers of the scaffold separately within the cell-laden hydrogel. Evaluation of the cell bioactivity in the bio-printed urethra revealed that UCs and SMCs maintained more than 80% viability even at 7 days after printing. Both cell types also showed active proliferation and maintained the specific biomarkers in the cell-laden hydrogel. These results provided a foundation for further studies in 3D bio-printing of urethral constructs that mimic the natural urethral tissue in mechanical properties and cell bioactivity, as well a possibility of using the bio-printed construct for *in vivo* study of urethral implantation in animal model [15].

Shee et al. published their experiences on a novel ex vivo trainer for robotic vesicourethral anastomosis. 10 surgical residents without prior robotics training were enrolled in the study: 5 residents received structured virtual reality (VR) training on the da Vinci Skills Simulator ("trained"), while the other 5 did not ("untrained"). 4 faculty robotic surgeons trained in robotic urologic oncology ("experts") were also enrolled. Mean (range) completion percentage was 20% (10–30%), 54% (40–70%), and 96% (85–100%) by the untrained, trained, and expert groups, respectively. Anastomosis integrity was rated as excellent (as opposed to moderate or poor) in

40%, 60%, and 100% of untrained, trained, and expert groups, respectively. Face validity (realism) was rated as 8 of 10 on average by the expert surgeons, each of whom rated the model as a superior training tool to digital VR trainers. Content validity (usefulness) was rated as 10 of 10 by all participants. The addition of 3D-printed ex vivo training to existing digital simulation technologies may augment and improve robotic surgical education in the future [16].

Tatar et al. produced four physical models related with bladder during the MedTRain3DModsim Erasmus+ European union project. The models were standard percutaneous suprapubic cystostomy, standard cystoscopy (flexible/rigid), standard transurethral resection of the bladder tumor and standard bladder neck incision. 290 trainees actively participated in the surgical training using 3D-printed or simulation models. General assessment of the courses was performed using the Likert scale questionnaire, with the median points for "Contribution to your knowledge", "Eligibility of the physical environment", "Satisfaction from the organization", "Education materials", "Eligibility of the training methods", "Suitability of the training period", "Suitability of the content of the education", and "Satisfaction from training" [13].

3.5 Prostate

Preister et al. developed a system for evaluating magnetic resonance imaging(MRI) of prostate cancer, using patient- specific 3D printed molds to facilitate MR-histology correlation. Prior to radical prostatectomy a patient receives a multiparametric MRI, which an expert genitourinary radiologist uses to identify and contour regions suspicious for disease. The same MR series is used to generate a prostate contour, which is the basis for design of a patient-specific mold. The 3D printed mold contains a series of evenly spaced parallel slits, each of which corresponds to a known MRI slice. After surgery, the patient's specimen is enclosed within the mold, and all whole-mount levels are obtained simultaneously through use of a multi-bladed slicing device. The levels are then formalin fixed, processed, and delivered to an expert pathologist, who identifies and grades all lesions within the slides. Finally, the lesion contours are loaded into custom software, which elastically warps them to fit the MR prostate contour. The suspicious regions on MR can then be directly compared to lesions on histology. Furthermore, the false-negative and false-positive regions on MR can be retrospectively examined, with the ultimate goal of developing methods for improving the predictive accuracy of MRI [17].

Khan et al. studied currently available simulators pertaining to prostate surgery and attempted to scientifically evaluate the evidence available, assessing their efficacy in terms of face, content, construct, concurrent and predictive validity. A total of 22 studies were identified, which carried out a validation study. Five validated models and/or simulators were identified for transurethral resection of the prostate (TURP), one for Green Light laser therapy, three for laparoscopic radical prostatectomy (LRP) and four for robotic surgery. Of the TURP simulators, all five demonstrated content validity, three demonstrated face validity and four construct validity. The Green Light laser simulator demonstrated face, content and construct validities. All three animal models for LRP demonstrated construct validity whilst The Chicken Skin Model was also content valid. Only two robotic simulators were identified with relevance to robot-assisted laparoscopic prostatectomy (RALP), both of which demonstrated construct validity [18].

Shin et al., 2016 reported firstly the concept for use of customized, patient-specific printed 3D models of the prostate gland and index cancer lesion to aid in prostate cancer surgery. Five patients with clinically localized prostate cancer were included. MRI was performed using a 3 T body coil (3 mm steps), followed by 3D MRI-transrectal ultrasound (TRUS) image-fusion targeted biopsy using Urostation system (Koelis, France). The index lesion in all 5 prebiopsy MRI scans was the MRI-visible dominant lesion, rated as Prostate Imaging Reporting and Data System (PI-RADS) 4 or 5 with a high probability of microscopic extra-capsular extension (ECE). Pathology examination of step-sectioned prostatectomy specimens revealed accurate concordance between the 3D printed model and the histologic location of the index lesion/ECE, resulting in negative surgical margins in all these challenging high-risk cases [19].

Wendler et al. published patient-specific pretreatment simulation by electric field measurement in a 3D bio-printed textured prostate cancer model to achieve optimal electroporation parameters for image-guided focal ablation. This is achieved by combining three aspects: First, modern commercially available plastic 3D printers make it possible to create accurate bodies for a wide variety of applications. Second, in vitro tissue models are useful platforms that can facilitate systematic laboratory investigations of complex culture systems. Third, irreversible electroporation ablation uses a series of brief but intense electric pulses delivered by paired needle-like electrodes into a targeted region of tissue, killing the cells by irreversibly disrupting cellular membrane integrity within a localized electric field with a critical potential at about 1500 V/cm or more [20].

Zhang et al. published the feasibility and safety evaluation of an individualized and reassemble three-dimensional (3D) printing navigation template for making accurate punctures during sacral neuromodulation (SNM). 24 patients undergoing SNM were enrolled. Conventional X-ray guidance was used in the control group, which included 14 patients, while the 3D printing template was used in the experimental group, which included 10 patients. When comparing the control group and the experimental group, the number of punctures were 9.6 ± 7.7 and 1.5 ± 0.7, respectively; the average puncture times were 35.4 ± 14.6 and 4.1 ± 2.2 min, respectively; and the X-ray exposure levels were 8.37 ± 4.83 mAs and 2.34 ± 0.54 mAs, respectively. The 3D printing template for SNM could help to perform accurate and quick punctures into the target sacral foramina, reduce X-ray exposure, and shorten the operation time [21].

Tatar et al. produced a standard physical 3D prostate bio-model for 3D prostate anatomy training and diagnosis for prostate cancer or nodule, a standard physical 3D bladder and prostate model for transurethral resection of the prostate, which filled with chicken liver- mimicking the real prostate tissue- to resect and a standard physical SNM model including sacrum, sacral plexus, sacrum's posterior surface gluteal muscles and SNM tool in Medtrain3DModsim Erasmus+ European union project [13].

3.6　Conclusion and Future

Urosimulation has made valuable progress in the last two decades, with increasing numbers of new physical and virtual models being developed and validated. High numbers of procedure- specific models have been reported for endourology, the majority of which are virtual and physical bench models. Training modalities for laparoscopic and robot-assisted urological surgery are mainly geared towards generic skills acquisition with a selected few procedure-specific dry-lab and animal models and VR and AR platforms, respectively. In contrast, very few simulators have been produced and validated for open urological surgery, with cadaveric simulation reported as the main modality of training. Furthermore, newer simulation modalities such as augmented reality and 3D printing of physical models are also rapidly gaining popularity. A final area of potential impact for 3DP in clinical medicine and urology is the bioengineering of tissue or even full-scale organs for possible implantation. The 3D-bioprinted tissue demonstrated similar mechanical properties and cell bioactivity compared to the animal models [22]. Efforts should continue to use the currently available models in a curricular approach, with the inclusion of nontechnical skills training. In light of the current evidence, the proposed generic and supplementary simulation curriculum for urological training will help to enhance operating-room experience and reduce many of its associated challenges.

References

1. Aydin A, Raison N, Khan MS, Dasgupta P, Ahmed K. Simulation-based training and assessment in urological surgery. Nat Rev Urol. 2016 Sep;13(9):503–19. https://doi.org/10.1038/nrurol.2016.147.
2. Colaco M, Igel DA, Atala A. The potential of 3D printing in urological research and patient care. Nat Rev Urol. 2018 Apr;15(4):213–21. https://doi.org/10.1038/nrurol.2018.6.
3. Silberstein JL, Maddox MM, Dorsey P, Feibus A, Thomas R, Lee BR. Physical models of renal malignancies using standard cross-sectional imaging and 3-dimensional printers: a pilot study. Urology. 2014 Aug;84(2):268–72. https://doi.org/10.1016/j.urology.2014.03.042.
4. Knoedler M, Feibus AH, Lange A, Maddox MM, Ledet E, Thomas R, Silberstein JL. Individualized physical 3-dimensional kidney tumor models constructed from 3-dimensional printers result in improved trainee anatomic understanding. Urology. 2015 Jun;85(6):1257–61. https://doi.org/10.1016/j.urology.2015.02.053.
5. Maddox MM, Feibus A, Liu J, Wang J, Thomas R, Silberstein JL. 3D-printed soft-tissue physical models of renal malignancies for individualized surgical simulation: a feasibility study. J Robot Surg. 2018 Mar;12(1):27–33. https://doi.org/10.1007/s11701-017-0680-6.

6. Libby RS, Silberstein JL. Physical model of clear-cell renal carcinoma with inferior vena cava extension created from a 3-dimensional printer to aid in surgical resection: a case report. Clin Genitourin Cancer. 2017 Oct;15(5):e867–9. https://doi.org/10.1016/j.clgc.2017.04.025.

7. Lee H, Nguyen NH, Hwang SI, Lee HJ, Hong SK, Byun SS. Personalized 3D kidney model produced by rapid prototyping method and its usefulness in clinical applications. Int Braz J Urol. 2018 Sep-Oct;44(5):952–7. https://doi.org/10.1590/S1677-5538.IBJU.2018.0162.

8. Fan G, Li J, Li M, Ye M, Pei X, Li F, Zhu S, Weiqin H, Zhou X, Xie Y. Three-dimensional physical model-assisted planning and navigation for laparoscopic partial nephrectomy in patients with endophytic renal tumors. Sci Rep. 2018 Jan 12;8(1):582. https://doi.org/10.1038/s41598-017-19056-5.

9. Adams F, Qiu T, Mark A, Fritz B, Kramer L, Schlager D, Wetterauer U, Miernik A, Fischer P. Soft 3D-printed phantom of the human kidney with collecting system. Ann Biomed Eng. 2017 Apr;45(4):963–72. https://doi.org/10.1007/s10439-016-1757-5.

10. Atalay HA, Ülker V, Alkan İ, Canat HL, Özkuvancı Ü, Altunrende F. Impact of three-dimensional printed Pelvicaliceal system models on Residents' understanding of Pelvicaliceal system anatomy before percutaneous Nephrolithotripsy surgery: a pilot study. J Endourol. 2016 Oct;30(10):1132–7.

11. Atalay HA, Canat HL, Ülker V, Alkan İ, Özkuvanci Ü, Altunrende F. Impact of personalized three-dimensional -3D- printed pelvicalyceal system models on patient information in percutaneous nephrolithotripsy surgery: a pilot study. Int Braz J Urol. 2017 May-Jun;43(3):470–5. https://doi.org/10.1590/S1677-5538.IBJU.2016.0441.

12. Akand M, Civcik L, Buyukaslan A, Altintas E, Kocer E, Koplay M, Erdogru T. Feasibility of a novel technique using 3-dimensional modeling and augmented reality for access during percutaneous nephrolithotomy in two different ex-vivo models. Int Urol Nephrol. 2019 Jan;51(1):17–25. https://doi.org/10.1007/s11255-018-2037-0.

13. Tatar İ, Huri E, Selçuk İ, Moon YL, Paoluzzi A, Skolarikos A. Review of the effect of 3D medical printing and virtual reality on urology training with 'MedTRain3DModsim' Erasmus + European Union project. Turk J Med Sci. 2019 Oct 24;49(5):1257–70. https://doi.org/10.3906/sag-1905-73.

14. Tatar İ, Huri E, Selçuk İ. Evaluation of a 3D printed female anatomical model for the hands on training of trans-obturator tape (TOT) and tension free vaginal tape (TVT) sling procedures. Int J Morphol. 2020;38(2):292–8. https://doi.org/10.4067/S0717-95022020000200292.

15. Zhang K, Fu Q, Yoo J, Chen X, Chandra P, Mo X, Song L, Atala A, Zhao W. 3D bioprinting of urethra with PCL/PLCL blend and dual autologous cells in fibrin hydrogel: an in vitro evaluation of biomimetic mechanical property and cell growth environment. Acta Biomater. 2017 Mar 1;50:154–64. https://doi.org/10.1016/j.actbio.2016.12.008.

16. Shee K, Koo K, Wu X, Ghali FM, Halter RJ, Hyams ES. A novel ex vivo trainer for robotic vesicourethral anastomosis. J Robot Surg. 2019 Jan 28; https://doi.org/10.1007/s11701-019-00926-1.

17. Priester A, Natarajan S, Le JD, Garritano J, Radosavcev B, Grundfest W, Margolis DJ, Marks LS, Huang J. A system for evaluating magnetic resonance imaging of prostate cancer using patient-specific 3D printed molds. Am J Clin Exp Urol. 2014 Jul 12;2(2):127–35.

18. Khan R, Aydin A, Khan MS, Dasgupta P, Ahmed K. Simulation-based training for prostate surgery. BJU Int. 2015 Oct;116(4):665–74. https://doi.org/10.1111/bju.12721.

19. Shin T, Ukimura O, Gill IS. Three-dimensional printed model of prostate anatomy and targeted biopsy-proven index tumor to facilitate nerve-sparing prostatectomy. Eur Urol. 2016 Feb;69(2):377–9. https://doi.org/10.1016/j.eururo.2015.09.024.

20. Wendler JJ, Klink F, Seifert S, Fischbach F, Jandrig B, Porsch M, Pech M, Baumunk D, Ricke J, Schostak M, Liehr UB. Irreversible electroporation of prostate cancer: patient-specific pretreatment simulation by electric field measurement in a 3D bioprinted textured prostate cancer model to achieve optimal electroporation parameters for image-guided focal ablation. Cardiovasc Intervent Radiol. 2016 Nov;39(11):1668–71. https://doi.org/10.1007/s00270-016-1390-6.

21. Zhang J, Zhang P, Wu L, Su J, Shen J, Fan H, Zhang X. Application of an individualized and reassemblable 3D printing navigation template for accurate puncture during sacral neuromodulation. Neurourol Urodyn. 2018 Nov;37(8):2776–81. https://doi.org/10.1002/nau.23769.
22. Parikh N, Sharma P. Three-dimensional printing in urology: history, current applications, and future directions. Urology. 2018 Nov;121:3–10. https://doi.org/10.1016/j.urology.2018.08.004.

Chapter 4
Cadaveric Models

Nuno Miguel Taipa Leandro Domingues, Diogo de Freitas Branco Pais, and João Erse de Goyri O'Neill

4.1 Introduction

Anatomy is the cornerstone of education for health professionals with the use of human material providing an excellent teaching tool [1].

Since the beginning of medicine the cadaver has been used to teach human anatomy by dissecting it. Dissection has been described by some anatomists as "a mainstay of properly rigorous basic science training" [2]. It is widely believed that the process of dissection adds a three dimensional view to the students' knowledge, and reinforces concepts introduced in lectures and tutorials [3].

For more than 3.000 years human beings have tried to stop after-death body decay to preserve the mortal frame for the afterlife or reanimation [4]. This process started with the Egyptians with the mummification and later on during nineteenth century, with embalming techniques [5].

Embalming is a chemical process that is used to preserve and sanitize the human body after death [6].

Since the beginning Anatomists tried to find an embalming technique that allows preserving human specimens to accurately resemble living tissue, preserve the cadaver for a long period of time and reduce health risk concerns related to working with cadavers [1].

The desired properties required for successful embalming of cadavers for anatomy and surgical teaching include a good long-term structural preservation of organs and tissues with minimal distortion, prevention of over-hardening or

N. M. T. L. Domingues (✉)
Department of Anatomy, Nova Medical School, NOVA University of Lisbon, Lisbon, Portugal

Hospital de Cascais & CUF Urology Department, Lisbon, Portugal

D. de Freitas Branco Pais · J. E. de Goyri O'Neill
Department of Anatomy, Nova Medical School, NOVA University of Lisbon, Lisbon, Portugal

© Springer Nature Switzerland AG 2021
E. Huri, D. Veneziano (eds.), *Anatomy for Urologic Surgeons in the Digital Era*,
https://doi.org/10.1007/978-3-030-59479-4_4

appearance alteration, while maintaining flexibility of internal organs and prevention of fungal or bacterial growth [7].

In modern medicine, the high requirement level in care, technical quality, surgical and microsurgical skills have recently demanded a degree of unprecedented excellence and technical mastery [8, 9].

Nowadays, minimally invasive surgery and especially, endoscopic, laparoscopic and robotic approach is the "Gold Standard" for numerous surgeries (i.e., Cholecystectomy, bariatric and anti-reflux surgery, nephrectomy) [10]. To achieve performances with excellence requires a high degree of skill, which is directly correlated with practice and exercise [11].

As a result, different international medical and surgical societies emphasizes the need to promote advances in technology through validated training programs, with measurement of performance, before moving to real situations, reducing in this way the advanced endoscopic and laparoscopic learning curve [12–14].

To mitigate this problem various techniques were introduced to teach and train young surgeons, from didactic lectures, video sessions, endo-trainer models, live demonstrations, hands-on sessions, wet lab with animals, virtual reality to cadavers.

The human cadaver is perhaps the best training model for all kinds of surgery, from open to endoscopic and laparoscopic to robotic. The cadaveric teaching model has the unique, irreplaceable advantage of human anatomy and real size experience that is the closest to reality you could have, making it the perfect model.

4.2   Human Preservation Techniques in Anatomy

An extensive literature review was performed to document different embalming techniques that are used to preserve human cadavers [1, 15]. The terms normally used for describing preservation techniques are considered to be ambiguous, so there was a need to define some terms that will be used [1].

The term "*fresh cadaver*" describes a human cadaver that has not been chemically treated (embalmed). When the embalming solution produces a cadaver with joint flexibility less than that of a fresh cadaver and with hard internal organs, this cadaver is described as "*hard fixed*." "*Soft preserved cadaver*" is used to describe cadavers that have equal or more joint flexibility than that of a fresh cadaver and with soft internal organs. "*Formalin based solution*" is used to describe solutions containing more than 0% formaldehyde while solutions containing 0% formaldehyde are described as "*Non-formalin based solution*".

4.2.1   *Formalin Based Solutions*

Hard-Fixed
Kaiserling, Jores, Neumann and Tutsch et al. represent the oldest embalming solutions, named after their authors, which use formaldehyde as the fixative in their formula [16–19]. Jores embalming technique, still used nowadays, results in

hard-fixation. Bacterial and fungal tests were performed on two formalin embalmed cadavers. Cadavers showed positive growth of microorganisms before embalming while 14 days after embalming tests showed that formaldehyde was able to kill the bacteria and fungus present in the pharynx, rectum, pleural fluids, and ascites [20].

Genelyn is a commercial product produced by Genelyn Pty. Ltd., Australia. Genelyn embalmed cadavers are generally less flexible compared to fresh cadavers [21]. The material safety data sheet (MSDS) provided by the company indicates that formaldehyde is an active ingredient of this solution [22]. Genelyn embalmed cadavers are also noted to be stiffer and more brittle compared to unembalmed tissue [23]. Ideally the cadaver would be placed in a flexed position for clinical training, but due to the lack of flexibility genelyn embalmed cadavers are used in prone position [24].

Soft Preservation
It is now over 20 years since Walter **Thiel** developed a novel preservation method that focused on tissue colour preservation that set the basis for a new photographic atlas of practical anatomy [25]. Cadavers embalmed by Thiel technique are preserved for over a year after being taken out of the tank of embalming fluid. This embalming technique includes a small percentage of formaldehyde compared to the commonly used formalin based recipes along with other salts such as ammonium nitrate, potassium nitrate and sodium sulfite [26].

Although cadavers embalmed by this technique have shown features close to fresh cadavers compared to formalin embalmed cadavers [21, 26], others have criticized some areas such as tendons [27], muscles [28] and bones [29]. On the technical level, the Thiel embalming technique is relatively expensive, time consuming and difficult to perform [30]. Some of the chemical used to prepare the Thiel solution is poisonous, very flammable, explosive, extremely hazardous to health and environmentally unfriendly [31]. To reduce the formation of furanes and dioxins, Thiel cadavers must be cremated at high temperature which is considered to be a disadvantage of this solution [31]. Thiel embalmed cadavers can be used to teach gross anatomy since it has some undeniable qualities, while it might not be ideal to use for some types of surgical training.

4.2.2 Non-formalin Based Solutions

Hard-Fixed
None of the non-formalin based solutions can be described as hard fixed.

Soft Preservation
There have been some efforts made to develop soft-preserving approaches with non-formalin-based solutions. The need for a formalin-free and fresh-like cadavers led anatomists to research for a new embalming technique. With the lack of criteria on whether an embalmed cadaver possesses the features of a fresh cadaver and as researchers are trying to avoid formaldehyde, no formalin-free solution was found in the literature that describes the preparation of hard fix cadavers.

Different solutions provided by The Embalmer's Supply Company, Ontario (**ESCO**), Canada have been used to embalm donated human cadavers [32]. The ESCO EPIC Conditioner is used as a humectant, plasticizer, preservative, and anti-dehydrant, and the main ingredient, according to the material safety data sheet of the product provided by the company, is methanol (8.6%) [33]. The other solution described by the article is the ESCO anticoagulant softener which, according to the material safety data sheet of the product provided by the company, has methanol, ethylene glycol, and EDTA Na_3 [33]. It states that cadavers would stay intact for 30 days after being thawed, or 45 days if they were never stored below zero. The removal of blood decreases the growth of bacteria and unlike other preservation techniques, mold growth was not observed during the period which the cadaver was used [32].

The **Nova Medical School** (**NMS**) technique described by Goyri-O'Neill uses aliphatic alcohols, diethylene glycol and monoethylene glycol (90:10), to prepare an embalming solution that is infused into the cadaver [34]. Cadavers embalmed with this solution showed no increase in skin resistance, detachment of skin layers, significant changes in coloration and joints remained movable without significant changes of passive range of motion. This quality of tissue was preserved for a period between 6 months to 1 year after embalming.

4.3   Nova Medical School Perfusion Technique

The NMS embalming solution is optimized in order to preserve the texture, volume, colour and shape of the body and its tissues as perfectly as possible, in order to allow the disinfection and sanitization of the process [34].

The resultant mixture solution is a clear liquid, practically odourless, colourless and denser than water. These properties, combined with adequate hygroscopic levels, good solubility in organic acids, are physiologically safe. Monoethylene glycol is toxic, the same being also true for diethylene glycol [35, 36]. Diethylene glycol can lead to serious complications that may prove fatal when ingested [37]. This substance produces no toxic vapours at room temperature and isn't harmful at touch, unless with direct contact with the product [38]. The cadaver embalming procedure involves a closed circuit of embalming fluid perfusion, from the machine itself to the closed vascular system of the preserved cadaver, without submersion of the entire body. These characteristics revealed this solution as a good choice, toxicologically comparable to glycerol, to achieve the intended goals [36, 37].

The technique consists of an incision in the right or left groin, with exposure of the femoral vessels. The femoral artery is injected bidirectionally with embalming solution using a 1 cm longitudinal cross or longitudinal section about 1 cm long, without any previous conservation intervention other than external washing with Chlorhexidine soap and cooling during transportation (in a temperature of approximately 4–6 ° C), sheathed in a simple cadaver plastic bag [34]. The injection is performed through an appropriate sized cannula at the proximal femoral artery, and a lower size cannula in the distal femoral artery, at room temperature [34].

The injection of the embalming solution is accomplished using a pulsed infusion at a pace between 60 to 70 pulses per minute, with the aim of mimicking normal physiological conditions, with recoil and variation of systolic and diastolic pressure, reducing the flow resistance and expanding the extent and scope of perfused tissues [34, 39].

The mean duration of cadaveric vascular infusion is 30–45 minutes, when performed with a perfusion rate of 70 pulses / minute. The average volume of the embalming solution injected is about 7 liters per body, varying with mass and stature [34].

The NMS perfusion technique of cadaveric embalming seems to be one of the best (Table 4.1), because it is formalin free, produces no toxic vapours at room temperature, is harmful at touch, looks and feels like real tissue and allows natural dissection similar to real surgery (Figs. 4.1 and 4.2).

Table 4.1 Comparison of different embalming techniques

Technique	Fixative used	Period of preservation	Quality of Tissue	Advantages	Disadvantages	References
Genelyn	Formalin based	N/A	Harder than fresh	Flexibility	Formalin based	(Jaung et al. [21])
Thiel	Formalin based	Over a year	Similar to fresh	Flexibility	Formalin based	(Benkhadra et al. [28])
				Realistic colors	Expensive	(Eisma et al. [26])
				Period of preservation	Complexity of embalming	(Thiel [25])
				Well researched		
ESCO	ESCO epic conditioner and	30 days	Similar to fresh	Flexibility	Short preservation period	(Messmer et al. [32])
	ESCO anticoagulant softener			Realistic colors	Not enough research	
Nova Medical School	Aliphatic alcohols, diethylene glycol	Six months to a year	Similar to fresh	Flexibility	Not enough research	(Goyri-O'Neill et al. [34])
	And Monoethylene glycol			Realistic colors		
				Period of preservation		
				No formalin		

Fig. 4.1 Cadaver upper
limb dissection

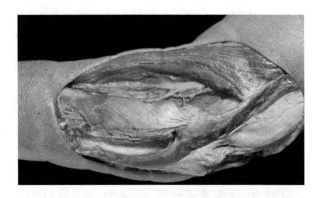

Fig. 4.2 Kidney—hilum

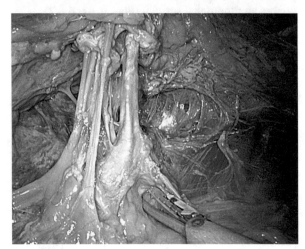

4.4 Present and Future Directions in Embalmed Cadaveric Use

Donation of the human body is a generous act that scientists and anatomists highly respect. Therefore, efforts should be made to make the most out of donation programs by maximizing the number of users.

Scientists are trying to develop an ideal embalming solution to preserve the human body. This solution would preserve the body in conditions comparable to that of an un-embalmed cadaver.

The chemicals used in this solution must be non-hazardous to eliminate any health risks that students, academics and researchers might encounter when dealing with the embalmed cadaver. The embalmed cadaver should be bacteria-free and the embalming solution should protect the body from being a host for any other microorganisms that will speed the decomposition process.

Finding an embalming technique that preserves the body in a realistic manner, not only serves the purpose of teaching anatomy as it should be taught, but also invites clinicians to research new surgical techniques.

In the twenty-first Century, medical schools need an embalming technique that preserves the body in a manner requiring the development of internationally recognized standards to allow comparison of the different embalming techniques.

The donated cadaver could be described as a shared resource used by academics, researchers and clinicians. The initial users should perform non-invasive clinical skills, which could be followed by different beneficiaries such as radiologists, minimal invasive surgeons, equipment testing companies, general/multidisciplinary surgeons and finally anatomy teaching.

The turning point in anatomy which was induced by the return of surgeons to the dissecting room for surgical training is remarkable.

The cadaver has the advantages of performing skills in real humans, where real-size experience and anatomy are much closer to a live patient in what pertains to handling instruments and tissues. Most importantly, surgeons gain valuable experience in operative laparoscopic surgery in an environment free of the limitations of the operating room.

The human cadaver embalmed with the NMS perfusion technique is perhaps the best training model for all kinds of surgery, from open to endoscopic and laparoscopic to robotic, you can get (Figs. 4.3, 4.4, and 4.5).

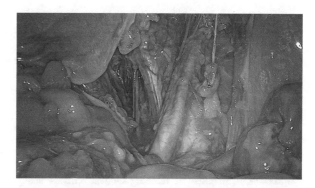

Fig. 4.3 Pelvic region (obturator fossa)

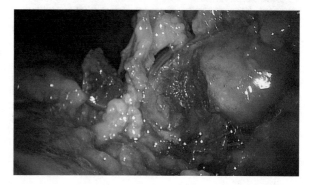

Fig. 4.4 Kidney_ laparoscopic parcial nephrectomy

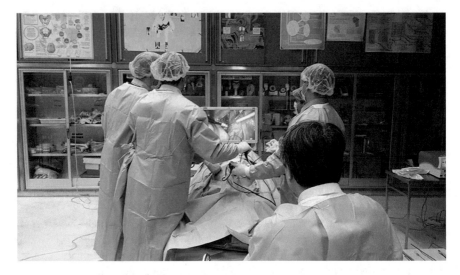

Fig. 4.5 Human Cadaveric Laparoscopic Course—Nova Medical School

References

1. Balta J, Cronin M, Cryan J. Human preservation techniques in anatomy: a 21st -century medical education perspective. Clin Anat. 2015;28:725–34.
2. McLachlan JC, Bligh J, Bradley P, Searle J. Teaching anatomy without cadavers. Med Educ. 2004;38:418–24.
3. Turner AJ, Mellington A, Ali F. Fresh cadaver dissection for training in plastic surgery. Br J Plast Surg. 2005;58:742–3.
4. Weiglein AH. Preservation and plastination. Clin Anat. 2002;15:445.
5. Jones D. Anatomy departments and anatomy education: reflections and myths. Clin Anat. 1997;10:34–40.
6. Bradbury SA, Hoshino K. An improved embalming procedure for long-lasting preservation of the cadaver for anatomical study. Acta Anat (Basel). 1978;101:97–103.
7. Coleman R, Kogan I. An improved low-formaldehyde embalming fluid to preserve cadavers for anatomy teaching. J Anat. 1998;192:443–6.
8. Reznick R, MacRae H. Teaching surgical skills — changes in the wind. N Engl J Med. 2006;355:2664–9.
9. Wolff KD, Kesting M, Mücke T, Rau A, Hölzle F. Thiel embalming technique: a valuable method for microvasular exercice and teaching of flap raising. Microsurgery. 2008;28:273–8.
10. Duchene DA, Rosso F, Clayman R, McDougall EM, Winfield HN. Current minimally invasive practice patterns among postgraduate urologists. J Endourol. 2011;25:1797–804.
11. Oliveira T, Cleynenbreugel B, Palmas A, Domingues N. Laparoscopic training in urology residency programs: a systematic review. Curr Urol. 2018;12:121–6.
12. Giger U, Frésard I, Häfliger A, Bergmann M, Krähenbühl L. Laparoscopic training on Thiel human cadavers: a model to teach advanced laparoscopic procedures. Surg Endosc. 2007;22:901–6.
13. Wein AJ, Kavoussi LR, Partin AW, Peters CA. Campbell-Walsh urology. 11th ed. Elsevier; 2016.
14. Aguilera Bazán A, Gómez Rivas J, Linares-Espinós E, Alvarez-Maestro M, Martínez-Piñeiro L. Training program in urological laparoscopic surgery. Future perspective. Arch Esp Urol. 2018;71:85–8.

15. Brenner E. Human body preservation–old and new techniques. J Anat. 2014;224(3):316–44. https://doi.org/10.1111/joa.12160.
16. Kaiserling C. Ueber Konservierung und Aufstellung pathologisch-anatomischer Praparate fur Schau-und Lehrsamm- lungen. Verhandl Deutsch Pathol Gesel. 1900;2:203–17.
17. Jores L. Ueber eine verbesserte methode der konservierung anatomischer objekte. Munch Med Wschr. 1913;60:976.
18. Tutsch H, Stahl G, Morike KD, Guckes H, Arnold M. Zur Aufbewahrung anatomischer Praparierobjekte, vol. 17. Bochum: Der Präparator; 1971. p. 85–95.
19. Neumann HG. Untersuchungen uber die Anwendungsmog-lichkeiten von, "Merphen" als Konservierungsmittel anatomischer Praparate, vol. 20. Bochum: Der Präparator; 1974. p. 30–5.
20. Hayashi S, Homma H, Naito M, Oda J, Nishiyama T, Kawamoto A, Kawata S, Sato N, Fukuhara T, Taguchi H, Mashiko K, Azuhata T, Ito M, Kawai K, Suzuki T, Nishizawa Y, Araki J, Matsuno N, Shirai T, Qu N, Hatayama N, Hirai S, Fukui H, Ohseto K, Yukioka T, Itoh M. Saturated salt solution method: a useful cadaver embalming for surgical skills training. Medicine (Baltimore). 2014;93:e196.
21. Jaung R, Cook P, Blyth P. A comparison of embalming fluids for use in surgical workshops. Clin Anat. 2011;24:155–61.
22. Genelyn. Material safety data sheet. 2010.
23. Norton-old KJ, Schache AG, Barker PJ, Clark RA, Harrison SM, Briggs CA. Anatomical and mechanical relationship between the proximal attachment of adductor longus and the distal rectus sheath. Clin Anat. 2013;26:522–30.
24. Belavy D, Ruitenberg MJ, Brijball RB. Feasibility study of real- time three–/four-dimensional ultrasound for epidural catheter insertion. Brit J Anaesth. 2011;107:438–45.
25. Thiel W. The preservation of the whole corpse with natural color. Ann Anat. 1992;174:185–95.
26. Eisma R, Lamb C, Soames RW. From formalin to Thiel embalming: what changes? One anatomy department's experiences. Clin Anat. 2013;26:564–71.
27. Fessel G, Frey K, Schweizer A, Calcagni M, Ullrich O, Snedeker JG. Suitability of Thiel embalmed tendons for biomechanical investigation. Ann Anat. 2011;193:237–41.
28. Benkhadra M, Gerard J, Genelot D, Trouilloud P, Girard C, Anderhuber F, Feigl G. Is Thiel's embalming method widely known? A world survey about its use. Surg Radiol Anat. 2011;33:359–63.
29. Unger S, Blauth M, Schmoelz W. Effects of three different preservation methods on the mechanical properties of human and bovine cortical bone. Bone. 2010;47:1048–53.
30. Wolff KD, Kesting M, Mucke T, Rau A, Holzle F. Thiel embalming technique: a valuable method for microvascular exercise and teaching of flap raising. Microsurgery. 2008;28:273–8.
31. Janczyk P, Weigner J, Luebke-Becker A, Kaessmeyer S, Plendl J. Nitrite pickling salt as an alternative to formaldehyde for embalming in veterinary anatomy–a study based on histo- and microbiological analyses. Ann Anat. 2011;193:71–5.
32. Messmer C, Kellogg RT, Zhang Y, Baiak A, Leiweke C, Marcus JR, Levin LS, Zenn MR, Erdmann D. A technique to perfuse cadavers that extends the useful life of fresh tissues: the Duke experience. Anat Sci Educ. 2010;3:191–4.
33. ESCO TESC. 2012. Material Safety Data Sheet. In European Commision. 2013. Guidance document on the evaluation of efficacy of embalming products (PT22). In: Environment, editor.
34. Goyri-O'Neill J, Pais D, Freire de Andrade F, Ribeiro P, Belo A, O'Neill A, Ramos S. Neves marques C. improvement of the embalming perfusion method: the innovation and the results by light and scanning electron microscopy. Acta Medica Port. 2013;26:188–94.
35. Brent J, McMartin K, Phillips S, Burkhart KK, Donovan JW, Wells M, et al. Fomepizole for the treatment of ethylene glycol poisoning. N Engl J Med. 1999;340:832–8.
36. O'Brien KL, Selanikio JD, Hecdivert C, Placide M-F, Louis M, Barr DB, et al. Epidemic of pediatric deaths from acute renal failure caused by diethylene glycol poisoning. JAMA. 1998;279:1175–80.

37. Schep LJ, Slaughter RJ, Temple WA, Beasley DM. Diethylene glycol poisoning. Clin Toxicol. 2009;47:525–35.
38. Sigma-Aldrich ®–Safety Information Diethylene glycol. https://www.sigmaaldrich.com/catalog/product/sigma/93171?lang=en&region=GB. Accessed 21 Nov 2019.
39. Gabrys E, Rybaczuk M, Kedzia A. Blood flow simulation through fractal models of circulatory system. Chaos, Solitons Fractals. 2006;27:1–7.

Chapter 5
Lab Animal Models and Analogies with Humans

İlyas Onbaşilar

Due to the anatomical and physiological similarities between humans and especially mammals, almost all medical information has been obtained by animal experiments so far [2]. Animal models are critical to understanding gene function and human disease. Many rodent models are used for this purpose [36]. Especially the use of animals such as rat and mouse seems indispensable in today's scientific world [2]. However, all results obtained from animal experiments shouldn't be directly adapted to humans. Animal models should be continually developed to be more reliable, reproducible and informative [2]. With the new generation models, limitations in existing animal models can be eliminated [28]. Simpler and effective models, especially transgenic mouse models that mimic human responses, should be used to understand and treat various medical studies [3].

Despite anatomical differences, rats are one of the most used species in kidney research in the world. For example; rat and mouse kidneys are much smaller than human kidney; they are unipapillary and have less renal tubule. Also, the pelvis of the rat and mouse kidney is much simpler and has a tiny urinary cavity. However, the ratio of the cortex and medulla (2:1) is very close to the human kidney. Species differences should be known well, while doing these studies. It should not be neglected that there may be strain and gender differences in studies. When it comes to the size of the stone produced by the kidney, these differences between the two kidneys become significant. In the rat and mouse kidneys with a simple and small pelvis, large stones cannot be formed, and only a miniature imitation of the human stone can be modeled in these kidneys [9, 38].

In rats, the possibility of spontaneous urinary tract stone formation is extremely low [9]. Therefore, in rodent models, some basic techniques are used

İ. Onbaşilar (✉)
Transgenic Animal Technologies Research and Application Center, Hacettepe University, Ankara, Turkey

Health Science Institute, Hacettepe University, Ankara, Turkey
e-mail: ilyas@hacettepe.edu.tr

© Springer Nature Switzerland AG 2021
E. Huri, D. Veneziano (eds.), *Anatomy for Urologic Surgeons in the Digital Era*,
https://doi.org/10.1007/978-3-030-59479-4_5

to experimentally inducing urine crystallization and stone formation in kidneys. These are manipulating urinary pH, increasing the urinary expression of crystallizable substances and preventing the expression of crystallization inhibitors [9]. For this purpose, many agents are used, especially ethylene glycol and hydroxy-L proline. Ethylene glycol has been used to induce hyperoxaluria in rats, and it is a perfect model for evaluating the metabolic effects [40]. Generally, ethylene glycol has been combined with ammonium chloride, vitamin D or calcium chloride to enhance the development of crystal deposition [11, 12, 21]. However, ethylene glycol can cause multi-organ failure and concentrations, and also use of above 0.75% may produce metabolic acidosis [16, 20]. Hydroxy-L-proline is given to rats in a two way with drinking water or mixed with food. Male Sprague-Dawley rats were given chow mixed with 5% HLP (weight/weight HLP/chow) for inducing the CaOx nephrolithiasis in rats [20].

Rodent urolithiasis models are not fully reliable and reproducible. The pathogenesis of the crystal formation in the rodent differs from humans. The presence of severe inflammation and cellular damage in many mouse models represent significant kidney damage, but this is significantly different from most human kidneys with urolithiasis [38].

Examining the genetically engineered urolithiasis models is useful in the study of the disease. Genetic hypercalciuric stone-forming rats have been inbred for over 95 generations to produce a strain in which urine calcium excretion is over ten times greater than that of controls, and all rats form kidney stones [26]. Slc7a9 KO mice, OPN KO mice, THP KO mice, NHERF-1 KO mice, Npt2a KO mice, and Sat1 KO mice should be used for urolithiasis models [38].

The rodent bladder cancer models have several advantages, such as small body size, short gestation, and easy manipulation of gene expression [5, 24, 35]. Rodents have a lower urinary tract that is homologous to that of humans. Also, bladder cancer is not very common in rodents unless a chemical carcinogen or oncogenes induce them [7, 19, 29]. Sensitivity to this type of cancer may vary among the rodent strains, for example, Brown Norway and DA/Han rats show a high incidence of spontaneous bladder tumors, and these strains can be used as rodent models without using the chemical carcinogens [19].

Rodent models of bladder cancer can be divided as a spontaneous and transplantable model [19]. In the spontaneous model is occurred with chemically induced such as N-methyl-N-nitrosurea, N-[4–5-nitro-2-furyl-2-thiazolyl]-formamide and N-butyl-N-(4-hydroxybuthyl) nitrosamine or genetically engineered [14]. The transplantable model is occurred as murine bladder cancer cells implanted into immunocompetent or transgenic mice (syngeneic) or human bladder cancer cells implanted into immune-deficient mice (xenografts) [19]. The commonly used rodent bladder cancer cell lines are MBT-2, MB49 and AY-27 for syngeneic modeling [14]. As tumors are rodent origin, tumor growth and metastasis may be different from those of human [35]. In the xenograft models, TCC cell lines, such as KU7, KU-19–19, UMUC1, UMUC3, UMUC13, and T24 have been used to develop tumors in immune deficient mice [37]. The disadvantage of this model is that the immune response cannot be assessed [35].

The rodent prostate and the human prostate are not entirely homologous. However, both prostate tissues originate from the wall of the urethra. The glands of both species have a histological similarity. Prostate tissue in rodents consists of a combination of many lobes called dorsal, ventral, lateral, and anterior lobes, and this differs from the human prostate. Also it is necessary to know very well which prostate pathology can be imitated in which lobe of rodent prostate. Usually, the ventral lobe is a most similar transition region of human is used in the benign prostatic hyperplasia studies, whereas dorsal and lateral lobes are most identical to the peripheral region of human are used in the prostate cancer studies. Due to these differences, an obstructive pattern cannot be created in prostate cancer models in mice and rats [1]. It should also be remembered that there are differences among rodent strains in terms of the probability of forming a disease model. To minimize this variation, spontaneous and genetically engineered models are used for prostate cancer. There are several rat models currently in use; however, not all models are valid for studies. For example, the ACI/Seg spontaneous rat model has limited usefulness due to its long latency, low tumor incidence, and low incidence of invasive prostate carcinoma [1, 4, 23].

The Dunning rat model is one of the first rat models that was established and The Dunning R-3327 tumor was a spontaneous adenocarcinoma that developed in an inbred Copenhagen rat [1, 15]. The Dunning model has the main advantage of not requiring exposure to chemical compounds for its execution, thus reducing the health risk for the investigator, the environmental effects and costs [27].

The Lobund–Wistar (L-W) prostate adenocarcinoma rat model is unique because it is the only rat model that spontaneously develops hormone-induced adenocarcinoma of the prostate with metastases. The spontaneous, metastatic, and hormone-refractory L-W model can be used to test chemo preventive and treatment for late stage and metastatic disease. Spontaneous rat models have some disadvantages such as long tumor latency, lack of reproducibility, and a low percentage of rats that spontaneously develop adenocarcinoma and metastasis [1].

Transgenic mouse models reproduce the different stages of prostate carcinoma associated with the typical human genetic mutation that allows tumor progression [10, 22, 32]. The first transgenic mouse models, C3(1)-Tag mice, for prostate cancer was established by expressing the simian virus (SV) 40 large T antigen (Tag) under the control of the C3(1) promoter [25, 30]. These mice on the background of FVB/N showed prostatic epithelial hyperplasia in the ventral and dorso-lateral lobes about 3 months of age and local adenocarcinoma about 7–11 months of age progression [1, 32]. It should be noted that the C3(1) promoter is not prostate specific, as it is expressed in non-prostate tissues such as urethral and mammary glands [1].

The TRAMP model (transgenic adenocarcinoma of the mouse prostate) was developed by linking the rat probasin promoter region to the SV40 early region [17, 30]. TRAMP mice developed epithelial hyperplasia by 8 weeks of age, progressed to prostatic intraepithelial neoplasia by 18 weeks of age, and after 28 weeks of age, 100% of the mice displayed lymphatic metastases, and approximately two-thirds displayed pulmonary metastases. This model displays castration-resistant disease [39]. TRAMP shows progression to extensively invasive neuroendocrine tumors that have metastatic potential [18]. However, the TRAMP model may not be the best suited for oncogenic studies, it is well purposed for studies of treatment and prevention. Studies conducted on this model suggest that many tumors show neuroendocrine differentiation, and this model is probably a small cell carcinoma model rather than adenocarcinoma [6, 8, 13].

The progression of prostate cancer in the FG/Tag (Fetal globin γ (Gγ)-SV40 large T/small t antigen model) mice is similar to that in humans. It originates from high-grade prostate intraepithelial neoplasia and progresses to advanced metastatic carcinomas [33]. This model is suitable for studies of the mechanisms of progression of aggressive and advanced prostate cancer. However, these mice also develop non-prostatic tumors including adrenocortical and brown adipose tumors [1, 31].

LPB-Tag (LADY) model uses only the large T antigen. This model group comprises several distinct mouse strains including the 12T-7f, 12T-7s, 12T-10 and 12T-11 models [18]. The LADY models more accurately mimic the majority of human prostate cancer because the cancer is slow growing and has a mostly epithelial phenotype. However, castration resistance and metastasis are not modeled well [39].

The PSP-TGMAP is generated by using the 3.8-kb promoter fragment of PSP94 (prostate secretory protein of 94 amino acids) to target T antigens to the prostate epithelium. A T antigen knockin model has been created by inserting the T antigen-coding sequence to the PSP94 locus (PSP-KIMAP) [41]. Compared with the original transgenic model, PSP-TGMAP, the PSP-KIMAP mice develop tumors at a younger age, and the tumor development is more predictive and has no founder line variations [41].

C-myc is an oncogene that is overexpressed in invasive and metastatic human prostate cancer samples [1]. Up to 30% of prostate tumors exhibit an increased c-Myc gene copy number or expression levels and elevated c-Myc expression is frequently observed in early stages of prostatic intraepithelial neoplasia lesions [41].

The tumor suppressor, PTEN (phosphatase and tensin homologue deleted from chromosome 10), is one of the most frequently mutated genes in human cancers, including prostate cancer [41]. The conditional knock-out PTEN model displays multistep carcinogenesis that mimics the initiation, progression, and metastasis of human prostate adenocarcinoma [1, 42]. Proliferation of the Pten null prostate cancer cells is not sensitive to androgen withdrawal. Androgen-independent growth observed in PTEN null prostate cancers may contribute to hormone-resistant prostate cancer formation [34].

Several animal models of prostate cancer have emerged including human prostate cancer xenograft models that are implanted in mice and other rodent models. These models are valuable for the mechanisms of prostate cancer [1].

Nowadays, patient-derived xenograft *in vivo* models are used for preclinical prostate cancer researches. Patient-derived xenograft models created by transferring the tumor tissue of the patient to immune-compromised mice without any manipulation in vitro, the microenvironment and heterogeneity of the original tumor are preserved; tumor prognosis and response to treatment can be evaluated more accurately. Patient-derived xenograft models are not widely used yet, because they have variable engraftment rates, long latency period after the engraftment, high costs of animal care and rare access to patient tissue samples. Xenograft mouse models represent a common "recipient" of human prostate cancer, generated through orthotopic or heterotopic implantation of human tumor tissues, cell lines, or primary cell cultures, in nude mice, SCID, NOD-SCID and etc. [32].

5.1 Conclusion

With the application of virtual reality applications and 3D models in the field of urology, the use of rodent and other vertebrates for education and training has been reduced. Due to the developing technology, it is inevitable that these applications will replace animal use for education and training in the future.

To date, almost all medical information has been obtained with animal use. After today, it is certain that animals will be used to develop treatment in biomedical research. In addition, genetically engineered mouse models that better mimic human diseases have been developed, especially after mapping the mouse genome. But today, there is no single genetically engineered mouse models that mimics the full spectrum of the human disease. With the development of genome editing technologies such as CRISPR-Cas9, more reliable and reproducible animal models will increase.

Patient-derived xenograft models are more promising compared to traditional or transgenic models in their research in the field of urooncology. In these models created by transferring the tumor tissue of the patient to immune-compromised mice, the microenvironment and heterogeneity of the original tumor are preserved; tumor prognosis and response to treatment can be evaluated more accurately. In this way, largely used in research has started to be used. There are variations in tumor engraftment rates in mouse lines such as nude mice, SCID, NOD-SCID, RAG, NOG/NSG, which are used as patient-derived models today. With the solution of this problem in the near future, the use of patient-derived xenograft models will become more widespread.

References

1. Alagbala AA, Foster BA. Animal models of prostate cancer. In: Conn PM, editor. Sourcebook of models for biomedical research. Totowa, NJ: Humana Press; 2008. p. 614–30. https://doi.org/10.1007/978-1-59745-285-4_66.
2. Barré-Sinoussi F, Montagutelli X. Animal models are essential to biological research: issues and perspectives. Future Sci OA. 2015;1:FSO63. https://doi.org/10.4155/fso.15.63.
3. Bartholomew I, Yasuhide F, Lucy O, Josiah H. Humanized mouse as an appropriate model for accelerated global HIV research and vaccine development: current trend. Immunopharm Immunot. 2016;38:395–407.
4. Bostwick DG, Ramnani D, Qian J. Prostatic intraepithelial neoplasia: animal models. Prostate. 2000;43:286–94.

5. Cekanova M, Rathore K. Animal models and therapeutic molecular targets of cancer: utility and limitations. Drug Des Devel Ther. 2014;8:1911–21.
6. Chiaverotti T, Couto SS, Donjacour A, Mao JH, Nagase H, Cardiff RD, et al. Dissociation of epithelial and neuroendocrine carcinoma lineages in the transgenic adenocarcinoma of mouse prostate model of prostate cancer. Am J Pathol. 2008;172:236–46. https://doi.org/10.2353/ajpath.2008.070602.
7. Clayson DB, Fishbein L, Cohen SM. Effects of stones and other physical factors on the induction of rodent bladder cancer. Food Chem Toxicol. 1995;33:771–84.
8. Cunningham D, You Z. In vitro and in vivo model systems used in prostate cancer research. J Biol Methods. 2015;2:e17.
9. Çakır ÖO, Yürük E, Binbay M. Üriner Sistem Taş Hastalığında Deneysel Modeller. Endoüroloji Bülteni. 2014;7:13–7.
10. DeCaprio JA, Ludlow JW, Figge J, Marsilio E, Paucha E, Livingston D. SV40 large tumor antigen forms a specific complex with the product of the retinoblastoma susceptibility gene. Cell. 1988;54:275–83.
11. de Bruijn WC, Boeve ER, van Run PR, van Miert PP, Romijin JC, Verkoelen CF, et al. Etiology of experimental calcium oxalate monohydrate nephrolithiasis in rats. Scanning Microsc. 1994;8:541–9.
12. de Water R, Boeve ER, van Miert PP, Deng G, Cao LC, Stijnen T, et al. Experimental nephrolithiasis in rats: the effect of ethylene glycol and vitamin D3 on the induction of renal calcium oxalate crystals. Scanning Microsc. 1996;10:591–601.
13. di Sant'Agnese PA. Neuroendocrine differentiation in carcinoma of the prostate. Diagnostic, prognostic, and therapeutic implications. Cancer. 1992;70:254–68.
14. Ding J, Xu D, Pan C, Ye M, Kang J, Bai Q, et al. Current animal models of bladder cancer: awareness of translatability (review). Exp Ther Med. 2014;8:691–9. https://doi.org/10.3892/etm.2014.1837.
15. Dunning WF. Prostate cancer in the rat. J Natl Cancer Inst Monogr. 1963;12:351–69.
16. Eder AF, McGrath CM, Dowdy YG, Tomaszewski JE, Rosenberg FM, Wilson RB, et al. Ethylene glycol poisoning: toxicokinetic and analytical factors affecting laboratory diagnosis. Clin Chem. 1998;44:168–77.
17. Greenberg NM, DeMayo F, Finegold MJ, Medina D, Tilley WD, Aspinall JO, et al. Prostate cancer in a transgenic mouse. Proc Natl Acad Sci USA. 1995;92:3439–43.
18. Ishii K, Shappell S, Matusik R, Hayward SW. Use of tissue recombination to predict phenotypes of transgenic mouse models of prostate carcinoma. Lab Investig. 2005;85:1086–103. https://doi.org/10.1038/labinvest.3700310.
19. John BA, Said N. Insights from animal models of bladder cancer: recent advances, challenges, and opportunities. Oncotarget. 2017;8:57766–81.
20. Khan SR, Glenton PA, Byer KJ. Modeling of hyperoxaluric calcium oxalate nephrolithiasis: experimental induction of hyperoxaluria by hydroxy-L-proline. Kidney Int. 2006;70:914–23.
21. Khan SR, Shevock PN, Hackett RL. Acute hyperoxaluria, renal injury and calcium oxalate urolithiasis. J Urol. 1992;147:226–30.
22. Lane DP, Crawford LV. T antigen is bound to a host protein in SV40-transformed cells. Nature. 1979;278:261–3.
23. Lucia MS, Bostwick DG, Bosland M, Cockett ATK, Knapp DW, Leaw I, et al. Workgroup I: rodent models of prostate cancer. Prostate. 1998;36:49–55.
24. Mak IW, Evaniew N, Ghert M. Lost in translation: animal models and clinical trials in cancer treatment. Am J Transl Res. 2014;6:114.
25. Maroulakou IG, Anver M, Garrett L, Green JE. Prostate and mammary adenocarcinoma in transgenic mice carrying a rat C3 (1) simian virus 40 large tumor antigen fusion gene. Proc Natl Acad Sci USA. 1994;91:11236–40.
26. Moe OW, Bushinsky DA, Kuiper JJ. Genetic hypercalciuria: a major risk factor in kidney stones. In: Thakker RV, Whyte MP, Eisman JA, Igarashi T, editors. Genetics of bone biology

and skeletal disease. 2nd ed. Oxford: Elsevier; 2018. p. 819–39. https://doi.org/10.1016/B978-0-12-804182-6.00043-5

27. Nascimento-Gonçalves E, Faustino-Rocha AI, Seixas F, Ginja M, Colaço B, Ferreira R, et al. Modelling human prostate cancer: rat models. Life Sci. 2018;203:210–24.

28. Okechukwu IB. Introductory chapter: animal models for human diseases, a major contributor to modern medicine. In: Okechukwu IB editor. Experimental animal models of human diseases: an effective therapeutic strategy. London:Intech Open; 2018. p. 1–9. https://doi.org/10.5772/intechopen.70745

29. Oliveira PA, Colaco A, De la Cruz PL, Lopes C. Experimental bladder carcinogenesis-rodent models. Exp Oncol. 2006;28:2–11.

30. Parisotto M, Metzger D. Genetically engineered mouse models of prostate cancer. Mol Oncol. 2013;7:190–205.

31. Perez-Stable C, Altman NH, Brown J, Harbison M, Cray C, Roos BA. Prostate, adrenocortical, and brown adipose tumors in fetal globin/T antigen transgenic mice. Lab Investig. 1996;74:363–73.

32. Rea D, Del Vecchio V, Palma G, Barbieri A, Falco M, Luciano A, et al. Mouse models in prostate cancer translational research: from xenograft to PDX. Biomed Res Int. 2016. https://www.hindawi.com/journals/bmri/2016/9750795. Accessed 10 May 2020.

33. Reiner T, De Las PA, Parrondo R, Perez-Stable C. Progression of prostate cancer from a subset of p63-positive basal epithelial cells in FG/Tag transgenic mice. Mol Cancer Res. 2007;5:1171–9.

34. Roy-Burman P, Wu H, Powell WC, Hagenkord J, Cohen MB. Genetically defined mouse models that mimic natural aspects of human prostate cancer development. Endoc-Relat Cancer. 2004;11:225–54.

35. Smolensky D, Rathore K, Cekanova M. Molecular targets in urothelial cancer: detection, treatment, and animal models of bladder cancer. Drug Des Devel Ther. 2016;10:3305–22. https://doi.org/10.2147/DDDT.S112113.

36. Sprengel R, Eshkind L, Hengstler J, Bockamp E. Improved models for animal research. In: Conn PM, editor. Sourcebook of models for biomedical research. Totowa, NJ: Humana Press; 2008. p. 17–24.

37. Teicher BA. Tumor models for efficacy determination. Mol Cancer Ther. 2006;5:2435–43.

38. Tzou DT, Taguchi K, Chi T, Stoller ML. Animal models to study urolithiasis. In: Animal models for the study of human disease. 2nd ed. London: Academic; 2017. p. 419–43.

39. Valkenburg KC, Williams BO. Mouse models of prostate cancer. Prostate Cancer. 2011. https://www.hindawi.com/journals/pc/2011/895238/. Accessed 12 May 2020.

40. Yuruk E, Tuken M, Sahin C, Kaptanagasi AO, Basak K, Aykan S, et al. The protective effects of an herbal agent tutukon on ethylene glycol and zinc disk induced urolithiasis model in a rat model. Urolithiasis. 2016;44:501–7.

41. Wang F. Modeling human prostate cancer in genetically engineered mice. Prog Mol Biol Transl Sci. 2011;100:1–49.

42. Wang S, Gao J, Lei Q, Rozengurt N, Pritchard C, Jiao J, et al. Prostate-specific deletion of the murine Pten tumor suppressor gene leads to metastatic prostate cancer. Cancer Cell. 2003;4:209–21.

Part II
Frontiers in Imaging-Acquisition Technologies

Chapter 6
Frontiers in Imaging-Acquisition Technologies: Ultrasound

Ahmet T. Turgut and Vikram Dogra

6.1 Introduction

Since the beginning of 1960s, ultrasound (US) has become the most commonly used imaging tool in clinical practice. Owing to the tremendous improvement in US technology and its diagnostic efficiency has resulted in increased number of US users. The innovation including contrast enhanced ultrasound (CEUS) and elastography has transformed US into a multiparametric imaging tool which allows the evaluation of different characteristics of the pathological conditions in the same session. The future of US seems even brighter thanks to the development of novel technologies which might potentially revolutionize modern medical diagnostics by expanding the field of its clinical applications. Apparently, urology is among the cardinal fields of medicine requiring the use of US both for diagnostic and therapeutic purposes. The complex nature of several urological disorders necessitates better understanding of the advanced and versatile US techniques working on different principles which enable analysis of the structure and morphology of tissues/organs and in addition can efficiently monitor the functions and molecular reactions at the cellular level.

A. T. Turgut (✉)
Department of Radiology, Yüksek Ihtisas University, Ankara, Turkey

V. Dogra
Department of Imaging Sciences, University of Rochester School of Medicine, Rochester, NY, USA
e-mail: Vikram_Dogra@URMC.Rochester.Edu

© Springer Nature Switzerland AG 2021
E. Huri, D. Veneziano (eds.), *Anatomy for Urologic Surgeons in the Digital Era*,
https://doi.org/10.1007/978-3-030-59479-4_6

6.2   Techniques

6.2.1   Three-Dimensional Ultrasound

6.2.1.1   Principles

Currently, three-dimensional (3D) US imaging is a widely available feature in many ultrasound machines. This technology with unlimited viewing perspectives and multiplanar capability allows the acquisition and storage of a dataset acquired from a specific region of interest, which can be further analyzed, either by multiplanar display, surface rendering, or volume calculation [1]. Compared to Gray scale US, this technique provides superior reliability, and consistency in end results for the morphological evaluation and disease processes [2].

6.2.1.2   Urological Applications

Bladder
3D US is extremely useful in planning and guiding prostate cancer treatment, measuring bladder urinary volume, and in imaging the urethral sphincter in pelvic floor disorders [3–5]. As a screening tool, it is superior to two dimensional (2D) US in tumor detection [1].

3D US enabling virtual sonographic cystoscopy is a non-invasive, innovative technique in detecting bladder tumors [1]. Thanks to the gradient between the bladder lumen and its wall, the surface rendering algorithm can usually reveal a detailed view of the bladder surface enabling display and characterization of bladder wall abnormalities at lower costs and with no radiation exposure [6]. Contrary to conventional cystoscopy, there is no risk of iatrogenic trauma or infection because the technique does not require catheterisation [7]. However, virtual cystoscopy has some inherent limitations, such as the inability to confirm the histopathologic nature of the mass detected [7].

Owing to the fact that the results of the virtual sonographic cystoscopy is comparable with computerized tomography (CT) and magnetic resonance (MR) imaging, the technology may be a useful alternative for screening and follow up of bladder cancer. However, it cannot preclude the need for conventional cystoscopy yet for the evaluation of mucosal abnormalities because of its inadequacy for demonstrating flat or intramural lesions (carcinoma in situ) appearing as subtle mucosal colour changes on a conventional cystoscopy [1]. Furthermore, this technology apparently cannot replace pathological staging, which might be future focus of interest with further improvement of 3D US technology.

Penis
3D US may also serve as a valuable complement of 2D US and enable better assessment of penile plaques in Peyronie disease with size, shape and location as it may enable the operator to visualize the organ in coronal axis. Technically, the probe

should be moved along the examined tissue at an optimal speed maintaining a constant direction and angle of displacement because even slight irregularities during the acquisition process may disturb the final image and result in inaccuracies for the assessment of plaque in the coronal view [8].

On 3D US, qualitative and quantitative evaluation of the plaques may be performed after the acquisition of images without the patient's participation, which reduces significantly the acquisition time and increases patient comfort [8]. This also transforms the subjective nature of 2D US to an objective examination which enables future appraisal by another physician during follow up, which may be a challenge in 2D US [8].

Furthermore, 3D US seems to be quite satisfactory for the evaluation of treatment outcomes as it allows imaging of the entire plaque, assessing the effect of treatment on the plaque size, shape and echogenicity and comparing the images before and after treatment [8]. However, the technique still has some limitations related to the individual skills of the examiner and variability of the severity of the cases, which affect the length and quality of the 2D and 3D US examinations.

6.2.2   Contrast-Enhanced Ultrasound

6.2.2.1   Principles

CEUS is always applied as an extension of conventional B-mode and color Doppler ultrasound (CDUS). The technique is mediated by ultrasound contrast agent(s) (UCA)s, mainly used for the evaluation of macro- and microvascular systems following intravenous injection which enhances the US signal from flowing blood, though they can also be instilled into body cavities such as the urinary bladder for the evaluation of vesicoureteral reflux [9]. Technically, contrast-specific US modes, involving the separation between non-linear response induced by microbubble UCA oscillations and linear US signal reflected by tissues are required for CEUS examinations [10]. In order to diminish non-linear harmonic US signals from the tissues, a low acoustic pressure is used, which is based on a low mechanical index (MI). For the sake of minimizing microbubble disruption besides reducing tissue harmonics and artifacts, an examination with MI value below 0.3 is preferred. However, most US systems are capable of performing CEUS examinations with lower MI values such as 0.08 or 0.05. Contrary to the recent widespread use of low MI specific modes, UCAs were initially developed to enhance the Doppler US signals, based on higher MI techniques [9].

Most US systems have a monitor with inherent dual split display feature, where the low MI CEUS image is shown alongside a conventional B-mode image. Thereby, CEUS window enables visualization of scarce signals from markedly reflective structures such as calcifications or interfaces with large acoustic impedance differences, depending on respective MI and gain settings [9].

From diagnostic point of view, the enhancement characteristics of each lesion should be noted. In this regard, the temporal behavior, degree of enhancement relative to surrounding tissues and the distribution pattern should be described. The flow kinetics for most organs having single arterial blood supply involve two phases; the arterial phase showing a progressive degree of enhancement and the venous phase showing a plateau followed by a progressive decrease [10, 11].

UCAs are used safely in various applications in both adult and pediatric populations, posing minimal risk to patients [9, 10, 12]. They can be safely used in patients with renal insufficiency with no risk of contrast-related nephropathy or nephrogenic systemic fibrosis as they are not excreted through the kidneys physiologically. Contrary to the iodinated CT agents and gadolinium-based MR contrast agents, the risk for anaphylactoid reactions is very low. The most frequent adverse effects include headache (2.1%), nausea (0.9%), chest pain (0.8%) and chest discomfort (0.5%), being mild in degree and transient in nature [9]. Owing to the fact that UCAs do not contain iodine, they don't have any effect on thyroid function.

6.2.2.2   Urological Applications

Kidney
After UCA administration, the arterial pedicle as well as the main branches enhance first, followed by the enhancement of the segmental, interlobar, arcuate and interlobular arteries and the entire cortex and medulla [13]. However, there is no UCA in the renal collecting system as UCAs are not excreted by the kidneys. The flow kinetics for kidney involve two phases; the cortical phase with cortical enhancement and parenchymal phase with cortical and medullar enhancement. Notably, contrast enhancement is less intense and fades earlier in patients with chronic renal disease [14].

CEUS can be used to diagnose ischemic renal disorders, such as infarction appearing as wedge shaped non-enhancing areas within an otherwise enhanced kidney [15]. In cases with equivocal conventional B-mode and Doppler US findings, CEUS can differentiate renal tumors from anatomical variants mimicking a renal tumor, namely "pseudotumors". The technique can also be used to characterize complex cysts according to the Bosniak criteria as benign or malignant with at least the same accuracy as CT imaging; it has also future potential to have a role in staging patients with malignant cystic lesions, though lesion calcification challenges the accuracy of CEUS evaluation [9, 16–18].

CEUS can be used for the follow-up of non-surgical renal lesions and to characterize indeterminate renal lesions because it is more sensitive than CT for detecting blood flow in hypovascularized lesions [16, 19]. Although heterogeneous enhancement implying rapid growth of the tumor and proneness to ischemic necrosis has been found to be a major CEUS characteristic for renal cell carcinoma (RCC) regardless of the subtype [20], tumors ≤3 cm have been reported to show predominantly homogeneous enhancement more frequently [21]. Recently, CEUS imaging features including fast wash out and perilesional rim-like enhancement around the tumor representing a fibrous pseudocapsule have been noted to be helpful for differentiating RCCs from renal angiomyolipoma, which would indeed have an impact on clinical treatment decision [22]. CEUS can be used for detecting and monitoring the resolution of renal abscess in complicated acute pyelonephritis, which appears as a non-enhancing area [23].

Contrast-enhanced voiding urosonography, where UCA can be administered intravesically via a transurethral bladder catheter or via suprapubic puncture, can be used as the initial examination for suspected vesicoureteral reflux in girls. The diagnosis of reflux involves the appearance of UCA in one or both ureters and/or the pelvicalyceal system. The technique can be used for the follow-up of the entity in girls and boys after conservative or surgical treatment [9].

Quantitative CEUS assessment of hemodynamic changes in transplanted kidney is still considered a research field in transplant assessment.

Bladder

Clinically, CEUS is very helpful for the differential diagnosis of intraluminal lesions in patients with hematuria as it can demonstrate the vascularization and enhancement of tumors, in contrast to non-enhancing hematomas [24, 25]. Sonographically, the bladder mucosa and submucosal layer exhibit early and intense enhancement after UCA administration contrary to the muscular layer having lesser and delayed enhancement. However, the role of CEUS for local staging and grading of bladder tumors is limited despite being superior to conventional B-mode US for identifying infiltration of the muscle layer [26, 27]. The role of CEUS in detecting both small (<1 cm) lesions and large flat, plaque-like tumors is limited [9].

Prostate

The most useful characteristics on CEUS for an area suspicious for prostate cancer are a rapid inflow and/or an increased maximal enhancement compared to the surrounding tissue. However, computer-aided quantification by contrast ultrasound dispersion imaging (CUDI) technique has been proposed to aid in the interpretation of CEUS, by estimating whether pixels belonged to a pre-defined malignant or benign prostate region [28–30]. Furthermore, 4 D contrast-enhanced transrectal ultrasound (TRUS) imaging has been introduced enabling objective quantification of the imaging data derived from CUDI [31].

Despite compressing CEUS in one image, incorporating quantitative analysis using CUDI maps has recently been reported to result in similar localization performance for clinically significant prostate cancer as qualitative analysis using 2D CEUS readings only [30] (Fig. 6.1). Additionally, CUDI compressing all the information of a CEUS video in a single image may shorten the reading time and enable low data consumption on storage devices/networks and easy file transfer [30]. On the other hand, a multiparametric ultrasound (mpUS) approach by combining CEUS/CUDI with complementary techniques such as elastography evaluating tissue stiffness, might improve the detection and diagnostic accuracy [32, 33].

CEUS has also been used to visualize perfusion defects during follow-up of patients who have undergone ablative treatments [34]. Interestingly, CEUS has also been reported to have a potential role in the assessment of the efficacy of prostatic artery embolisation (PAE) at the early post-interventional period or even on-site when prostatic infarctions could be delineated [35]. The authors speculated that the

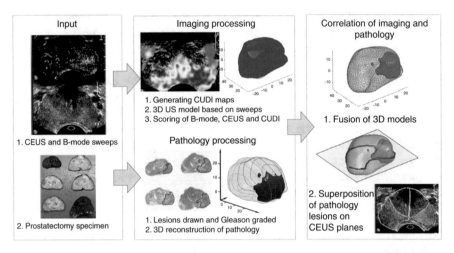

Fig. 6.1 Study procedures. *CEUS* contrast-enhanced ultrasound, *CUDI* contrast ultrasound dispersion imaging, *US* ultrasound (Reprinted from Postema AW, Gayet MCW, van Sloun RJG et al. (2020) Contrast-enhanced ultrasound with dispersion analysis for the localization of prostate cancer: correlation with radical prostatectomy specimens. World J Urol doi: https://doi.org/10.1007/s00345-020-03103-4. [Epub ahead of print] with permission)

technique can be used to document the technical success of PAE and predict the relevant clinical benefit [35].

Recently, a novel high frame US framework for imaging intra-urethral urinary flow, namely contrast-enhanced urodynamic vector projectile imaging has been developed to assess the functional impact of uropathological factors such as benign prostatic hyperplasia (BPH) on voiding, which might help in developing treatment strategies that are personalized for patients with lower urinary tract symptoms [36].

Scrotum

The flow kinetics for scrotum involves the arterial enhancement followed within seconds by complete parenchymal enhancement and decline of enhancement over a variable period of time resulting in minimal residual enhancement by almost 3 min. CEUS can identify segmental infarction by demonstrating one or more ischemic parenchymal lobules separated by normal testicular vessels [37, 38]. Subacute segmental infarction characteristically exhibits a perilesional rim of enhancement, which diminishes over time and is eventually lost with changes in lesion shape and shrinkage [37, 39].

Testicular CEUS can delineate non-viable regions in testicular trauma enabling organ-sparing treatment, which may be difficult to evaluate with conventional Doppler US because the injured testis is often hypovascular even in viable regions, as a consequence of testicular edema compromising vascular flow. CEUS also offers a clear delineation of fracture lines and intratesticular hematomas [40, 41].

In patients with severe epididymo-orchitis, CEUS can not only identify abscess formation at an earlier stage of development but also helps in assessing the complete extent of a large abscess, thereby allowing for prompt treatment [38, 42, 43]. CEUS can aid in differentiation of vascularized from non-vascularized focal testicular lesions with a diameter of less than 1.5 cm showing no flow on color Doppler US, which is critical to exclude malignancy [9]. In spite of the fact that, wash-in and washout time-intensity curves may help distinguish malignant from benign tumors, both qualitative and quantitative CEUS analyses of different histological types may overlap (Fig. 6.2). Also, CEUS is not routinely used for the management of incidentally discovered testicular lesions [44].

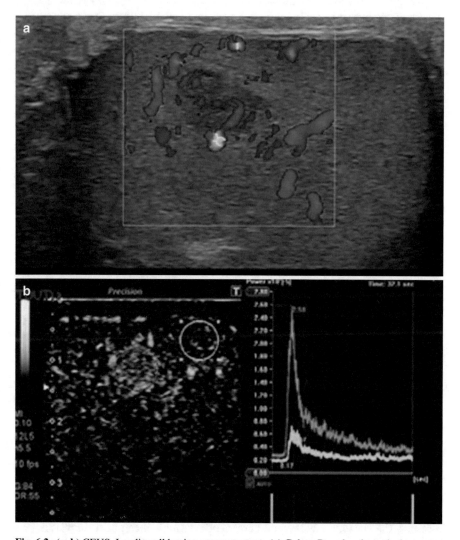

Fig. 6.2 (**a, b**) CEUS, Leydig cell benign proven tumour. (**a**) Colour Doppler showed a hypervascular, hypoechoic solid tumour. (**b**) CEUS with times-intensity curves showed strong enhancement and rapid wash-out (purple curve). The green curve corresponded to the enhancement of the adjacent normal parenchyma (Reprinted from Rocher L, Ramchandani P, Belfield J (2016) Incidentally detected non-palpable testicular tumours in adults at scrotal ultrasound: impact of radiological findings on management Radiologic review and recommendations of the ESUR scrotal imaging subcommittee. Eur Radiol 26:2268–2278 with permission)

6.2.3   Elastography

6.2.3.1   Principles

US elastography is a cutting-edge imaging modality which allows the measurement and display of the biomechanical characteristics of soft tissues under the influence of an applied force [45]. Technically, the signal processing within the scanner for all elastography methods begins with the measurement of tissue displacement as a function of spatial position and time, which is performed by cross-correlation tracking, Doppler, or other signal processing methods [46]. Based on the relevant displacement data revealing tissue stiffness under the influence of a shear waves, different elastography methods create an elastogram or perform elasticity measurement displayed either qualitatively as a black-and-white or colour image, or as numerical quantification of some parameters correlated with the shear wave [45]. Accordingly, the ultrasound elastography techniques can be classified as either qualitative ("Strain Elastography", SE) or quantitative ("Shear Wave Elastography", SWE).

Strain elastography (SE) involves the application of a force to the tissue within the region of interest by manual compression where the applied force varies slowly relative to the shear propagation time to the depth of interest and the image acquisition demonstrates qualitative tissue properties [47].

On shear-wave elastography (SWE), an acoustic radiation force used to generate low-frequency mechanical (shear) waves that induce tissue displacement is used for assessing tissue stiffness. Contrary to SE, SWE allows more precise standardization of tissue compression because the compression of the textures can be achieved using repeatable and equalized electronic acoustic waves by multiple focused ultrasound beams [48]. SWE technology based on measurements of shear wave speed through target tissues, can be used to dynamically map and reflect tissue stiffness properties in regions of interest quantitatively and in real time [47]. Compared with strain elastography, SWE has the advantages of quantitative evaluation of soft tissue stiffness based on true elasticity values of tissues, strong repeatability and higher clinical application value. Thus, it is a more useful method for investigating the elasticity of visceral organs. Overall, SWE is considered the most cutting-edge ultrasonic elastography technology at present.

SWE methods include transient elastography (TE), point shear wave elastography (pSWE) and multidimensional SWE (2D-SWE and 3D-SWE), which are based on either a transient shear deformation induced by a controlled applied force (TE) or by quantification of tissue displacement induced by acoustic radiation force impulse (ARFI) [49, 50]. Depending on the location where the tissue stiffness is assessed, the elastography method may involve a single location, as in pSWE, or a larger area within a sample box, as in 2D-SWE. On acoustic radiation force impulse (ARFI) elastography, which is an up-to-date shear-wave technique capable of measuring the velocity of tissue strain wave scatter perpendicular to compression direction generated by the compression of ARFI, the level of tissue stiffness is proportional to the relevant SW velocity value [48].

On most SE ultrasound systems, a real time displayed indicator (quality index) serving to confirm that the degree of compressions/decompressions is appropriate to generate repeatable and reproducible SE images is available [46]. Quality factors used for shear wave speed estimate are available also for the 2D-SWE methods. For ARFI-based methods, an assessment approach for the measurement quality similar to that of TE is used where the interquartile range (IQR) values (i.e. the difference between the 75th and 25th percentile) less than 30% of the median is considered reliable [49, 50].

6.2.3.2 Urological Applications

Kidney
Except for the use as an additional tool for the diagnosis of chronic allograft nephropathy, the current role of US renal elastography for native kidney abnormalities is limited. The use of SE, which is mainly a qualitative technique supposing uniform deformation of the tissue of interest, is usually limited to renal transplants with superficial location due to the challenges associated with the depth of the organ, applying reproducible homogeneous external deformation and having absolute stiffness measurements [51].

Renal elastography has been used for the noninvasive assessment of chronic kidney disease (CKD), particularly for the early stages when renal function is not yet significantly affected, or for disease monitoring [52]. As for SWE, conflicting results have been reported in the literature regarding the correlation between renal stiffness and fibrosis or renal function [46, 53–56]. Anisotropic delineation of the kidney as well as renal perfusion changes associated with the progression of fibrosis in the progression CKD have been speculated to have an impact on renal stiffness and explain some discrepancies between results [57, 58].

Among further applications of renal elastography are stiffness assessment in the presence of reflux nephropathy and tumor. The technique might also have a role in the detection and characterization of renal masses by improving the identification of ill-defined lesions and assessment of tumor stiffness [59]. Notably, overlaps in elastography values among different types of renal lesions has been attributed to heterogeneity of the lesions [58].

Bladder
A combination of high-frequency US, SWE and Duplex Doppler for obtaining control reference data regarding structural, biomechanical and hemodynamic changes in bladder wall has been shown to have a potential for assessing bladder wall changes associated with lower urinary tract disorders, differentiating bladder pathology in clinical practice as a diagnostic test and even for identifying individuals at high risk of developing bladder pathology [60].

Prostate

As a potential alternative to multiparametric MRI, real-time TRUS elastography of the prostate can be used reliably to detect suspicious regions for targeted biopsy. On SE where slight compressions are induced by the transrectal transducer, hypoechoic stiff lesions of the prostate are typically considered suspicious for malignancy [61, 62]. The technique also enables stiffness comparison between suspicious lesions and the adjacent normal prostatic tissue and provides semi-quantitative information by measuring the strain ratio between two regions of interest. In this regard, strain ratio has been reported to improve the detection of prostatic cancer with high sensitivity (100%) and high negative predictive value (100%) [63]. The use of SE-guided targeted biopsy complements the use of conventional systematic biopsy especially for patients with smaller prostate volume, owing to the fact that the gland size may affect elastography results [63].

On SWE, which requires no compression on the rectal wall contrary to SE, hypoechoic stiff lesions imply malignancy, similar to SE [64]. The technique has been found useful for differentiating prostate cancer and benign tissue with a high degree of diagnostic accuracy [2–47]. The technology can also reliably predict the grade of cancer. Moreover, quantitative US SWE-measured tissue stiffness has been found to have a role in predicting postoperative biochemical recurrence following radical prostatectomy for clinically localized prostate cancer [63].

The diagnostic accuracy of real-time elastography, which seems to be a useful tool in systematic, shows quite correspondence with the elevation of prostate specific antigen level and may help avoid unnecessary biopsy in the future [65]. Importantly, the use of elastography as a triage test followed by CEUS during mpUS or incorporating the technique to MR imaging-TRUS fusion increases the accuracy for prostate cancer diagnosis [46].

Recently, multiparametric machine learning involving the development of a random forest-based classifier for multiparametric classification of PCa based on co-registered B-mode, SWE, and CEUS has been shown to have technical feasibility for improving upon single US modalities for the localization [66]. Thus, computer-aided mpUS has been concluded to be promising for clinicians in biopsy targeting [66] (Fig. 6.3).

Scrotum

Although elastography techniques enabling the assessment of stiffness of abnormal areas of the testis is considered promising in the assessment of focal testicular lesions, there is an overlap in tissue stiffness findings by both SE and SWE techniques between benign and malignant neoplasms. In this regard, the role of elastography in the evaluation of testicular tumors remains in evolution [44]. However, elastography has been recommended to be used in conjunction with CEUS during mpUS for characterizing incidental focal testicular lesions, rather than being employed as a standalone technique [67].

On elastography, tissue stiffness has been reported to increase due to neoplastic testicular lesions and to decrease in benign testicular processes, such as orchitis and infarction (Fig. 6.4). On the other hand, the role of SWE for evaluating testicular pathologies has been investigated for neoplastic processes, infarction, torsion, or

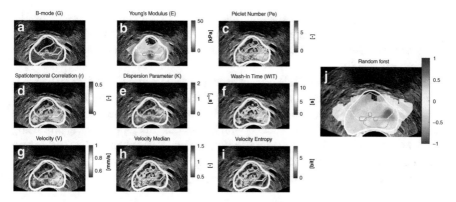

Fig. 6.3 Image plane example, showing the B-mode (**a**), Young's modulus (SWE) (**b**), Péclet number (**c**), spatiotemporal correlation (**d**), dispersionrelated parameter (**e**), wash-in time (**f**), velocity (**g**), velocity relative to image median (**h**), 2-mm entropy of velocity (**i**), and resulting multiparametric map (**j**). In each map, the prostate and zonal segmentations are depicted in white, the calcifications are encircled in blue, and histopathologically confirmed malignant and benign ROIs are indicated in red and green, respectively (Reprinted from Wildeboer RR, Mannaerts CK, van Sloun RJG et al. (2020) Automated multiparametric localization of prostate cancer based on B-mode, shear-wave elastography, and contrast-enhanced ultrasound radiomics. Eur Radiol 30:806–815 with permission)

orchitis, and the evaluation of spermatogenesis after torsion [68–72]. The technique may also enable differentiating seminomas from non-seminomatous lesions [73]. Notably, SWE has been reported to suggest elevated stiffness values for background parenchyma in testicular microlithiasis, infertility, undescended testis [48, 74–76].

Among the challenges associated with the assessment of focal lesions adjacent to tunica albuginea is the fibrosis adjacent to this region, the variability of SWE measurements between the center and peripheral zones and the lack of standardization for the point of relevant measurement [77–79].

Penis
Recently, a 2D penile ultrasound vibro-elastography (PUVE) technique for producing the shear wave speed map over an area of regional of interest (ROI) in the penis has been reported to have a potential for assessing patients with erectile dysfunction/Peyronie disease and their future cardiovascular risk [65].

6.2.4 Ultrasound-Enhanced Chemiluminescence

6.2.4.1 Principles

Contrary to the shallow organs where tissue imaging can be performed with adequate spatial resolution, imaging of deep tissues is still challenging due to energy loss in case magnetic field or traditional US is used. Bioluminescence (BL), which is an optical imaging method acting at the molecular level, is unique in that it involves the production and release of light from the live cells by an enzymatic reaction. On the other hand, chemiluminescence (CL) technique, precluding the need for external light sources similar to BL, is an advanced form of luminescence imaging where luminescent enhancers are used to increase the intensity of low-level light emissions [80].

In spite of the fact that CL is widely used in tissue imaging, a major challenge is the increased noise due to scattering light. US, especially focused US, that can increase the intensity of CL by reducing light scattering while enhancing spatial resolution, can be used in conjunction with CL for dual imaging which is promising for deeper imaging of biological tissues [80]. Indeed, US enhanced CL will have a significant impact on practical medical imaging in future by providing high resolution images, which will aid in more accurate diagnosis.

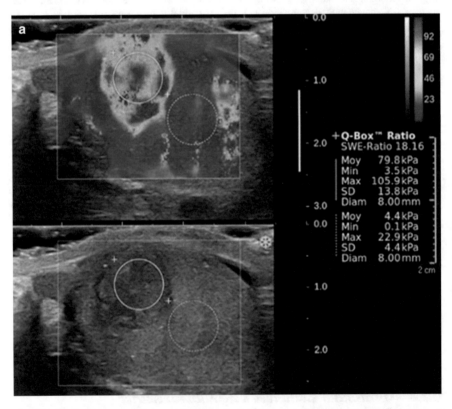

Fig. 6.4 (**a, b**) Shearwave elastography (Aixplorer, Supersonic Imaging, Aix en Provence) of several tumours. (**a**) Non-seminomatous germ cell tumour, strong stiffness of the lesion compared to adjacent pulp (79.8 kPa/4.4 kpa). (**b**) Benign Leydig cell tumour: the stiffness is mildly increased (6.7 kPa+/−1.9 kPa) (Reprinted from Rocher L, Ramchandani P, Belfield J (2016) Incidentally detected non-palpable testicular tumours in adults at scrotal ultrasound: impact of radiological findings on management Radiologic review and recommendations of the ESUR scrotal imaging subcommittee. Eur Radiol 26:2268–2278 with permission)

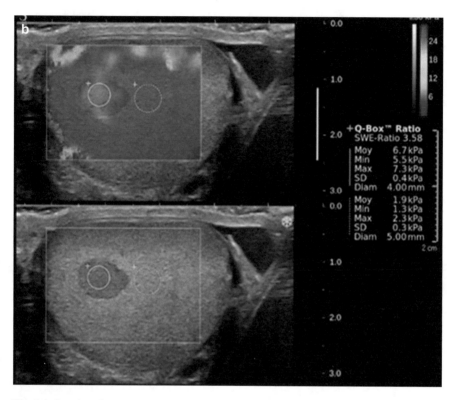

Fig. 6.4 (continued)

6.2.5   Endoluminal Ultrasound

6.2.5.1   Principles

The endoluminal imaging procedure involved the introduction of a 45 MHz 3.5 Fr (1.7 mm) intravascular ultrasound probe with an axial resolution of 200 μm and a lateral resolution of 200–250 μm. through the ureteral orifice followed by image acquisition performed by retracting and repositioning the imaging probe along the entire renal pelvis and ureter using an automatic pullback system [81, 82].

6.2.5.2   Urological Applications

Endoluminal ultrasound (ELUS) may be of value for the evaluation of upper urinary tract tumors as an alternative to diagnostic ureterorenoscopy combined with biopsy as the diagnostic standard. In ex-vivo setting where optical coherence tomography (OCT) and ELUS datasets coregistered with 3D CT were compared with the histology of a complete nephroureterectomy specimen, ELUS capable of distinguishing all anatomical layers of the ureter identified suspect lesions, although it was not possible to determine the presence of any invasion for a tumor and hence make a proper staging [81]. Compared to OCT, ELUS was noted to have an increased imaging depth for normal ureter and ureter lesions while producing images of lower resolution. The authors concluded that the combination of OCT and ELUS allows for high-resolution imaging of the upper urinary tract and greater imaging depth information at the same time [81].

6.2.6 Micro-ultrasound

6.2.6.1 Principles and Urological Applications

Micro-ultrasound, as a novel high-resolution real-time imaging method for prostate biopsy has been found to be promising in detecting clinically significant prostate cancer [83]. The technique involving a novel high-resolution 29-MHz US with three times greater resolution as compared with conventional US resolution enables the detailed evaluation of related prostate tissue characteristics [84]. Despite offering real-time biopsies targeted to suspicious areas detected with high sensitivity, micro-ultrasound has been noted to have low specificity which is a limitation for its clinical application as a diagnostic tool for clinically significant prostate cancer [83].

6.2.7 Photoacoustic Imaging

6.2.7.1 Principles and Urological Applications

Photoacoustic imaging (PAI) is a new, noninvasive soft tissue medical imaging modality based on the photoacoustic (PA) effect, referring to production of acoustic waves from an object illuminated by pulsed laser light [85]. Accordingly, PAI involves the combination of optical imaging yielding high-contrast imaging and US imaging producing high resolution in deep tissue imaging by PA effect [86, 87]. In spite of the fact that currently available medical imaging modalities used for cancer diagnosis such as US, CT, and MR imaging are well established and widely used in practice, they have inherent problems related to low sensitivity and specificity for cancer diagnosis [88]. More importantly, they are not efficient for early detection of cancer tissue.

However, PAI has the potential to detect cancer in the early stage thanks to it capability at multiple wavelengths for extracting chromophore (oxyhemoglobin, deoxyhemoglobin, lipid, water) signature of a tissue specimen [89]. The abundance of deoxy content as well as the paucity of oxy content in the cancerous tissue make the PA imaging system competent for imaging optical biomarkers for cancer tissue detection [89, 90]. As the chromophore has different absorption features at a different wavelength, the PA imaging at the given wavelength can produce high-contrast optically active corresponding chromophore images.

In multispectral photoacoustic (MPA) imaging, tissue angiogenesis associated with rapid tumor growth in the early stages can be detected by means of the difference in light absorption coefficient between blood and other tissue constituents which makes the PA imaging capable of functional imaging [91].

Overall, the PA image acquisition with a US transducer produces robust and less error-prone co-registered images enabling both structural and functional imagings compared to current imaging techniques such as MRI with the US [92]. Besides, PA imaging is also safe due to its non-ionizing radiation properties which make it very promising for cancer detection in the near future. Recently, an automated deep learning model to detect the presence of cancer in excised thyroid and prostate tissue of humans at once based on PA imaging has been proposed (Figs. 6.5 and 6.6) [88]. The authors speculated that the model may also be a starting point for in vivo PA image analysis for cancer diagnosis [88].

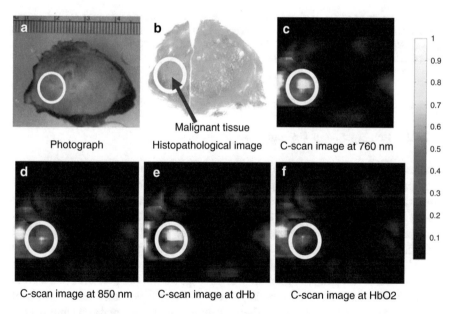

Fig. 6.5 (a) Tissue specimen, (b) histopathology of the prostate with malignant region encircled, (c) PA image acquired at 760 nm wavelength, (d) PA image acquired at 850 nm wavelength, (e) PA image showing absorption of dHb, (f) PA image showing absorption of HbO2 [3]. The encircled region taken at the deoxyhemoglobin channel of the PAimage (e) shows the presence of malignant region because deoxyhemoglobin absorbs more light to generate a higher pixel intensity region. The presence of deoxyhemoglobin is a strong indicator of the presence of cancer [3]. The encircled region with the malignant tissue in the PA image at 760 nm wavelength corresponds to the higher pixel intensity [3]. Previous works required humans to extract the encircled region of interest corresponding to cancer and non-cancer regions by the co-registration of the histopathological slide, photograph-based image, and PA-based image. This manual process was very labor-intensive and time-consuming (Reprinted from Jnawali K, Chinni B, Dogra V, Rao N (2020) Automatic cancer tissue detection using multispectral photoacoustic imaging. Int J Comput Assist Radiol Surg 15:309–320 with permission)

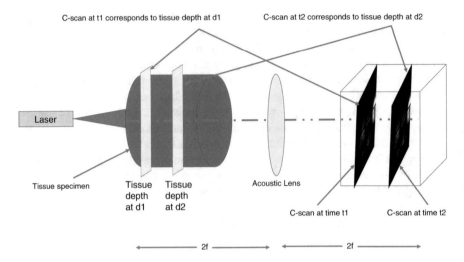

Fig. 6.6 Schematic of the PA signal data acquisition setup. An acoustic lens was used to focus the photoacoustically generated US waves and detect it by a linear US transducer array (not shown in figure) (Reprinted from Jnawali K, Chinni B, Dogra V, Rao N (2020) Automatic cancer tissue detection using multispectral photoacoustic imaging. Int J Comput Assist Radiol Surg 15:309–320 with permission)

6.2.8   Photoacoustic Tomography

6.2.8.1   Principles and Urological Applications

Photoacoustic tomography (PAT), which uses US transducer arrays for signal collection, has been proposed as a potential alternative MR imaging-fusion biopsy for improving prostate biopsy [93]. PAT involves the interaction between an absorber and pulsed light where the energy is converted to heat with the resultant local thermodynamic expansion releasing an acoustic wave, which is detectable by an US transducer [94]. This enables deeper imaging of major endogenous absorbers, such as deoxygenated and oxygenated hemoglobin, lipid, and water [94, 95]. The authors concluded that lowering the total number of biopsy cores per prostate compared to the currently used systemic sampling protocols would be possible by means of using 1064 nm PAT and US texture-based feature analysis as a real-time multimodal imaging technique which requires future in-vivo research [93].

6.2.9   Super-Resolution Ultrasound Microvessel Imaging

6.2.9.1   Principles and Clinical Applications

Microbubble-based super-resolution ultrasound microvessel imaging (SR-UMI) or super-resolution ultrasound localization microscopy (ULM), has been developed to overcome compromise in conventional US imaging between spatial resolution and penetration depth [96, 97]. It is a next-generation US imaging modality relying on the localization and tracking of individual contrast microbubbles in vasculature. This novel imaging tool provides approximately tenfold improvement in imaging resolution at clinically relevant penetration depths. It has been being successfully applied to a wide range of clinical applications including cancer imaging [96]. However, clinical translation of SR-UMI may be challenging due limited number of microbubbles detected within a given accumulation time is limited.

Recently, a Kalman filter-based method has been proposed for robust MB tracking and more precise blood flow speed measurements with reduced numbers of MBs which provided improved imaging performance [96]. Based on the presented SR-UMI images and the quantitative results obtained, the relevant method has been found to substantially improve the robustness of SR-UMI which is crucial for its clinical translation [96].

On the other hand, another technique has been developed by Huang et al. to ease the clinical translation of ULM by breaking the inherent tradeoff between acquisition time and MB concentration [97]. Owing to the fact that the number of MBs in circulation should be sufficient to fully traverse all vasculature of interest for a successful reconstruction of microvasculature on ULM, the authors proposed a post-processing technique separating spatially overlapping MB events into sub-populations with sparser MB concentrations which lessened the need for dilute MB injections, and shortened the long acquisition time of ULM imaging required for the reconstruction of microvasculature [97].

References

1. Tawfeek AM, Mostafa D, Radwan A, Hamza IH. The role of 3-dimensional sonography and virtual sonographic cystoscopy in the detection of bladder tumors. Afr J Urol. 2018;24:73–8.
2. Downey DB, Fenster A, Williams JC. Clinical utility of three-dimensional US. Radiographics. 2000;20:559–71.
3. Shen F, Shinohara K, Kumar D, et al. Three-dimensional sonography with needle tracking: role in diagnosis and treatment of prostate cancer. J Ultrasound Med. 2008;27:895–905.
4. Riccabona M, Fritz G, Ring E. Potential applications of three-dimensional ultrasound in the pediatric urinary tract: pictorial demonstration based on preliminary results. Eur Radiol. 2003;13:2680–7.
5. Digesu GA, Robinson D, Cardozo L, Khullar V. Three-dimensional ultrasound of the urethral sphincter predicts continence surgery outcome. Neurourol Urodyn. 2009;28:90–4.
6. Moon MH, Kim SH, Lee YH, et al. Diagnostic potential of three-dimensional ultrasound-based virtual cystoscopy: an experimental study using pig bladders. Investig Radiol. 2006;41:883–9.
7. Song JH, Francis IR, Platt JF, et al. Bladder tumor detection at virtual cystoscopy. Radiology. 2020;218:95–100.
8. Tyloch JF, Tyloch DJ, Adamowicz J, et al. Application of three-dimensional ultrasonography (3D ultrasound) to pretreatment evaluation of plastic induration of the penis (Peyronie's disease). Med Ultrason. 2020. https://doi.org/10.11152/mu-2132
9. Sidhu PS, Cantisani V, Dietrich CF, et al. The EFSUMB guidelines and recommendations for the clinical practice of contrast-enhanced ultrasound (CEUS) in non-hepatic applications: update 2017 (Long Version). Ultraschall Med. 2018;39:e2–e44.

10. Piscaglia F, Nolsoe C, Dietrich CF, et al. The EFSUMB guidelines and recommendations on the clinical practice of contrast enhanced ultrasound (CEUS): update 2011 on non-hepatic applications. Ultraschall Med. 2012;32:33–59.
11. Claudon M, Dietrich CF, Choi BI, et al. Guidelines and good clinical practice recommendations for contrast enhanced ultrasound (CEUS) in the liver – update 2012. Ultraschall Med. 2013;34:11–29.
12. Tang C, Fang K, Guo Y, et al. Safety of sulfur hexafluoride microbubbles in sonography of abdominal and superficial organs: retrospective analysis of 30222 cases. J Ultrasound Med. 2017;36:531–8.
13. Correas JM, Claudon M, Tranquart F, et al. The kidney: imaging with microbubble contrast agents. Ultrasound Q. 2006;22:53–66.
14. Tsuruoka K, Yasuda T, Koitabashi K, et al. Evaluation of renal microcirculation by contrast-enhanced ultrasound with SonazoidTM as a contrast agent comparison between normal subjects and patients with chronic kidney disease. Int Heart J. 2010;51:176–82.
15. Bertolotto M, Martegani A, Aiani L, et al. Value of contrast-enhanced ultrasonography for detecting renal infarcts proven by contrast enhanced CT. A feasibility study. Eur Radiol. 2008;18:376–83.
16. Barr RG, Peterson C, Hindi A. Evaluation of indeterminate renal masses with contrast-enhanced US: a diagnostic performance study. Radiology. 2014;271:133–42.
17. Quaia E, Bertolotto M, Cioffi V, et al. Comparison of contrast-enhanced sonography with unenhanced sonography and contrast-enhanced CT in the diagnosis of malignancy in complex renal masses. Am J Roentgenol. 2008;191:1239–49.
18. Clevert DA, Minaifar N, Weckbach S, et al. Multislice computed tomography versus contrast-enhanced ultrasound in evaluation of complex cystic renal masses using the Bosniak classification system. Clin Hemorheol Microcirc. 2008;39:171–8.
19. Bertolotto M, Cicero C, Perrone R, et al. Renal masses with equivocal enhancement at CT: characterization with contrast-enhanced ultrasound. Am J Roentgenol. 2015;205:W557–65.
20. Xu ZF, Xu HX, Xie XY, Liu GJ, Zheng YL, Lu MD. Renal cell carcinoma and renal angiomyolipoma: differential diagnosis with real-time contrast-enhanced ultrasonography. J Ultrasound Med. 2010;29:709–17.
21. Xue LY, Lu Q, Huang BJ, Li CX, Yan LX, Wang WP. Differentiation of subtypes of renal cell carcinoma with contrast-enhanced ultrasonography. Clin Hemorheol Microcirc. 2016;63:361–71.
22. Cao H, Fang L, Chen L, et al. The independent indicators for differentiating renal cell carcinoma from renal angiomyolipoma by contrast-enhanced ultrasound. BMC Med Imaging. 2020;20:32.
23. Fontanilla T, Minaya J, Cortes C, et al. Acute complicated pyelonephritis: contrast-enhanced ultrasound. Abdom Imaging. 2012;37:639–46.
24. Drudi FM, Cantisani V, Liberatore M, et al. Role of low-mechanical index CEUS in the differentiation between low and high grade bladder carcinoma: a pilot study. Ultraschall Med. 2010;31:589–95.
25. Wang XH, Wang YJ, Lei CG. Evaluating the perfusion of occupying lesions of kidney and bladder with contrast-enhanced ultrasound. Clin Imaging. 2011;35:447–51.
26. Caruso G, Salvaggio G, Campisi A, et al. Bladder tumor staging: comparison of contrast-enhanced and gray-scale ultrasound. Am J Roentgenol. 2010;194:151–6.
27. Drudi FM, Di Leo N, Maghella F, et al. CEUS in the study of bladder, method, administration and evaluation, a technical note. J Ultrasound. 2014;17:57–63.
28. Postema A, Idzenga T, Mischi M, Frinking P, de la Rosette J, Wijkstra H. Ultrasound modalities and quantification: developments of multiparametric ultrasonography, a new modality to detect, localize and target prostatic tumors. Curr Opin Urol. 2015;25:191–7.
29. Mischi M, Kuenen MP, Wijkstra H. Angiogenesis imaging by spatiotemporal analysis of ultrasound contrast agent dispersion kinetics. IEEE Trans Ultrason Ferroelectr Freq Control. 2012;59:621–9.

30. Postema AW, Gayet MCW, van Sloun RJG et al. Contrast-enhanced ultrasound with dispersion analysis for the localization of prostate cancer: correlation with radical prostatectomy specimens. World J Urol. 2020. https://doi.org/10.1007/s00345-020-03103-4
31. Schalk SG, Demi L, Smeenge M, et al. 4-D spatiotemporal analysis of ultrasound contrast agent dispersion for prostate cancer localization: a feasibility study. IEEE Trans Ultrason Ferroelectri Freq Control. 2015;62:839–51.
32. Grey A, Ahmed HU. Multiparametric ultrasound in the diagnosis of prostate cancer. Curr Opin Urol. 2016;26:114–9.
33. Postema A, Mischi M, de la Rosette J, et al. Multiparametric ultrasound in the detection of prostate cancer: a systematic review. World J Urol. 2015;33:1651–9.
34. Smeenge M, Barentsz J, Cosgrove D, et al. Role of transrectal ultrasonography (TRUS) in focal therapy of prostate cancer: report from a consensus panel. BJU Int. 2012;110:942–8.
35. Moschouris H, Stamatiou K, Kalokairinou Motogna M, et al. Early post-interventional sonographic evaluation of prostatic artery embolization. A promising role for contrast-enhanced ultrasonography (CEUS). Med Ultrason. 2018;20:134–40.
36. Ishii T, Nahas H, Yiu BYS, Chee AJY, Yu ACH. Contrast-enhanced urodynamic vector projectile imaging (CE-UroVPI) for urethral voiding visualization: principles and phantom studies. Urology. 2020. https://doi.org/10.1016/j.urology.2020.03.005
37. Bertolotto M, Derchi LE, Sidhu PS, et al. Acute segmental testicular infarction at contrast-enhanced ultrasound: early features and changes during follow-up. Am J Roentgenol. 2011;196:834–41.
38. Lung PF, Jaffer OS, Sellars ME, et al. Contrast enhanced ultrasound (CEUS) in the evaluation of focal testicular complications secondary to epidiymitis. Am J Roentgenol. 2012;199:W345–54.
39. Patel K, Huang DY, Sidhu PS. Metachronous bilateral segmental testicular infarction: multi-parametric ultrasound imaging with grey-scale ultrasound, Doppler ultrasound, contrast enhanced ultrasound (CEUS) and real-time tissue elastography (RTE). J Ultrasound. 2014;17:233–8.
40. Valentino M, Bertolotto M, Derchi L, et al. Role of contrast enhanced ultrasound in acute scrotal diseases. Eur Radiol. 2011;21:1831–40.
41. Lobianco R, Regine R, De Siero M, et al. Contrast-enhanced sonography in blunt scrotal trauma. J Ultrasound. 2011;14:188–95.
42. Yusuf T, Sellars ME, Kooiman GG, et al. Global testicular infarction in the presence of epididymitis. Clinical features, appearances on grayscale, color Doppler, and contrat-enhanced sonography, and histologic correlation. J Ultrasound Med. 2013;32:175–80.
43. Rafailidis V, Robbie H, Konstantatou E, et al. Sonographic imaging of extra-testicular focal lesions: comparison of grey-scale, colour Doppler and contrast-enhanced ultrasound. Ultrasound. 2016;24:23–33.
44. Rocher L, Ramchandani P, Belfield J. Incidentally detected non-palpable testicular tumours in adults at scrotal ultrasound: impact of radiological findings on management radiologic review and recommendations of the ESUR scrotal imaging subcommittee. Eur Radiol. 2016;26:2268–78.
45. Shiina T, Nightingale KR, Palmeri ML, et al. WFUMB guidelines and recommendations for clinical use of ultrasound elastography: Part 1: basic principles and terminology. Ultrasound Med Biol. 2015;41:1126–47.
46. Săftoiu A, Gilja OH, Sidhu PS, et al. The EFSUMB guidelines and recommendations for the clinical practice of elastography in non-hepatic applications: update 2018. Ultraschall Med. 2019;40:425–53.
47. Yang Y, Zhao X, Zhao X, Shi J, Huang Y. Value of shear wave elastography for diagnosis of primary prostate cancer: a systematic review and meta-analysis. Med Ultrason. 2019;21:382–8.
48. Yavuz A, Yokus A, Taken K, Batur A, Ozgokce M, Arslan H. Reliability of testicular stiffness quantification using shear wave elastography in predicting male fertility: a preliminary prospective study. Med Ultrason. 2018;20:141–7.

49. Dietrich CF, Bamber J, Berzigotti A, et al. EFSUMB guidelines and recommendations on the clinical use of liver ultrasound elastography, Update 2017 (Long Version). Ultraschall Med. 2017;38:E16–47.
50. Dietrich CF, Bamber J, Berzigotti A, et al. EFSUMB guidelines and recommendations on the clinical use of liver ultrasound elastography, update 2017 (Short Version). Ultraschall Med. 2017;38:377–94.
51. Franchi-Abella S, Elie C, Correas JM. Ultrasound elastography: advantages, limitations and artefacts of the different techniques from a study on a phantom. Diagn Interv Imaging. 2013;94:497–501.
52. Correas JM, Anglicheau D, Joly D, et al. Ultrasound-based imaging methods of the kidney-recent developments. Kidney Int. 2016;90:1199–210.
53. Derieppe M, Delmas Y, Gennisson JL, et al. Detection of intrarenal microstructural changes with supersonic shear wave elastography in rats. Eur Radiol. 2012;22:243–50.
54. Guo LH, Xu HX, Fu HJ, et al. Acoustic radiation force impulse imaging for noninvasive evaluation of renal parenchyma elasticity: preliminary findings. PLoS One. 2013;8:e68925.
55. Sasaki Y, Hirooka Y, Kawashima H, et al. Measurements of renal shear wave velocities in chronic kidney disease patients. Acta Radiol. 2018;59:884–90.
56. Asano K, Ogata A, Tanaka K, et al. Acoustic radiation force impulse elastography of the kidneys: is shear wave velocity affected by tissue fibrosis or renal blood flow? J Ultrasound Med. 2014;33:793–801.
57. Marticorena GSR, Guo J, Dürr M, et al. Comparison of ultrasound shear wave elastography with magnetic resonance elastography and renal microvascular flow in the assessment of chronic renal allograft dysfunction. Acta Radiol. 2018;59:1139–45.
58. Aydin S, Yildiz S, Turkmen I, et al. Value of shear wave elastography for differentiating benign and malignant renal lesions. Med Ultrason. 2018;1:21–6.
59. Clevert DA, Stock K, Klein B, et al. Evaluation of acoustic radiation force impulse (ARFI) imaging and contrast-enhanced ultrasound in renal tumours of unknown etiology in comparison to histological findings. Clin Hemorheol Microcirc. 2009;43:95–107.
60. Volikova AI, Marshall BJ, Yin JMA, Goodwin R, Chow PE, Wise MJ. Structural, biomechanical and hemodynamic assessment of the bladder wall in healthy subjects. Res Rep Urol. 2019;11:233–45.
61. Onur R, Littrup PJ, Pontes JE, et al. Contemporary impact of transrectal ultrasound lesions for prostate cancer detection. J Urol. 2004;172:512–4.
62. Salomon G, Köllerman J, Thederan I, et al. Evaluation of prostate cancer detection with ultrasound real-time elastography: a comparison with step section pathological analysis after radical prostatectomy. Eur Urol. 2008;54:1354–62.
63. Emara DM, Naguib NN, Yehia M, El Shafei MM. Ultrasound elastography in characterization of prostatic lesions: correlation with histopathological findings. Br J Radiol. 2020. https://doi.org/10.1259/bjr.20200035
64. Wei C, Zhang Y, Malik H, et al. Prediction of postprostatectomy biochemical recurrence using quantitative ultrasound shear wave elastography imaging. Front Oncol. 2019;9:572.
65. Zhang X, Zhou B, Kopecky SL, Trost LW. Two dimensional penile ultrasound vibroelastography for measuring penile tissue viscoelasticity: a pilot patient study and its correlation with penile ultrasonography. J Mech Behav Biomed Mater. 2020;103:103570.
66. Wildeboer RR, Mannaerts CK, van Sloun RJG, et al. Automated multiparametric localization of prostate cancer based on B-mode, shear-wave elastography, and contrast-enhanced ultrasound radiomics. Eur Radiol. 2020;30:806–15.
67. Sidhu PS. Multiparametric ultrasound (MPUS) imaging: terminology describing the many aspects of ultrasonography. Ultraschall Med. 2015;36:315–7.
68. Aigner F, De Zordo T, Pallwein-Prettner L, et al. Real-time sonoelastography for the evaluation of testicular lesions. Radiology. 2012;263:584–9.
69. Marsaud A, Durand M, Raffaelli C, et al. Elastography shows promise in testicular cancer detection. Prog Urol. 2015;25:75–82.

70. Sun Z, Xie M, Xiang F, et al. Utility of real-time shear wave elastography in the assessment of testicular torsion. PLoS One. 2015;10:e0138523.
71. Zhang X, Lv F, Tang J. Shear wave elastography (SWE) is reliable method for testicular spermatogenesis evaluation after torsion. Int J Clin Exp Med. 2015;8:7089–97.
72. Xue E, Yu Y, Lin L, Li Z, Su H. Application value of real-time shear wave elastography in differential diagnosis of testicular torsion. Med Ultrason. 2020;22:43–8.
73. Dikici AS, Er ME, Alis D, et al. Is there any difference between seminomas and nonseminomatous germ cell tumours on shear wave elastography? A preliminary study. J Ultrasound Med. 2016;35:2575–80.
74. Pedersen MR, Møller H, Osther PJS, et al. Comparison of tissue stiffness using shear wave elastography in men with normal testicular tissue, testicular microlithiasis and testicular cancer. Ultrasound Int Open. 2017;3:E150–5.
75. Rocher L, Criton A, Gennisson JL, et al. Testicular shear wave elastography in normal and infertile men: a prospective study on 601 patients. Ultrasound Med Biol. 2017;43:782–9.
76. Ucar AK, Alis D, Samanci C, et al. A preliminary study of shear wave elastography for the evaluation of unilateral palpable undescended testes. Eur J Radiol. 2017;86:248–51.
77. De Zordo T, Stronegger D, Pallwein-Prettner L, et al. Multiparametric ultrasonography of the testicles. Nat Rev Urol. 2013;10:135–48.
78. D'Anastasi M, Schneevoigt BS, Trottmann M, et al. Acoustic radiation force impulse imaging of the testes: a preliminary experience. Clin Hemorheol Microcirc. 2011;49:105–14.
79. Trottmann M, Marcon J, D'Anastasi M, et al. Shear-wave elastography of the testis in the healthy man – determination of standard values. Clin Hemorheol Microcirc. 2016;62:273–81.
80. Le D, Dhamecha D, Gonsalves A, Menon JU. Ultrasound-enhanced chemiluminescence for bioimaging. Front Bioeng Biotechnol. 2020;8:25.
81. Bus MTJ, Cernohorsky P, de Bruin DM, et al. Ex-vivo study in nephroureterectomy specimens defining the role of 3-D upper urinary tract visualization using optical coherence tomography and endoluminal ultrasound. J Med Imaging (Bellingham). 2018;5:017001.
82. Mintz GS, Nissen SE, Anderson WD, et al. American College of Cardiology Clinical Expert Consensus Document on standards for acquisition, measurement and reporting of intravascular ultrasound studies (IVUS). A report of the American College of Cardiology Task Force on Clinical Expert Consensus Documents. J Am Coll Cardiol. 2001;37:1478–92.
83. Zhang M, Wang R, Wu Y, et al. Micro-ultrasound imaging for accuracy of diagnosis in clinically significant prostate cancer: a meta-analysis. Front Oncol. 2019;9:1368.
84. Rohrbach D, Wodlinger B, Wen J, Mamou J, Feleppa E. High-frequency quantitative ultrasound for imaging prostate cancer using a novel micro-ultrasound scanner. Ultrasound Med Biol. 2018;44:1341–54.
85. Valluru KS, Chinni BK, Rao NA, Shweta B, Dogra VS. Basics and clinical applications of photoacoustic imaging. Ultrasound Clin. 2009;4:403–29.
86. Valluru KS, Chinni BK, Rao NA. Photoacoustic imaging: opening new frontiers in medical imaging. J Clin Imaging Sci. 2011;1:24.
87. Jnawali K, Chinni B, Dogra V, Rao N. Photoacoustic simulation study of chirp excitation response from different size absorbers. In: Medical imaging 2017: ultrasonic imaging and tomography, vol 10139. International Society for Optics and Photonics, 2017. p. 101391L.
88. Jnawali K, Chinni B, Dogra V, Rao N. Automatic cancer tissue detection using multispectral photoacoustic imaging. Int J Comput Assist Radiol Surg. 2020;15:309–20.
89. Dogra VS, Chinni BK, Valluru KS, et al. Multispectral photoacoustic imaging of prostate cancer: preliminary ex-vivo results. J Clin Imaging Sci. 2013;3:41.
90. Sinha S, Dogra VS, Chinni BK, Rao NA. Frequency domain analysis of multiwavelength photoacoustic signals for differentiating among malignant, benign, and normal thyroids in an ex vivo study with human thyroids. J Ultrasound Med. 2017;36:2047–59.
91. Lashkari B, Mandelis A. Linear frequency modulation photoacoustic radar: optimal bandwidth and signal-to-noise ratio for frequency-domain imaging of turbid media. J Acoust Soc Am. 2011;130:1313–24.

92. Agarwal A, Huang SW, O'donnell M, et al. Targeted gold nanorod contrast agent for prostate cancer detection by photoacoustic imaging. J Appl Phys. 2007;102:064701.
93. Bungart BL, Lan L, Wang P, et al. Photoacoustic tomography of intact human prostates and vascular texture analysis identify prostate cancer biopsy targets. Photo-Dermatology. 2018;11:46–55.
94. Wang LV, Yao J. A practical guide to photoacoustic tomography in the life sciences. Nat Methods. 2016;13:627–38.
95. Hui J, Li R, Phillips EH, Goergen CJ, Sturek M, Cheng JX. Bond-selective photoacoustic imaging by converting molecular vibration into acoustic waves. Photo-Dermatology. 2016;4:11–21.
96. Tang S, Song P, Trzasko JD, et al. Kalman filter-based microbubble tracking for robust super-resolution ultrasound microvessel imaging. IEEE Trans Ultrason Ferroelectr Freq Control. 2020. https://doi.org/10.1109/TUFFC.2020.2984384
97. Huang C, Lowerison MR, Trzasko JD, et al. Short acquisition time super-resolution ultrasound microvessel imaging via microbubble separation. Sci Rep. 2020;10:6007.

Chapter 7
CT Scan

Antonio Bottari, Giuseppe Cicero, Salvatore Silipigni, Alberto Stagno, Francesca Catanzariti, Antonella Cinquegrani, and Giorgio Ascenti

7.1 History

Radiological techniques have always played a pivotal role in the study of renal diseases.

In the past, intravenous urography (IVU), also known as "excretory urography" and/or "intravenous pyelography", has been largely performed for assessment of the urinary tract.

This technique includes a first X-ray plain film followed by the intravenous administration of a water-soluble contrast (1.5 ml/kg body weight). Afterwards, a series of images are obtained at specific timepoints: 1–2 min for renal parenchyma visualization, 3 min for the pyelocaliceal system and 10–15 min for ureters and bladder [1]. Moreover, additional images obtained on oblique planes, prone decubitus, delayed or after bladder emptying can be obtained for a more accurate assessment [1]. Principal limitations of this technique include the two-dimensional appraisal and the absent evaluation of the adjacent anatomical structures.

After the introduction of computed tomography, IVU has widely fallen out of favour.

A. Bottari (✉) · G. Cicero
Department of Biomedical, Dental, Morphological and Functional Imaging Sciences,
University of Messina, Messina, Italy
e-mail: bottaria@unime.it; gcicero@unime.it

S. Silipigni · A. Stagno · F. Catanzariti · A. Cinquegrani
Department of Imaging and Radiotherapy, University Hospital "G. Martino", Messina, Italy

G. Ascenti
Department of Biomedical, Dental, Morphological and Functional Imaging Sciences,
University of Messina, Messina, Italy

President of the Board of Genitourinary Imaging of the Italian Society of Medical and Interventional Radiology, Milan, Italy
e-mail: gascenti@unime.it

© Springer Nature Switzerland AG 2021
E. Huri, D. Veneziano (eds.), *Anatomy for Urologic Surgeons in the Digital Era*,
https://doi.org/10.1007/978-3-030-59479-4_7

However, only during the 90s, with the introduction of spiral technology, the scanning times were considerably sped up, so that a study of large areas of the body, such as the abdomen, was performable in few seconds. With the advent of multi-detector technology in 2000s, the spatial resolution has been upgraded such that the urothelium of the upper urinary tract and bladder can be appreciated. Moreover, isotropic voxels enabled the creation of equal spatial resolution images in any plane resulting into three-dimensional reconstructions, useful in a more accurate evaluation of anatomic relationships. Consequently, the administration of intravenous contrast medium has been improved as well, leading to the establishment of a specific protocol for urinary tract assessment.

"CT-Urography" (CTU) was established with the aim of a simultaneous morphologic and functional assessment of kidneys, ureters and bladder and therefore consisting in corticomedullary, nephrographic and excretory phases.

Nowadays, CTU is widely performed in the assessment of the kaleidoscopic scenario of urologic diseases, from urolithiasis detection to malignancies staging.

Since the beginnings of CT inception, it was already known that X-ray spectra at different energies were able in differentiating materials with different atomic numbers. Only in 2006, this principle has been successfully applied to the study of human tissues and the first Dual-Energy CT (DECT) system was finally introduced in the daily clinical practice.

DECT has immediately demonstrated its suitableness in evaluation of pathologic conditions of the urinary tract, from material decomposition of urinary stones to iodine uptake of urinary malignancies.

7.2   Technical Background

The worldwide availability, the anatomic detail resolution and the functional information yielded by the dynamic study led to make CTU the technique of choice in urologic imaging.

Clinical indications for CTU performance include urolithiasis (without contrast medium), trauma, surgical planning or transplantation, vascular damage and iatrogenic complications, characterization of benign lesions from malignancies [2–6].

CTU study must include the whole abdominal cavity preferably using thin slice with a high collimation of the X-ray beam in order to improve spatial resolution, to avoid partial volume artifacts and to obtain multiplanar reconstructions [7].

The 2007 European Society of Urogenital Radiology (ESUR) group meeting underlined the role of CTU in daily clinical practice and led to the creation of an official expert-based guideline for a study protocol standardization [8]. However, this document was not specifically focused on CTU and addressed all indications for abdominopelvic CT.

In October 2018 the French Society of Genitourinary Imaging decided to set up a conference aimed at achieving consensus on patient preparation and CTU imaging protocols for different types of indications [9, 10]. First of all, a strong consensus was reached on patient preparation by recommending only an intravenous injection of 20 mg of furosemide before contrast medium administration. Indeed, the furosemide induces hyper-diuresis within minutes after its injection, which accelerates the opacification of the urinary tract and improves the distension and visualization of the middle and distal ureters. It also induces a dilution of the excreted contrast medium thereby reducing streaking artefacts and improving the visualization of the ureteral wall and the detection of filling defects. The only contraindications to its use are dehydration and acute urinary tract obstruction. Hyper-diuresis can also be obtained by oral or intravenous hydration. A consensus was reached against systematic patient hydration because it seems less effective and reproducible.

Contrast medium (CM) intravenous injection should be tailored according to patient weight and iodine concentration, usually 1.7–2.0 ml/kg of 300 mgI/ml and 1.4–1.6 ml/kg of 370 mgI/ml [8]. Injection rate conventionally employed ranges from 2 to 3.5 ml/s.

According to the clinical suspicion and the information required, CTU can be mainly obtained through two different protocols: conventional multiphasic single-bolus study and biphasic split-bolus technique [8, 11].

The former includes, as a first step, an unenhanced phase meant as a baseline for contrast enhancement assessment, essential in stone detection and hyperdense or hypodense components within masses appraisal. Afterwards, the cortical-medullary phase (obtained at 35–40 s) allows the enhancement of renal cortex and vessels, useful for bleeding detection in trauma cases, hypervascular lesions appraisal, surgical or pre-transplantation assessment. During the nephrographic phase (90–120 s) a homogeneous enhancement of cortical and medullary components of renal parenchyma is obtained, helpful in displaying hypodense nodules. Finally, the excretory phase (7–8 min) permits the opacification of the collecting system, allowing the recognition of filling defects such as stones or urothelial malignancies. Leaks of urinary tract with fluid collections (urinomas) can be detected as well.

For best identification of these findings is mandatory to perform multiplanar reconstruction of excretory phase on coronal view.

As conventional study foresees at least four scans, a considerable radiation dose is delivered to the patient, an important issue especially for young patients. Depending on the clinical scenario, multiple phase imaging may not be required, and some phases may be omitted in order to reduce the amount of radiation delivered to the patient. In this sense, the efforts to further decrease radiation dose led to the development of the so-called "split bolus" technique.

This protocol requires that the CM be administered in two separate injections: after the unenhanced scan, a first CM bolus is followed, after a delay of 8–9 min by a second one.

Currently, a univocal consensus about the amount of contrast agent administered during the first and the second injection has not been reached yet. However, a consensus was reached in favor of injecting two-thirds of the bolus first and using the remaining third for the second injection [10]. A cortico-medullary phase can be performed 30s after the first bolus, whereas a combined nephrographic–excretory phase can be obtained with a delay of 90s after the second contrast bolus [8, 12].

Although different studies have demonstrated high sensitivity and specificity for collecting system and bladder neoplasm detection, this technique seems to be less sensitive for the detection of smaller renal cell carcinomas (RCCs) [12].

Some authors have also proposed a triple-bolus technique [13], with a small bolus of 30 ml was used for opacification of the excretory system followed by 7 min delayed second bolus of 50 ml for parenchyma and veins enhancement and a third 20 s delayed bolus of 65 ml for arterial enhancement.

The choice between different technical approaches should depend on the context. Indeed, if reducing the amount of radiation exposure is crucial for young patients with benign disease, it is less important in patients with severe conditions or malignant tumors.

In conclusion the study by Renard-Penna et al. [10] brings a consensus on CTU technique and strengthen the role of corticomedullary phase. They show that urothelial tumors avidly enhance and in fact may sometimes be better seen with an earlier phase of imaging on a background of normal urothelium and nonopacified urine (Fig. 7.1 and Fig. 7.2). Moreover, small or 'en plaque' urothelial lesions may be masked at excretory phase imaging and better detected at corticomedullary or nephrographic phase imaging.

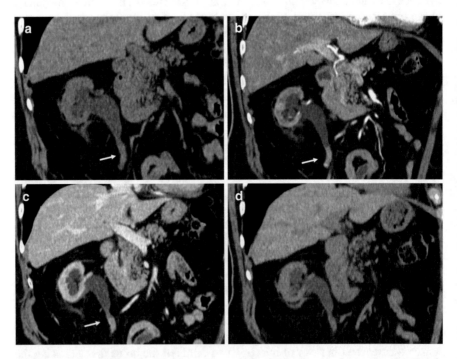

Fig. 7.1 Four-phase CTU after injection of furosemide. (**a**) Baseline acquisition showing slightly hyperdense material inside the ureter (arrow); (**b**) Cortico-medullary phase showing pathologic tissue with strong enhancement (arrow) also visible in nephrographic phase (**c**); (**d**) Delayed phase show no excretion of urine

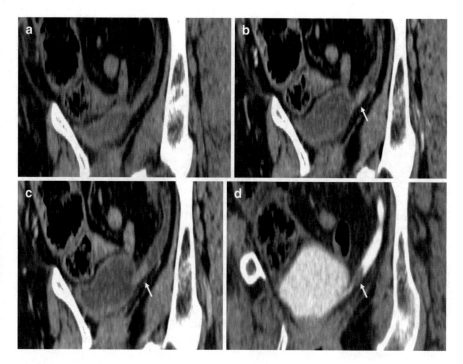

Fig. 7.2 Four-phase CTU after injection of furosemide. (**a**) Baseline acquisition; (**b**) Cortico-medullary phase showing pathologic tissue with strong enhancement (arrow) also visible in nephrographic phase (**c**); (**d**) Excretory phase show filling defect (arrow) in the distal portion of the ureter

7.2.1 Dual-Energy CT (DECT)

In the last decade the dual energy technology has been extensively employed in urologic imaging [14–17]. Briefly, DECT technology exploits the exposure of body tissues at two different energy radiation levels, obtained at the time of radiation beam creation and delivery (i.e., "dual sources" or "rapid switching" scanners) or during photon absorption ("double layer" technology) [18]. Hence, DECT is capable to distinguish materials with different atomic number, the so-called "material decomposition", which results in several advantages.

The first one is achieving image datasets with noise correction and better iodine appraisal, thanks to linear/non-linear blending images and virtual monoenergetic reconstructions. The improved iodine visualization brings the opportunity of reducing injected CM volumes and therefore the risk of renal damage [19].

Moreover, the possibility of virtual non-contrast (VNC) reconstructions, namely the creation of unenhanced scan from the enhanced ones, permits to avoid baseline acquisition with consequent dose reduction [14, 17].

Nevertheless, iodine quantification within lesions can be obtained through quantitative (mg/mL per region of interest, ROI) or qualitative (Colour coded iodine

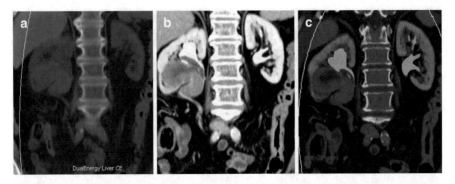

Fig. 7.3 Dual Energy application in URO-CT performed with "split bolus" technique. (**a**) Unenhanced scan reconstruction from enhanced one (VNC) (**b**) Combined nephrographic-excretory phase showing a mass growth inside the collecting system of the right kidney (**c**) Color coded iodine overlay map better shows the iodine uptake of the lesion

overlay maps) assessment. This is particularly helpful in the evaluation of complex cysts or low attenuating masses and for pseudo-enhancement phenomenon recognition [20] (Fig. 7.3).

Finally, material specific analysis of nephrolithiasis, with differentiation of uric acid stones from other types, can provide useful information for the subsequent patient management.

7.3 Benefits

Although ultrasound is usually performed as the first line imaging modality and its diagnostic potential can be significantly improved through the injection of intravenous contrast medium (CEUS) CT scan is currently considered the gold standard due to the wide availability, the fast scan times, and the comprehensive evaluation. Dedicated diagnostic renal imaging aids in the appropriate treatment planning for renal tumors and may avoid an unnecessary operation.

A conventional CT protocol routinely includes pre- and multiphasic post-contrast images. Volumetric datasets provided by modern CT scanners can be reconstructed in multiple planes and be of variable slices thickness preserving excellent image quality.

CT urography (CTU) also relies on the multiphase principle to focus on an "excretory" phase after the contrast has filtered into the collecting system and bladder, essentially creating an IV urogram with vastly improved tissue contrast.

7.4 Limitations

Even tough contrast-enhanced computed tomography is the reference standard for primary imaging of urinary tract, intrinsic limitations should be addressed.

Radiation exposure and contrast media nephrotoxicity are considered the main ones.

In a phantom study Vrtiska et al. showed that the range of effective doses for the evaluated CT urography protocols was 20.1–66.3 mSv using 4, 16, and 64 MDCT scanners. The number of phases, anatomic coverage per phase, and scanning parameters all contributed to this variation in dose [21]. The mean effective radiation dose that was reported in vivo in association with four-phase CT scan ranged from 15 to 35 mSv [22, 23].

Radiation dose reduction is extremely important specially in younger patients.

In these cases, first, the use of alternative imaging modalities as ultrasound and MRI must be always kept in consideration. If these techniques cannot provide the requested information than will be necessary to act on CT protocol.

In previous section was already described how radiation dose can be reduced by limiting the number of phases using dual-energy CT or split bolus technique. Radiation dose can be also reduced using low dose unenhanced scan as first step of CTU because the increased image noise is not a problem in stone detection thanks to the marked differences of attenuation between calculi and surrounding soft tissues [22, 24, 25]. Low dose protocol can be also applied on post-contrast phases thanks to machine-related dose reduction algorithms that allow a lower radiation exposure without a significant image quality worsening.

Contrast-enhanced CT studies are contraindicated in patients with an allergy to radiographic contrast media and in patients with impaired renal function.

To minimize contrast-induced nephropathy, contrast material should not be given to patients with Glomerular Filtration Rate (GFR) below 30 ml/min without carefully weighing the risks and benefits and it should be used with caution in patients with GFR ranging from 30 to 60 ml/min [26].

Beyond merely technical limits, other issues can come from image interpretation.

For instance, detection of smaller tumors can especially pose a challenge and differentiation among solid lesions is frequent unclear because of heterogeneous presentation of different histologic subtypes [27].

Distinguish between simple and complex cystic lesions could be also difficult because of low accuracy of CT on thin septa appraisal.

In such cases, different imaging approaches, through US and MRI, can be helpful in obtaining more detailed information about lesion features.

Response assessment following ablative therapies, anti-angiogenic and immunotherapies remains challenging, as reduction in tumor size may not occur. The pattern of enhancement on CT may be a more reliable indicator of treatment success. However, a number of emerging techniques have been investigated.

CT texture analysis using an image processing algorithm to assess heterogeneity in tumor morphology has been proposed as a marker of response. Functional imaging has been investigated, including dynamic contrast-enhanced (DCE) CT, DCE-MRI, DCE-ultrasound and PET. DCE imaging follows the bio-distribution of a contrast agent injected intravenously and then absorbed into the tumor microcirculation, providing information on the tumor microenvironment and vascularity pre- and post-anti-angiogenic therapy [28].

7.5 Future

In the new era of *precision medicine*, the ability to extrapolate, from radiological images, quantitative data is the challenge of the present and the next future. This process, known as *radiomics*, was first invented by Lambin in 2012, it is based on the concept that clinical images contain quantitative features, which may reflect the underlying pathophysiology of a tissue [29, 30].

Machine-Learning (ML) algorithms are emerging tools that may support radiomics. They lead to the selection of appropriate features that can be analysed by dedicated software.

The use of these assays can improve medical decision-making and it finds space especially in oncology, for example, allowing an evaluation of cancer microenvironment and influencing treatment choice. In the last few years, many studies have been carried out on the application of this method even for the evaluation of urothelial cancer, but it is still a prerogative of research.

In a review Zhang et al. summarize their studies and literature about radiomics applied in urothelial cancer to predict pathological grade, clinical stage, lymph node metastasis and treatment response. These studies demonstrate the capability of radiomics to assist more precise characterization and stratification of patients with urothelial cancer.

In particular Zhang et al., Mammen et al., Wang et al. in their papers revealed that texture features extracted from CT or MRI images could reflect the difference between low- and high-grade urothelial carcinoma [31–34].

Despite the huge potentiality, radiomics still needs improvements such as standardized data collection and evaluation criteria to become applicable in clinical practice.

References

1. Dyer RB, Chen MY, Zagoria RJ. Intravenous urography: technique and interpretation. Radiographics. 2001;21(4):799–821.
2. WSES-AAST Expert Panel, Coccolini F, Moore EE, et al. Kidney and uro-trauma: WSES-AAST guidelines. World J Emerg Surg. 2019;14:545.
3. Ali O, Fishman EK, Sheth S. Correction to: upper urinary tract urothelial carcinoma on multidetector CT: spectrum of disease. Abdom Radiol. 2020;45:889.
4. Gray Sears CL, Ward JF, Sears ST, et al. Prospective comparison of computerized tomography and excretory urography in the initial evaluation of asymptomatic microhematuria. J Urol. 2002;168:2457–24607.
5. Albani JM, Ciaschini MW, Streem SB, et al. The role of computerized tomographic urography in the initial evaluation of hematuria. J Urol. 2007;177:644–8.
6. Ascenti G, Zimbaro G, Mazziotti S, et al. Doppler power with contrast media in the characterization of renal masses. Radiol Med (Torino). 2000;100:168–74.
7. Fried JG, Morgan MA. Renal imaging: core curriculum 2019. Am J Kidney Dis. 2019;73:552–65.

8. CT Urography Working Group of the European Society of Urogenital Radiology (ESUR), Van Der Molen AJ, Cowan NC, et al. CT urography: definition, indications and techniques. A guideline for clinical practice. Eur Radiol. 2008;18:4–17.
9. Hiram Shaish. Making sense of the CT Urogram European. Radiology. 2020;30:1385–6.
10. Renard Penna R, Rocher L, Roy C, et al. Imaging protocols for CT urography: results of a consensus conference from the French society of genitourinary imaging. Eur Radiol. 2020;30(3):1387–96.
11. Noroozian M, Cohan RH, Caoili EM, et al. Multislice CT urography: state of the art. Br J Radiol. 2004;77:S74–86.
12. Cheng K, Cassidy F, Aganovic L, et al. CT urography: how to optimize the technique. Abdom Radiol. 2019;44:3786–99.
13. Kekelidze M, Dwarkasing RS, Dijkshoorn ML, et al. Kidney and urinary tract imaging: triple-bolus multidetector CT urography as a one-stop shop—protocol design, opacification, and image quality analysis. Radiology. 2010;255:508–16.
14. Graser A, Johnson TRC, Hecht EM, et al. Dual-energy CT in patients suspected of having renal masses: can virtual nonenhanced images replace true nonenhanced images? Radiology. 2009;252:433–40.
15. Ascenti G, Mileto A, Gaeta M, et al. Single-phase dual-energy CT urography in the evaluation of haematuria. Clin Radiol. 2013;68:e87–94.
16. Mileto A, Marin D. Dual-energy computed tomography in genitourinary imaging. Radiol Clin N Am. 2017;55:373–91.
17. Marino MA, Silipigni S, Barbaro U, et al. Dual energy CT scanning in evaluation of the urinary tract. Curr Radiol Rep. 2017;5:46.
18. Cicero G, Ascenti G, Albrecht MH, Blandino A, Cavallaro M, D'Angelo T, Carerj ML, Vogl TJ, Mazziotti S. Extra-abdominal dual-energy CT applications: a comprehensive overview. Radiol Med. 2020;125(4):384–97.
19. Mileto A, Ramirez-Giraldo JC, Marin D, et al. Nonlinear image blending for dual-energy MDCT of the abdomen: can image quality be preserved if the contrast medium dose is reduced? AJR Am J Roentgenol. 2014;203:838–45.
20. Wang ZJ, Coakley FV, Fu Y, et al. Renal cyst pseudoenhancement at multidetector CT: what are the effects of number of detectors and peak tube voltage? Radiology. 2008;248:910–6.
21. Vrtiska TJ, Hartman RP, Kofler JM, Bruesewitz MR, King BF, McCollough CH. Spatial resolution and radiation dose of a 64-MDCT scanner compared with published CT urography protocols AJR. Am J Roentgenol. 2009;192(4):941–8.
22. O'Connor OJ, Maher MM. CT urography. Am J Roentgenol. 2010;195:W320–4.
23. Caoili EM, Inampudi P, Cohan RH, Ellis JH. Optimization of multi-detector row CT urography: effect of compression, saline administration, and prolongation of acquisition delay. Radiology. 2005;235:116–23.
24. O'Connor OJ, McSweeney SE, Maher MM. Imaging of hematuria. Radiol Clin N Am. 2008;46:113–32.
25. Graser A, Johnson TR, Chandarana H, Macari M. Dual energy CT: preliminary observations and potential clinical applications in the abdomen. Eur Radiol. 2009;19:13–2.
26. Wymer DC. Imaging. Comp Clin Nephrol. 2010;2010:56–74.
27. van Oostenbrugge TJ, Fütterer JJ, Mulders PFA. Diagnostic imaging for solid renal tumors: a pictorial review. Kidney Cancer. 2018;2(2):79–93.
28. Rossi SH, Prezzi D, Kelly-Morland C, Goh V. Imaging for the diagnosis and response assessment of renal tumours. World J Urol. 2018;36(12):1927–42.
29. Lambin P, Rios-Velazquez E, Leijenaar R, Carvalho S, van Stiphout RG, Granton P, et al. Radiomics: extracting more information from medical images using advanced feature analysis. Eur J Cancer. 2012;48(4):441–6.
30. Lambin P, Leijenaar RTH, Deist TM, Peerlings J, de Jong EEC, van Timmeren J, et al. Radiomics: the bridge between medical imaging and personalized medicine. Nat Rev Clin Oncol. 2017;14(12):749–62.

31. Zhang G, Xu L, et al. Current applications and challenges of radiomics in urothelial cancer. Chin J Acad Radiol. 2020;2:56–62.
32. Mammen S, Krishna S, Quon M, Shabana WM, Hakim SW, Flood TA, et al. Diagnostic accuracy of qualitative and quantitative computed tomography analysis for diagnosis of pathological grade and stage in upper tract urothelial cell carcinoma. J Comput Assist Tomogr. 2018;42(2):204–10.
33. Zhang X, Xu X, Tian Q, Li B, Wu Y, Yang Z, et al. Radiomics assessment of bladder cancer grade using texture features from diffusion-weighted imaging. J Magn Reson Imaging. 2017;46(5):1281–8.
34. Wang H, Hu D, Yao H, Chen M, Li S, Chen H, et al. Radiomics analysis of multiparametric MRI for the preoperative evaluation of pathological grade in bladder cancer tumors. Eur Radiol. 2019.

Chapter 8
Use of Multiparametrric Magnetic Resonance Imaging (mpMRI) for Prostate Cancer: A Journey from 1.5 to 10 Tesla

Giovanni E. Cacciamani ⓘ, Andre L. De Castro Abreu, Andrew Chen, Mihir Saha, Ugo Falagario, Eduardo B. Zukovksi, and Riccardo Autorino

8.1 Brief History of mpMRI for Prostate Cancer (PCa) Detection

Historically, the imaging modality of choice for the prostate was transrectal ultrasound. With the advent of MRI in the early 1970s [1], clinical application of imaging of the whole body and later of the prostate followed quickly. While the first imaging of the prostate used a 0.08 Tesla (T) magnet in 1982, advances in technology have validated 1.5 T and 3 T MRI scanners in the clinical diagnosis of prostate cancer (PCa) [2–4]. The development of the endorectal coil in 1989 also improved spatial resolution and reduced local motion of the prostate during imaging in initial studies, although has recently begun to diminish in popularity [5]. A multiparametric MRI (mpMRI) approach is a growing technique for prostate cancer detection [6]. Early publications described visualization and characterization of subglandular structures

G. E. Cacciamani (✉) · A. L. De Castro Abreu · A. Chen · M. Saha
Catherine and Joseph Aresty Department of Urology, USC Institute of Urology, Keck School of Medicine, University of Southern California, Los Angeles, CA, USA
e-mail: Giovanni.cacciamani@med.usc.edu

U. Falagario
Division of Urology, VCU Health, Richmond, VA, USA

Urology and Renal Transplantation Unit, Department of Medical and Surgical Sciences, University of Foggia, Foggia, Italy

E. B. Zukovksi
Department of Radiology, Hospital Sirio Libanes, São Paulo, Brazil

R. Autorino
Division of Urology, VCU Health, Richmond, VA, USA

© Springer Nature Switzerland AG 2021
E. Huri, D. Veneziano (eds.), *Anatomy for Urologic Surgeons in the Digital Era*,
https://doi.org/10.1007/978-3-030-59479-4_8

of the prostate using T2-weighted imaging (T2WI). T2WI serves as the primary assessment of the transition zone and detects cancer as focal regions of moderately low signal intensity [7, 8]. T1-weighted imaging (T1WI) can determine the presence and location of hemorrhage, which can also appear as hypointensity on T2WI [9]. In addition to the anatomical information provided by T1 and T2WI, mpMRI includes functional information. Diffusion-weighted imaging (DWI) of the prostate is useful for identification of the peripheral zone of the prostate. It can be sampled with different b-values, with lower b-values combining more DWI and T2WI information, and higher b-values showing DWI effects alone [10]. Additionally, calculation of the apparent diffusion coefficient (ADC) can be used to identify suspicious lesions with lower ADC values demonstrating higher correlation with cancer cells [11]. Another sequence, dynamic contrast-enhanced imaging (DCE), contributes to diagnosis and captures abnormal vascularity. And while magnetic resonance spectroscopic imaging (MRSI) can be used to assess metabolic characteristics within the prostate, it is not included in the PI-RADS v2 guidelines [3, 12]. Prior to the development of a standardized system, pooled analysis showed that mpMRI had a high sensitivity (0.74) and specificity (0.88) for prostate cancer [5]. Currently, interpretation of mpMRI is most widely based on the PI-RADS v2 grading system. In further meta-analysis, the PI-RADS v2 grading system has shown a pooled sensitivity of 0.89 and specificity of 0.73 in detection of prostate cancer, an improvement over PI-RADS v1 [13]. While guidelines differ in detail in recommending mpMRI, the National Comprehensive Cancer Network (NCCN), American Urological Association (AUA), and the United Kingdom National Institute of Health and Care Excellence (NICE) agree that mpMRI should be offered or considered prior to initial biopsy. The European Association of Urology (EAU) strong recommends mpMRI in both the biopsy-naïve and repeat negative biopsy patient. PI-RADS v2, the EAU Prostate Guidelines, and the AUA Standard Operating Procedure for mpMRI state that 1.5 T and 3Ta are suitable for detection of prostate cancer, while acknowledging that 3 T provide improved signal-to-noise ratio and increased spatial and temporal resolution [3, 14–17]. Clinical trials have shown that mpMRI-guided diagnostic pathways are superior to ultrasound-guided diagnostic pathways with fewer overall biopsies needed, more clinically significant and fewer clinically insignificant prostate cancer detected [18–22].

8.2 Limitations and Pitfalls of the 3 T mpMRI in Terms of PCa Detection

While 3 T mpMRI has been shown to improve diagnostic pathways for prostate cancer and is generally recommended over 1.5 T, it is not without limitations [3, 23]. 3 T has been shown to have increased signal to noise ratio (SNR) when compared to 1.5 T but the increase in magnetic field strength is accompanied by susceptibility artifacts, blurring, and geometric distortion [24, 25]. Sensitivity for extra-prostatic extension (EPE) and seminal vesicle invasion (SVI) remains moderate (0.61 and 0.57, respectively) although 3 T improved detection sensitivity and overall stage T3 on meta-analysis [26]. Thus, mpMRI is not recommended for local staging in low-risk patients [14]. Inter-reader concordance is also moderate when averaged across institutions and studies [27]. However, closer examination of single institutions unmasks underlying significant variability across individual radiologists. The clinical implications of these findings would lead to variability in the percentage of avoided biopsies by a factor of 2, with up to 13–60% of PI-RADS <3 lesions containing clinically significant disease [28]. Analysis advises interpretation by subspecialists to improve NPV and PPV and greater training of radiologists in prostate mpMRI [29]. Multiple experts have identified diagnostic pitfalls to be avoided on 3 T mpMRI [30–32]. Within the prostate, there are a number of anatomic mimics of PCa. On T2WI, hypertrophic anterior fibromuscular stroma appears as an area of homogeneous low signal intensity as well as low ADC. The junction between the transition and peripheral zone, the surgical capsule, can present with similar findings. The central zone of the prostate can be misinterpreted as a lesion extending from either the peripheral zone or transition zone and be deemed high suspicion for tumor. Interpreters must also take care to avoid the "pitfall of a pitfall", when tumor mimics the central zone, where less than 5% of prostate cancers originate from [33, 34]. Benign prostatic hyperplasia can mimic PCa as either a stroma-rich nodule or as bilateral benign prostatic hyperplasia proliferation. In addition, the anatomy surrounding the prostate can also lead to confusion. The periprostatic venous complex rounds laterally around the prostate before communicating anterior to the prostate and draining into the internal iliac vein. Depending on the velocity and turbulence of blood, veins can have low signal intensity of T2WI and ADC maps. The neurovascular bundle also lies in close proximity to the peripheral zone and can be misinterpreted instead as a lesion within the peripheral zone. Similarly, periprostatic lymph nodes, may appear to have restricted diffusion and to be intraprostatic due to low spatial resolution on DWI.

   In addition to patient anatomy, certain disease states cause diagnostic uncertainty as well. Focal prostatitis in the peripheral zone is a common benign pathology that can be difficult to differentiate from prostate cancer. Granulomatous prostatitis is another entity that can present with a firm nodule on digital rectal examination and elevated prostate-specific antigen. It too can have an abnormal T2WI and ADC with involvement of periprostatic fat which can be misdiagnosed as extraprostatic extension. Therefore, histopathology remains the only definitive method of diagnosis. Depending on the timing of mpMRI, post-biopsy hemorrhage can either mimic or obscure tumor. Although T1WI can be used to discern hemorrhage from tumor, it can limit interpretation of DCE. The extent and dimensions of tumor can remain difficult to localize. While diagnosis can be improved with further education and updates in guidelines, the limitations of 3 T restrict the widespread adoption of mpMRI as the primary diagnostic modality of PCa.

8.3   7 Tesla MRI

Since the beginning of the magnetic resonance imaging (MRI) era there has been a push by scientists and engineers to achieve the highest possible magnetic field in clinical practice [35, 36]. The benefit of a higher magnetic field is that it provides a higher field strength for the imaging leading to higher signal-to-noise ratio (SNR), contrast-to-noise ratio (CNR), and spatial resolution. Additionally, if higher resolution is not needed, the higher field strength also allows for faster scanning at the lower resolution (equivalent to 1.5 T or 3 T). The scientific community has therefore over the years transitioned from first generation MRI scanners (less than or equal to 0.5 T) to the conventional (1.0–1.5 T) and then to high field 3 T scanners. The push towards higher magnetic field continues as several ultra-high field MRI (UhFMRI) systems ranging from 7 T to 11.7 T have been developed over past several years [36]. Significant strides have been made in regards to safety, susceptibility associated artifacts, inhomogeneities, other technical issues and relative cost related to the 7 T MRI scanner to allow for its use in clinical setting, but more research in these areas is needed prior to its widespread adoption in clinical practice [37]. For context, transition from 1.5 T to 3.0 T in clinical practice took close to 15 years for its widespread acceptance.

Most the early research geared towards clinical applicability of 7 T MRI has been focused on studying the anatomy of the human brain but also the functional aspects of the human brain. The ability of UhFMRI to achieve very high resolution in T1-weighted imaging, high CNR in fluid attenuation inversion recovery (FlAIR) imaging, and time-of-flight MR angiography (TOF-MRA), as well as its ability to detect microbleeds in T2-weighted sequences lends well to evaluation of the anatomical aspects of the human brain. With regards to the functional imaging of the brain, the 7 T offers advantages relative to 1.5 T–3 T imaging in its ability to provide an increased SNR to measure the BOLD effect of functional MRI (fMRI), which allows for more accurate localization of brain activity due to a specific task as well as improved magnetic resonance spectroscopy (MRS) [37]. Due to such advantages, 7 T MRI has been used to study the brain and its activity in diseases such as Multiple Sclerosis, cerebrovascular diseases, degenerative brain diseases such as Alzheimer's dementia and Parkinson's disease, brain tumors and epilepsy [38, 39]. In addition to its application in neuroradiology, the UhFMRI is being studied in musculoskeletal, breast, abdominal, and prostate imaging. The results of 7 T MRI in imaging all of the aforementioned body parts and organs is very promising and further investigative work by the scientific community continues.

8.4   New Evidences of 7 Tesla MRI in Prostate Cancer Detection

Multiparametric MR imaging for prostate cancer has been adopted by radiologist in clinical practice to allow for improved accuracy and diagnosis of prostate cancer. Multiparametric MRI includes various imaging sequences such as T2 weighted MR image plus functional MR imaging such as dynamic contrast agent-enhanced MR imaging, diffusion-weighted (DW) imaging, and MR spectroscopic imaging. Over the past decade the emergence of 3 Tesla MRI systems has allowed for significant improvement in quality of these aforementioned sequences compared to its predecessor, the 1.5 Tesla MR system [40].

The improvement in quality of prostate imaging with 3 Tesla MRI has been so substantial, such that 3 T systems are now routinely used at many centers. With the emergence of 7 Tesla MR imaging systems, given its potential benefits over the 3 Tesla systems, there is great optimism in its ability to more accurately image the prostate gland.

Moving to an UhFMRI system such as the 7 T from the current 1.5 T and 3 T MR systems provides clinical advantages because of its ability to provide an increase signal-to-noise ratio, which in theory could be used to increase spatial resolution for improved anatomic evaluation of the prostate gland or reduce imaging time. Additionally, MR spectroscopy for prostate gland at a higher field has advantages of increased separation of spectral peaks as well as option to image new metabolites such as choline, creatine, citrate, phosphorus, and spermine [41, 42]. Moreover, 7 T system offers the possibility of imaging prostate cancer using contrast techniques previously not been possible with 1.5 T and 3 T systems, such as arterial spin labeling [43] and multinuclear imaging [44]. These functional sequences could provide in-vivo insight into tumor biology and metabolism such as to improve our ability to detect clinically significant and aggressive tumors. Such functional sequences would be used in conjunction with adequate anatomic reference imaging in a multiparametric MRI of the prostate. A small study by Kobus and colleagues has shown promise in the area of MR spectroscopy using Phosphorous to image the prostate gland and identify potential tumors [42]. Additionally, study by Durand et al. has looked to evaluate the role of 7 T MR system in its ability to evaluate the prostate at a microscopic level in-vivo and shows promising results (ref).

Imaging the prostate gland at ultra-high magnetic field however has numerous challenges, such as radiofrequency (RF) inhomogeneity, increased tissue heating, reduced RF field penetration. Due to such challenges created by its deep-seated location in the pelvis, adequate MR imaging of the prostate gland requires transmit-receiver coils. There is ongoing progress in this arena as several researchers have created such coil arrays needed for adequate quality imaging [45–47]. Advent of such coils has led to satisfactory to good quality T2W imaging of the prostate using 7 T MRI.

The UhFMRI systems offer great potential in improved prostate imaging and while great strides have been made in our ability to image the prostate gland using 7 T MR system, more work is needed to standardize technique, image sequences, and external coils prior to widespread adaptation in clinical practice.

8.5 7 Tesla MRI and Beyond

Prostate MRI is currently performed in clinical setting with 1.5 or 3 Tesla (T) Scanner. 7-T MRIs have been used in research labs around the world, and in 2017, the first 7-T model was approved for clinical use and it is currently employed mainly for brain Imaging.

However, ultra-high-field scanners (beyond 7-T) are on the rise. A few institutions have performed the first in-vivo Body-MRI using 10.5 T devices. 11.7-T MRI have been extensively tested on animals and it is ready for first tests on people. Germany, China and South Korea are considering building 14-T human scanners. Finally, a 21-T MRI is available with an interior space just 10.5 cm in diameter, too small to be used on man [48].

The development of ultra-high-field scanners is primarily driven by the associated increase in the signal to noise ratio (SNR) that can lead to improved spatial and/or temporal resolution. This means that stronger magnet can capture higher resolution images or same resolution but with shorter acquisition time. Additionally, the higher temporal resolution has potential to improve the performance of dynamic contrast-enhanced MRI [49, 50].

Even if most of the studies on 7-T MRI have been performed on brain diseases, few reports are available on abdominal imaging. Laader et al. compared 1.5, 3 and 7-T MRI for abdominal imaging in 10 healthy volunteers. The increase of the field strength from 1.5 to 3-T offered imaging at increased spatial resolution with comparable image quality and no relevant exacerbation of artifacts. Further increase of the field strength to 7 Tesla demonstrated its high imaging potential for T1 sequences offering a more accurate diagnosis of abdominal parenchymatous and vasculature disease. However, 7-T MRI was also shown to be more impaired by artifacts, including residual B1 inhomogeneities, susceptibility and chemical shift artifacts, resulting in reduced diagnostic quality of T2w sequences [51].

Rosenkrantz et al. reported similar findings on two patients with biopsy proven prostate cancer who underwent radical prostatectomy. Using whole section of the prostate as comparison, the tumors were readily visible as a hypointense lesion on T2w at 7-T in both patients. In addition, while both lesions abutted the capsule, the 7-T T2w correctly indicated the absence of extra prostatic extension in both patients. However, tumor-to-PZ contrast and PZ heterogeneity were slightly decreased at 7-T, indicating the need for continued sequence optimization in a clinical setting [52].

In another study, three radiologists independently scored images of 17 prostate cancer patients who underwent T2w imaging at 7-T with only an external transmit/receive array coil. T2w sequences with satisfactory to good quality could be routinely acquired, and cancer lesions were visible [53]. Last, 7-T MRI provide high-resolution imaging of pelvic lymph nodes to accurately visualize their size and morphology as well as the relation to their surrounding tissue [54].

One must keep in mind that hardware engineering at ultra-high-field scanners is under continuous development. So far, limited data is available on abdominal imaging, only on 7-T MRI. If local power deposition is mitigated at 7-T, higher SNRs can indeed be achieved, which could be used for higher spatial resolution or even further reduction in imaging time. Further research is needed to optimize protocols for imaging acquisition. Additionally, none of the studies mentioned have tested functional imaging techniques such as DWI with ADC maps, DCE sequences, and possibly MRI spectroscopy, that can have a strong impact on diagnosis of suspicious prostate lesions.

References

1. Lauterbur PC. Progress in NMR zeugmatographic imaging. Philos Trans R Soc Lond B, Biol Sci. 1980;289(1037):483–7.
2. Steyn JH, Smith FW. Nuclear magnetic resonance imaging of the prostate. Br J Urol. 1982;54(6):726–8.
3. Weinreb JC, Barentsz JO, Choyke PL, Cornud F, Haider MA, Macura KJ, Margolis D, Schnall MD, Shtern F, Tempany CM, Thoeny HC. PI-RADS prostate imaging–reporting and data system: 2015, version 2. Eur Urol. 2016;69(1):16–40.
4. Drost FJ, Osses DF, Nieboer D, Steyerberg EW, Bangma CH, Roobol MJ, Schoots IG. Prostate MRI, with or without MRI-targeted biopsy, and systematic biopsy for detecting prostate cancer. Cochrane Database Syst Rev. 2019;4
5. Schnall MD, Lenkinski RE, Pollack HM, Imai Y, Kressel HY. Prostate: MR imaging with an endorectal surface coil. Radiology. 1989;172(2):570–4.
6. de Rooij M, Hamoen EH, Fütterer JJ, Barentsz JO, Rovers MM. Accuracy of multiparametric MRI for prostate cancer detection: a meta-analysis. Am J Roentgenol. 2014;202(2):343–51.
7. Poon PY, McCallum RW, Henkelman MM, Bronskill MJ, Sutcliffe SB, Jewett MA, Rider WD, Bruce AW. Magnetic resonance imaging of the prostate. Radiology. 1985;154(1):143–9.
8. Hricak H, Dooms GC, Jeffrey RB, Avallone A, Jacobs D, Benton WK, Narayan P, Tanagho EA. Prostatic carcinoma: staging by clinical assessment, CT, and MR imaging. Radiology. 1987;162(2):331–6.
9. White S, Hricak H, Forstner R, Kurhanewicz J, Vigneron DB, Zaloudek CJ, Weiss JM, Narayan P, Carroll PR. Prostate cancer: effect of postbiopsy hemorrhage on interpretation of MR images. Radiology. 1995;195(2):385–90.
10. Padhani AR. Integrating multiparametric prostate MRI into clinical practice. Cancer Imaging. 2011;11(1A):S27.
11. Yoshizako T, Wada A, Uchida K, Hara S, Igawa M, Kitagaki H, Maier SE. Apparent diffusion coefficient of line scan diffusion image in normal prostate and prostate cancer—comparison with single-shot echo planner image. Magn Reson Imaging. 2011;29(1):106–10.
12. Hegde JV, Mulkern RV, Panych LP, Fennessy FM, Fedorov A, Maier SE, Tempany CM. Multiparametric MRI of prostate cancer: an update on state-of-the-art techniques and their performance in detecting and localizing prostate cancer. J Magn Reson Imaging. 2013;37(5):1035–54.
13. Woo S, Suh CH, Kim SY, Cho JY, Kim SH. Diagnostic performance of prostate imaging reporting and data system version 2 for detection of prostate cancer: a systematic review and diagnostic meta-analysis. Eur Urol. 2017;72(2):177–88.
14. Mottet N, Bellmunt J, Briers E, Bolla M, Bourke L, Cornford P, De Santis M, Henry A, Joniau S, Lam T, Mason MD, Van den Poel H, Van den Kwast TH, Rouvière O, Wiegel T, Members of the EAU – ESTRO – ESUR –SIOG Prostate Cancer Guidelines Panel. EAU – ESTRO – ESUR – SIOG Guidelines on Prostate Cancer. Retrieved from: https://uroweb.org/guideline/prostate-cancer/. Accessed 27 Mar 2020.
15. Fulgham PF, Rukstalis DB, Rubenstein JN, Taneja SS, Carroll PR, Pinto PA, Bjurlin MA, Eggener S, Turkbey IB, Margolis DJ, Rosenkrantz AB. Standard operating procedure for multiparametric magnetic resonance imaging in the diagnosis, staging and management of prostate cancer. Retrieved from: https://www.auanet.org/guidelines/mri-of-the-prostate-sop/. Accessed 27 Mar 2020.
16. National Institute for Health and Care Excellence. Prostate cancer: diagnosis and management; 2019. Retrieved from: https://www.nice.org.uk/guidance/ng131/chapter/Recommendations#assessment-and-diagnosis/. Accessed 27 Mar 2020.
17. National Comprehensive Cancer Network. Prostate Cancer Version 1.2020. March 16, 2020. Retrieved from: https://www.nccn.org/professionals/physician_gls/pdf/prostate.pdf/. Accessed 27 Mar 2020.

18. Ahmed HU, Bosaily AE, Brown LC, Gabe R, Kaplan R, Parmar MK, Collaco-Moraes Y, Ward K, Hindley RG, Freeman A, Kirkham AP. Diagnostic accuracy of multi-parametric MRI and TRUS biopsy in prostate cancer (PROMIS): a paired validating confirmatory study. Lancet. 2017;389(10071):815–22.
19. Siddiqui MM, Rais-Bahrami S, Turkbey B, George AK, Rothwax J, Shakir N, Okoro C, Raskolnikov D, Parnes HL, Linehan WM, Merino MJ. Comparison of MR/ultrasound fusion–guided biopsy with ultrasound-guided biopsy for the diagnosis of prostate cancer. JAMA. 2015;313(4):390–7.
20. Baco E, Rud E, Eri LM, Moen G, Vlatkovic L, Svindland A, Eggesbø HB, Ukimura O. A randomized controlled trial to assess and compare the outcomes of two-core prostate biopsy guided by fused magnetic resonance and transrectal ultrasound images and traditional 12-core systematic biopsy. Eur Urol. 2016;69(1):149–56.
21. Schoots IG, Roobol MJ, Nieboer D, Bangma CH, Steyerberg EW, Hunink MM. Magnetic resonance imaging–targeted biopsy may enhance the diagnostic accuracy of significant prostate cancer detection compared to standard transrectal ultrasound-guided biopsy: a systematic review and meta-analysis. Eur Urol. 2015;68(3):438–50.
22. Kasivisvanathan V, Rannikko AS, Borghi M, Panebianco V, Mynderse LA, Vaarala MH, Briganti A, Budäus L, Hellawell G, Hindley RG, Roobol MJ. MRI-targeted or standard biopsy for prostate-cancer diagnosis. N Engl J Med. 2018;378(19):1767–77.
23. van der Leest M, Cornel E, Israel B, Hendriks R, Padhani AR, Hoogenboom M, Zamecnik P, Bakker D, Setiasti AY, Veltman J, van den Hout H. Head-to-head comparison of transrectal ultrasound-guided prostate biopsy versus multiparametric prostate resonance imaging with subsequent magnetic resonance-guided biopsy in biopsy-naïve men with elevated prostate-specific antigen: a large prospective multicenter clinical study. Eur Urol. 2019;75(4):570–8.
24. Soher BJ, Dale BM, Merkle EM. A review of MR physics: 3T versus 1.5 T. Magn Reson Imaging Clin N Am. 2007;15(3):277–90.
25. Mazaheri Y, Vargas HA, Nyman G, Akin O, Hricak H. Image artifacts on prostate diffusion-weighted magnetic resonance imaging: trade-offs at 1.5 Tesla and 3.0 Tesla. Acad Radiol. 2013;20(8):1041–7.
26. de Rooij M, Hamoen EH, Witjes JA, Barentsz JO, Rovers MM. Accuracy of magnetic resonance imaging for local staging of prostate cancer: a diagnostic meta-analysis. Eur Urol. 2016;70(2):233–45.
27. Richenberg J, Løgager V, Panebianco V, Rouviere O, Villeirs G, Schoots IG. The primacy of multiparametric MRI in men with suspected prostate cancer. Eur Radiol. 2019;29(12):6940–52.
28. Sonn GA, Fan RE, Ghanouni P, Wang NN, Brooks JD, Loening AM, Daniel BL, To'o KJ, Thong AE, Leppert JT. Prostate magnetic resonance imaging interpretation varies substantially across radiologists. Eur Urol Focus. 2019;5(4):592–9.
29. Hansen NL, Koo BC, Gallagher FA, Warren AY, Doble A, Gnanapragasam V, Bratt O, Kastner C, Barrett T. Comparison of initial and tertiary centre second opinion reads of multiparametric magnetic resonance imaging of the prostate prior to repeat biopsy. Eur Radiol. 2017;27(6):2259–66.
30. Panebianco V, Giganti F, Kitzing YX, Cornud F, Campa R, De Rubeis G, Ciardi A, Catalano C, Villeirs G. An update of pitfalls in prostate mpMRI: a practical approach through the lens of PI-RADS v. 2 guidelines. Insights Imaging. 2018;9(1):87–101.
31. Rosenkrantz AB, Taneja SS. Radiologist, be aware: ten pitfalls that confound the interpretation of multiparametric prostate MRI. Am J Roentgenol. 2014;202(1):109–20.
32. Kitzing YX, Prando A, Varol C, Karczmar GS, Maclean F, Oto A. Benign conditions that mimic prostate carcinoma: MR imaging features with histopathologic correlation. Radiographics. 2016;36(1):162–75.
33. Vargas HA, Akin O, Franiel T, Goldman DA, Udo K, Touijer KA, Reuter VE, Hricak H. Normal central zone of the prostate and central zone involvement by prostate cancer: clinical and MR imaging implications. Radiology. 2012;262(3):894–902.

34. Barrett T, Rajesh A, Rosenkrantz AB, Choyke PL, Turkbey B. PI-RADS version 2.1: one small step for prostate MRI. Clin Radiol. 2019;22
35. Brown RW, Cheng YN, Haacke EM, Thompson MR, Venkatesan R. Magnetic resonance imaging: physical principles and sequence design. 2nd ed. New Jersey: Wiley; 2014.
36. Schmitt F, Potthast A, Stoeckel B, Triantafyllou C, Wig-Gins CJ, Wiggins G, Wald LL. Aspects of clinical imaging at 7T. In: Robitaille PM, Berliner L, editors. Ultra HighField magnetic resonance imaging, vol. 26. New York: Springer Science; 2006. p. 59–104.
37. Opportunities and Challenges of 7 Tesla Magnetic Resonance Imaging: A Review. Karamat, Muhammad Irfan; Darvish-Molla, Sahar; Santos-Diaz, Alejandro ISSN: 0278-940X, 1943-619X. https://doi.org/10.1615/CritRevBiomedEng.2016016365. (Critical reviews in biomedical engineering. 2016; 44(1–2):73–89).
38. Balchandani P, Naidich TP. Ultra-high-field MR neuroimaging. Am J Neuroradiol. 2015;36(7):1204–15.
39. Van der Kolk AG, Hendrikse J, Zwanenburg JJM, Visser F, Luijten PR. Clinical applications of 7T MRI in the brain. Eur J Radiol. 2013;82:708–18.
40. Bonekamp D, Jacobs MA, El-Khouli R, Stoianovici D, Macura KJ. Advancements in MR imaging of the prostate: from diagnosis to interventions. Radiographics. 2011;31:677–703.
41. Wu C-L, Jordan KW, Ratai EM, Sheng J, Adkins CB, De-feo EM, Jenkins BG, Ying L, McDougal WS, Cheng LL. Metabolomic imaging for human prostate cancer detection. Sci Transl Med. 2010;2(16):16ra8.
42. Kobus T, Bitz AK, van Uden MJ, Lagemaat MW, Rothgang E, Orzada S, et al. In vivo (31) P MR spectroscopic imaging of the human prostate at 7 T: safety and feasibility. Magn Reson Med. 2012;68(6):1683–95.
43. Li X, de Moortele V, Ugurbil U, Metzger G. Dynamically applied multiple B1þ shimming scheme for arterial spin labelling of the prostate at 7T. In: Proceedings of the 19th Annual Meeting of ISMRM, Montreal, 2011 (abstract 593).
44. van Uden MJ, Veltien A, Scheenen TW, Heerschap A. Design of a double tuned TxRx 1H/31P endorectal prostate coil for 7T. In: Proceedings of the 18th Annual Meeting of ISMRM, Stockholm, Sweden, 2010 (abstract 3904).
45. Raaijmakers AJE, Italiaander M, Voogt IJ, et al. The fractionated dipole antenna: a new antenna for body imaging at 7 Tesla. Magn Reson Med. 2016;75:1366–74. https://doi.org/10.1002/mrm.25596.
46. Metzger GJ, Snyder C, Akgun C, Vaughan T, Ugurbil K, Van De Moortele PF. Local B1 + shimming for prostate imaging with transceiver arrays at 7T based on subject-dependent transmit phase measurements. Magn Reson Med. 2008;59:396–409.
47. Rosenkrantz AB, Zhang B, Ben-Eliezer N, et al. T2-weighted prostate MRI at 7 Tesla using a simplified external transmit-receive coil array: correlation with radical prostatectomy findings in two prostate cancer patients. J Magn Reson Imaging. 2015;41:226–32.
48. Nowogrodzki A. The world's strongest MRI machines are pushing human imaging to new limits. Nature. 2018;563(7729):24–6. https://doi.org/10.1038/d41586-018-07182-7.
49. Mönninghoff C, Maderwald S, Theysohn JM, Kraff O, Ladd SC, Ladd ME, Forsting M, Quick HH, Wanke I. Evaluation of intracranial aneurysms with 7 T versus 1.5 T time-of-flight MR angiography – initial experience. Rofo. 2009;181(1):16–23. https://doi.org/10.1055/s-2008-1027863.
50. Kollia K, Maderwald S, Putzki N, Schlamann M, Theysohn JM, Kraff O, Ladd ME, Forsting M, Wanke I. First clinical study on ultra-high-field MR imaging in patients with multiple sclerosis: comparison of 1.5T and 7T. AJNR Am J Neuroradiol. 2009;30(4):699–702. https://doi.org/10.3174/ajnr.A1434.
51. Laader A, Beiderwellen K, Kraff O, Maderwald S, Wrede K, Ladd ME, Lauenstein TC, Forsting M, Quick HH, Nassenstein K, Umutlu L. 1.5 versus 3 versus 7 Tesla in abdominal MRI: a comparative study. PLoS One. 2017;12(11):e0187528. https://doi.org/10.1371/journal.pone.0187528.

52. Rosenkrantz AB, Zhang B, Ben-Eliezer N, Le Nobin J, Melamed J, Deng FM, Taneja SS, Wiggins GC. T2-weighted prostate MRI at 7 Tesla using a simplified external transmit-receive coil array: correlation with radical prostatectomy findings in two prostate cancer patients. J Magn Reson Imaging. 2015;41(1):226–32. https://doi.org/10.1002/jmri.24511.
53. Vos EK, Lagemaat MW, Barentsz JO, Fütterer JJ, Zámecnik P, Roozen H, Orzada S, Bitz AK, Maas MC, Scheenen TW. Image quality and cancer visibility of T2-weighted magnetic resonance imaging of the prostate at 7 Tesla. Eur Radiol. 2014;24(8):1950–8. https://doi.org/10.1007/s00330-014-3234-6.
54. Philips BWJ, Fortuin AS, Orzada S, Scheenen TWJ, Maas MC. High resolution MR imaging of pelvic lymph nodes at 7 Tesla. Magn Reson Med. 2017;78(3):1020–8. https://doi.org/10.1002/mrm.26498.

Chapter 9
Prostate Specific Membrane Antigen Based Imaging

Murat Tuncel [ORCID]

9.1 Introduction

Prostate cancer (Pca) is the most common cancer and the second leading cause of death among men. An estimated 174,650 new cases of Pca will be diagnosed in the US by 2019, and unfortunately, 31,620 Pca-related deaths are expected [1]. Imaging plays a crucial role in therapy decisions. Several new imaging technologies were available for PCa. Routine clinical application and endorsement of these new techniques occur with a delay due to availability & cost concerns, and more importantly, lack of randomized control trials. Current *National Comprehensive Cancer Network* (*NCCN*) guideline recommended bone scan (BS) and computed tomography (CT) scan as an initial staging procedure in patients with intermediate and high-risk patients [2]. The role of multiparametric magnetic resonance imaging (mpMRI) is well established in patients with high-risk patients prior negative systematic biopsy or patients on active-surveillance. Although mpMRI detects more lesion with ISUP-grade > 2 than systemic biopsy, its recommendation before an initial biopsy has weak strength in European Association of Urology (EAU) guidelines [3–5].

Positron emission tomography-computed tomography (PET-CT) performed with new radiopharmaceuticals has revolutionized the imaging area in Pca. Over decades several radiopharmaceuticals, like ^{18}F-Flourodexyglucose (FDG), ^{18}F/^{11}C Choline, ^{68}Ga-DOTATATE,^{18}F-Florocyclovine,and ^{68}Ga-labeled prostate-specific membrane antigen (PSMA) have been used for staging and restaging of Pca (Table 9.1). Each radiotracer targets different metabolic substrate, receptor, or antigen. ^{68}Ga-PSMA-PET-CT imaging has the highest sensitivity and specificity among these radiotracers [6], and replaced most of the PET-tracers and also BS in several clinical situations

M. Tuncel (✉)
Faculty of Medicine, Department of Nuclear Medicine, Hacettepe University, Ankara, Turkey
e-mail: murat.tuncel@hacettepe.edu.tr

© Springer Nature Switzerland AG 2021
E. Huri, D. Veneziano (eds.), *Anatomy for Urologic Surgeons in the Digital Era*,
https://doi.org/10.1007/978-3-030-59479-4_9

Table 9.1 Radiopharmaceuticals for prostate cancer

Imaging target	PET radiotracer	SPECT radiotracer
Tumor metabolism		
Glucose metabolism	^{18}F-FDG	
Aminoacid	^{11}C-methionine, ^{18}F-Fluciclovine	
Nucleic acid	^{18}F-Flohymidine	
Sterol synthesis	^{11}C-acetate	
Hypoxia	^{18}F-MISO, ^{18}F-FAZA	
Tumor receptor		
Androgen	^{18}F-Dihydrotestosterone	
Bombesin	^{68}Ga-RM2	
Tumor antigen		
PSMA small molecule	^{68}Ga-PSMA-11 ^{68}Ga-PSMA-617 ^{68}Ga-PSMA I&T ^{18}F-DCFBC ^{18}F-DCFPyL ^{18}F-PSMA-1007 ^{124}I- MIP-1095	^{99m}Tc-MIP-1040 ^{99m}Tc-PSMA I&S ^{123}I-MIP-1072 ^{123}I-MIP-1095
PSMA antibody	^{89}Z-anti-PSMA minibody ^{89}Z-J591	^{111}In-Capromab Pendetide ^{111}In-radiolabeled anti-PSMA Nanobody
Osteoblastic response	^{18}F-NaF ^{68}Ga-DOTA-zoledronate	^{99m}Tc-MDP, HDP

[7]. PSMA-based imaging not only detects early disease recurrence but also guides the surgeon intraoperatively. This chapter mainly focuses on PSMA-based imaging and discuss the potential benefits and limitations.

9.2 Prostate-Specific Antigen as a Target in Prostate Cancer

PSMA is a type-II transmembrane glycoprotein with a 707-amino-acid extracellular domain [8]. After binding to the extracellular domain, novel PSMA-ligands are internalized and undergo endosomal recycling, leading to enhanced uptake and retention in tumor cells.

Although PSMA is highly specific for the prostatic tissue, it is also expressed in several healthy tissues, including salivary glands, neuroendocrine tissue, small bowel, and kidney (Fig. 9.1) [9]. Physiological uptake in parasympathetic ganglia, most commonly the celiac, cervical, and presacral ganglia, may mimic lymph node (LN) metastases. Knowledge of the locations, uptake pattern, intensity, and anatomic appearance on CT may guide the identification of this normal variants [10, 11]. Although there is a slight difference in the biodistribution of the PSMA-based radiotracers, ^{68}Ga-labeled-PSMA agents are mainly excreted via kidney, and physiological uptake in ureters is also seen. Activity in ureters may mimic LN metastases if the route of the ureter is not well tracked. Halo artifacts due to high radiotracer uptake or excretion in kidney and bladder may artifactually decrease the activity of

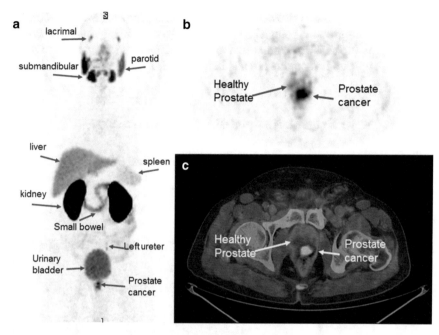

Fig. 9.1 A 70-year-old patient suffering from prostate cancer (Gleason score 4 + 4 and PSA: 14 ng/ml) underwent ^{68}Ga-PSMA-PET-CT imaging for primary staging showed (**a**) Maximum intensity projection (MIP) PET image showed physiological uptake in salivary glands, liver, spleen, kidney, small bowel, ureter, urinary bladder and increased uptake in primary prostate cancer. (**b**) and (**c**) Axial PET and PET-CT fusion images showed increased uptake in the primary prostate cancer located at the mid-portion of the left peripheric zone (SUV$_{max}$: 5)

neighboring activities like LNs[12]. Several techniques, including administration of furosemide and delay in imaging was introduced to differentiate physiologic urinary activity from pathologic uptake[12].

In PCa, PSMA is overexpressed in the order of 100–1000 times compared with healthy prostate tissue. Overexpression occurs in greater than 90% of PCa lesions [12, 13]. Moreover, its expression is increased with Gleason grade. The transition to androgen-independent PCa eventually leads to further PSMA-expression [14]. PSMA expression also has a prognostic value; tumors with strong PSMA-expression had a higher risk of biochemical recurrence (BCR) [15].

Although PSMA imaging is sensitive in Pca imaging, <10% of prostate carcinomas exhibit no or minimal uptake at PSMA-PET/CT, reflecting low PSMA expression [16]. Most of the PSMA-negative lesions are observed in heavily treated patients with several lines of chemotherapy & androgen deprivation therapy (ADT), patients with poorly differentiated tumors with neuroendocrine differentiation, dedifferentiated acinar PCa [17, 18]. Other radiotracers like FDG can be useful in these PSMA negative metastatic lesions. The relationship between PSMA uptake and previous ADT has to be considered in the interpretation of PSMA-PET imaging. PSMA expression was also found to be increased by short term application of ADT [19, 20].

PSMA expression was also detected in the neovasculature of several tumors [21] and several non-prostatic, benign and malign uptake sites might be seen on PSMA-scans (Fig. 9.2). Table 9.2 summarizes the brief examples of non-prostatic benign and malign uptake sites reported in the literature [22, 23].

9.3 Prostate-Specific Antigen-Based Radiotracers

Several PSMA-based radiotracers were produced (Table 9.1), ^{68}Ga PSMA-HBED-CC (also known as ^{68}Ga-PSMA-11) is the most widely used radiotracer in clinical practice. There has been an increasing interest in the clinical use of ^{18}F-labeled, PSMA-targeted PET imaging agents (e.g.,[18]F-DCFBC,[18]F-DCFPyL,[18]F-PSMA-1007),due

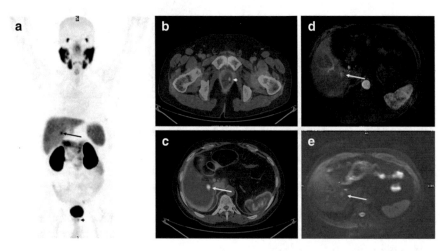

Fig. 9.2 A 55-year-old patient who has hepatocellular cancer (HCC), recently diagnosed as having secondary primary cancer in the prostate with Gleason score of 4 + 3. The patient underwent ^{68}Ga-PSMA-PET-CT imaging for primary staging. (**a**) Maximum intensity projection PET image showed increased uptake in the prostate primary (SUV_{max}: 3) (arrow head) and a focal uptake in liver segment 6 (SUV_{max}: 5). (arrow) which was diagnosed as residual HCC. (**b**) and (**c**) Axial PET-CT fusion images showed increased uptake in the primary prostate cancer (arrow-head) and focal uptake in liver segment 6 (arrow) (**d**) axial contrast enhanced and (**e**) diffusion-weighted MRI images showed residual HCC with increased vascularity and diffusion restriction respectively (arrows)

Table 9.2 Non-prostatic PSMA uptakes in benign and malign diseases

Benign diseases	Malign diseases
Schwannoma [24]	Breast cancer [25, 26]
Paget disease [27]	Thyroid cancer [28]
Osteoid osteoma [29]	Colon cancer [30]
Fibrous dysplasia [31]	Brain tumor [32]
Adrenal adenoma [33]	Hepatocellular cancer [34]
Benign liver hemangioma [35]	Renal cell cancer [36]
Amyloidosis [37]…	Gastric cancer [38]…

to their favorable physical properties, higher production capacity by cyclotron, and improved imaging characteristics. ^{18}F-PSMA-1007 is has a primarily hepatobiliary clearance, when compared to other PSMA-ligands. It shows significantly lower uptake in the kidneys, urinary bladder, and lacrimal glands and higher uptake in the liver, gallbladder, spleen, pancreas, muscle and salivary glands [39] Nonurinary excretion of ^{18}F-PSMA-1007 might be advantageous for delineation of local recurrence or pelvic LN metastases. Studies proved that ^{18}F-labeled PSMA ligands perform similarly, even better when compared to ^{68}Ga-labelled PSMA ligands [40].

PSMA PET is commonly done by PET-CT scanners however the introduction of PET-MRI hybrid devices had provided an one-stop-shop imaging of Pca. The multiparametric data and superior soft-tissue resolution provided by MRI has increased the accuracy in local staging.

9.4   Primary Staging

9.4.1   Detection of Primary, T Stage

According to the NCCN and European Association of Urology (EAU) guidelines, T staging is mainly done by rectal examination and biopsy results. mpMRI is the method of choice for prediction of T stage and usage is increased tremendously. Accuracy of imaging modality is especially crucial in the primary therapy selection (active surveillance, focal therapy or definitive therapy) [2].

In primary PCa, the diagnostic accuracy and interpretation methods of ^{68}Ga-PSMA-ligand PET/CT is studied by several study groups. Some authors used an increased uptake above the background in the peripheral zone as a positive criterion, and others used several SUV_{max} values (commonly around a value of 3.2) [41, 42]. In order to resolve these discrepancies in image evaluation, two interpretation models were suggested; PSMA-RADS, is a 5-point scale interpretation system, with higher numbers indicating a greater probability of PCa [43]. Prostate Cancer Molecular Imaging Standardized Evaluation (PROMISE) interpretation criteria is a more complex interpretation algorithm that takes into account the clinical situation and the other imaging modalities' results. Briefly for the primary tumor, if the patient a not have previous mpMRI, any focal uptake above liver was accepted as a primary tumor. If the patient has focal uptake above blood pool uptake and a corresponding PIRADS > 4 lesion on mpMRI, then this uptake was also interpreted as positive for primary Pca [44] (Fig. 9.3).

There are several predictors of increased uptake in the primary. In their study Uprimny C et al. found that ^{68}Ga-PSMA-11 PET/CT detected the primary tumor of eighty-two patients (91.1%). Tumors with GS of 6, 7a(3 + 4) and 7b(4 + 3) showed significantly lower ^{68}Ga-PSMA-11 uptake, with median SUV_{max} of 5.9, 8.3 and 8.2, respectively, compared to patients with GS > 7 (median SUV_{max}: 21.2; p<0.001). PCa patients with PSA $\geq$ 10.0 ng/ml exhibited significantly higher uptake than

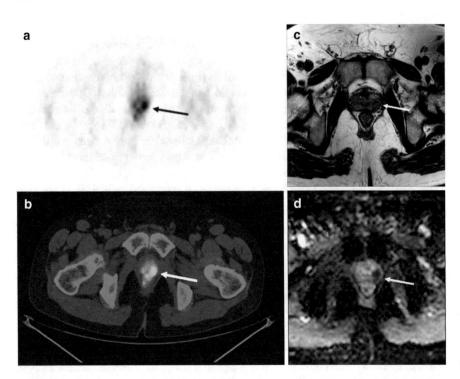

Fig. 9.3 A 65-year-old patient with PCa underwent ^{68}Ga-PSMA-PET-CT imaging for primary staging. (**a**) Axial PET and (**b**) PET-CT fusion images showed increased uptake in prostate primary located at the mid-portion of the left peripheric zone (arrow) (**c**) axial T2 weighted and (**d**) diffusion-weighted (ADC map) MRI images showed hypointense lesion with diffusion restriction (PIRADS: 5) (arrows)

those with lower (median SUV_{max}: 17.6 vs. 7.7; $p < 0.001$) [45]. Many institutions used mpMRI as the method of choice for the evaluation of T stage. Eiber M et al. found that mpMRI, PET, and PET/MRI detected cancer in 66%, 92%, and 98% of the 53 patients, respectively. Simultaneous PET/MRI statistically outperformed mpMRI (area under the curve [AUC]: 0.88 vs. 0.73; $p < 0.001$) and PET imaging (AUC: 0.88 vs. 0.83; $p = 0.002$) for localization of PCa. Compared with mpMRI, PET imaging was more accurate (AUC: 0.83 vs. 0.73; $p = 0.003$) [46]. Kalapara AA et al. compared the accuracy of ^{68}Ga-PSMA-PET/CT with mpMRI in detecting and localizing primary Pca when compared with RP pathology. There was no significant difference between ^{68}Ga-PSMA-PET/CT and mpMRI in the detection of any tumor (94% vs. 95%, $p > 0.9$), localization of index tumors (91% vs. 89%, $p = 0.47$), clinically significant index tumors (96% vs. 91%, $p = 0.15$), or transition zone tumors (85% vs. 80%, $p > 0.9$) [47]. Detection and delineation of tumor volume is critical for local therapies like radiation therapy. In a study with direct correlation with histopathology. Bettermann AS et al. compared accuracy of mpMRI vs. PSMA-PET in delineation of tumor volume. Median gross tumor volume (GTV) for histology was 10.4 ml, 10.8 ml for PSMA-PET and 4.5 ml for mpMRI (p < 0.05). The authors concluded that mpMRI underestimate tumor volume significantly and PSMA-PET may be complementary for GTV delineation in focal therapies [48]. ^{68}Ga-PSMA PET/CT also performed better than the nomograms used for the prediction of PCa in high-risk patients. ^{68}Ga-PSMA-PET/CT exhibited a higher AUC (0.867) than those of European Randomized study of Screening for Prostate Cancer (ERSPC)-RC3 (0.855) and Prostate Cancer Prevention Trial (*PCPT*) (0.770). Among the 58 patients, 11(19%) biopsies suggested by ERSPC-RC3 were unnecessary and could have been avoided if decided after the ^{68}Ga-PSMA PET/CT results [49]. Accuracy of ^{68}Ga-PSMA PET/CT for the detection of actual tumor volume and invasion of seminal vesicle and extracapsular invasion was also studied (Fig. 9.4). Christoph-Alexander J. von Klo investigated the role of ^{68}Ga-PSMA I&T PET/CT in presurgical local staging of prostate cancer prior to radical prostatectomy. The authors have found that SUV_{mean} was higher in tumors with ECE than in organ-confined tumors (13.8 ± 11.0 vs. 5.6 ± 3.2, p = 0.029). Sensitivity, specificity, PPV and NPV were, respectively, 94.7%, 75.0%, 97.3% and 60.0% for tumor infiltration of an individual prostate lobe, 75.0%, 100.0%, 100.0% and 97.4% for SVI, and 90.0%, 90.9%, 90.0% and 90.9% for ECE, using an angulated contour of the prostate as the criterion. Tumor volume derived from ^{68}Ga-PSMA I&T PET/CT was significantly correlated with preoperative prostate-specific antigen value (r_p = 0.75, *p* < 0.001), tumor volume on histopathology (r_p = 0.45, p = 0.039) and Gleason score (r_s = 0.49, p = 0.025) [50]. In a study by Fendler WP et al. ^{68}Ga-PSMA PET/CT evaluated the accuracy of PET/CT with ^{68}Ga-PSMA to localize cancer in the prostate and surrounding tissue at initial

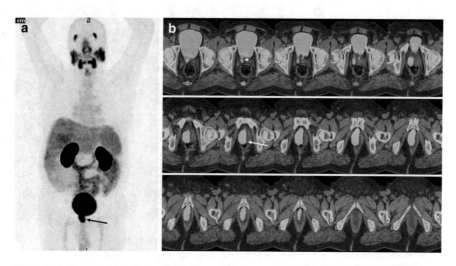

Fig. 9.4 A 62-year-old patient suffering from prostate cancer with Gleason score 4 + 4 and PSA levels of 24 ng/ml underwent ^{68}Ga-PSMA-PET-CT imaging for primary staging. (**a**) MIP PET showed increased uptake in the primary Pca (arrow) (**b**) axial PET-CT fusion images showed increased uptake in the primary Pca located at the right side of prostate (arrow). PCa extends from apex to base and invades right seminal vesicle (arrow head)

diagnosis. PET/CT correctly detected invasion of seminal vesicles (n = 11 of 21 patients; 52%) with 86% accuracy and tumor spread through the capsule (n = 12; 57%) with 71% accuracy [46].

9.4.2   N Staging

N staging is critical for surgery planning both in staging and restaging. Abdominopelvic-CT and T1-T2-weighted-MRI assess nodal involvement by using LN diameter and morphology. Usually, LNs with a short axis >8 mm in the pelvis and >10 mm outside the pelvis are considered malignant. Using these thresholds the sensitivities of CT/MRI are less than 40% [51]. Decreasing these thresholds improves sensitivity but decreases specificity [52]. Diffusion-weighted MRI may detect metastases in normal-sized nodes, but the sensitivity per node is limited up to 26% [53]. Several groups studied the accuracy of PSMA-PET-CT in LN detection. As done with the primary (T stage) several authors proposed SUV_{max} values (SUV_{max}: 2) for discrimination of normal and metastatic LNs [54]. According to PROMISE interpretation criteria, any pelvic/retroperitoneal LN with uptake above blood-pool was interpreted as positive for LN involvement [44] (Fig. 9.5). Maurer T et al. studied the accuracy of ^{68}Ga-PSMA scans compared to CI in the detection of LNs by using histopathology as a reference. On patient-based analysis the sensitivity, specificity, and accuracy of ^{68}Ga-PSMA-PET were 65.9%, 98.9%,

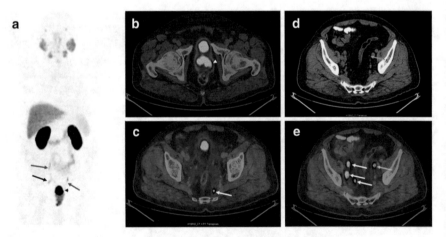

Fig. 9.5 A 72-year-old patient suffering from prostate cancer with Gleason score 4 + 4 and PSA levels of 21 ng/ml underwent ^{68}Ga-PSMA-PET-CT imaging for primary staging (**a**) MIP PET (**b**) axial PET-CT fusion images showed increased uptake in the primary Pca (arrow head) and right parailliac lymph nodes (black arrow) and ureters (red arrows) (**c, d, e**) axial PET/CT fusion and CT images showed lymph node metastases in perirectal, right parailliac lymph nodes (white arrows) and activity in left ureter (green arrows)

and 88.5%, and those of CI were 43.9%, 85.4%, and 72.3%, respectively. On template-based analysis the sensitivity, specificity, and accuracy of ^{68}Ga-PSMA-PET were 68.3%, 99.1%, and 95.2%, and those of CI were 27.3%, 97.1%, and 87.6%, respectively. On ROC-analysis, ^{68}Ga-PSMA-PET performed significantly better than CI alone on a patient and template-based analyses (p = 0.002 and <0.001, respectively) [55]. Petersen LJ et al. compared the diagnostic accuracy of ^{68}Ga-PSMA-PET/CT with conventional cross-sectional imaging for detecting LN metastasis (LNM). The patient-based analysis showed that the sensitivity and specificity for detecting LNM were 39% and 100% with ^{68}Ga-PSMA PET/CT, 8% and 100% with MRI/CT, and 36% and 83% with DW-MRI, respectively. The positive and negative PVs were 100% and 49% with ^{68}Ga-PSMA PET/CT, 100% and 37% with MRI/CT, and 80% and 42% with DW-MRI. True-positive LNM on ^{68}Ga-PSMA PET/CT was 9–11 mm in diameter, whereas false-negative LNM had a median diameter of 4 mm. Some false-positive findings with DW-MRI reduced its specificity and PPV compared with those of ^{68}Ga-PSMA-PET/CT and MRI/CT [56]. In a study for staging intermediate- and high-risk PCa, Van Leeuwen PJ et al. found that ^{68}Ga-PSMA-PET/CT had a sensitivity of 64% for the detection of LNMs, its specificity was 95%, the PPV was 88%, and the NPV was 82% in patient-bases. In the LN-region-based analysis, the sensitivity of ^{68}Ga-PSMA-PET/CT for detection of LNMs was 56%, the specificity was 98%, the PPV was 90% and the NPV was 94%. The mean size of missed LNMs was 2.7 mm. ROC curve analysis showed a high accuracy of SUV_{max} for the detection of LNMs, with an AUC of 0.915; the optimum SUV_{max} was calculated as 2.0 [54]. Some authors also investigated possible PET findings that may predict LN involvement. Upprimny C et al. found that the median SUV_{max} of tumors in patients with LNMs was higher than in patients without malignant LN involvement (18.7 vs. 9.7) (p = 0.001) [45]. In the primary staging PET positivity in prostate gland or metastatic involvement differs with PSA levels. In the primary staging of newly diagnosed PCa. The rate of detection of primary tumor by ^{68}Ga-PSMA for patients with serum PSA less than 5 ng/ml was 73%. The corresponding rate was 90% for patients with PSA 5–10 ng/ml and 97% for patients with PSA more than 10 ng/ml. The rate of detection of metastatic PCa was greater in patients with GS 9 or more (48%) relative to those with GS 8 (32%) or GS ≤7 (18%). There was a low rate of detection of PSMA-avid metastases in low-grade disease (GS 7 or less and PSA <5 ng/ml), suggesting a limited role for this modality in such cases [57]. Several nomograms were available for the prediction of LN metastases. The value of PSMA-PET compared to these nomograms also has been investigated. Thalgott M et al. compared the diagnostic potential of ^{68}Ga-PSMA-11 PET/MRI with preoperative staging nomograms in patients with high-risk Pca. Imaging revealed a higher specificity (100%) for LNM and a comparable sensitivity (60%) to the MSKCC nomogram (68%) and Partin tables (60%) [58]. In addition to nomograms or prediction formulas PSMA-PET/CT provides anatomic localization of LNM that tailored treatment planning [59].

9.4.3 M Stage

BS has been the most widely used method for evaluating bone metastases of PCa. A recent meta-analysis showed combined sensitivity and specificity of 79% and 82% at the patient level and 59% and 75% at lesion level [60]. BS diagnostic yield is influenced by the PSA level, the clinical stage, and the tumor ISUP grade. The mean BS positivity rate was 2.3% in patients with PSA levels <10 ng/ml and 16.2% in patients with PSA levels of 20.0–49.9 ng/ml. Detection rates were 5.6% and 29.9% for ISUP grade 2 and >3, respectively [61].

BS and PSMA-PET were compared in several studies; Pyka T et al. compared BS and PET-PSMA in a total of 75 of 126 patients with PCa. Sensitivities and specificities regarding overall bone involvement were 98.7–100% and 88.2–100% for PET, and 86.7–89.3% and 60.8–96.1% (p < 0.001) for BS. The cohort was further divided into clinical subgroups (primary staging,BCR and metastatic castration-resistant PCa [mCRPC]). PSMA PET also performed better in all subgroups, except patient-based analysis in mCRPC. These heavily treated patient group present with predominantly osteoblastic metastases with low PSMA uptake and evident uptake on BS [62]. The avidity of PSMA-PET also correlated with findings on CT as reported with ^{11}C-choline PET-CT [63]. The highest clinical impact on treatment was seen on patients with negative or suspicious bone scan and positive on Choline/^{68}Ga-PSMA uptake (Fig. 9.6). Sclerotic lesions in heavily treated patients have less ^{11}C-choline/^{68}Ga-PSMA uptake, whereas showed high uptake with bone-seeking agents like ^{99m}Tc-MDP and ^{18}F-NaF. Janssen JC et al. evaluated potential differences in PSMA uptake in osteolytic (OL), osteoblastic (OB), mixed (M), and bone marrow (BM) metastases in Pca patients. SUV_{max} and mean Hounsfield units (HU_{mean}) of each metastasis were measured. The SUV_{max} for the different types of metastases were 10.6 ± 7.07 osteoblastic (OB), 24.0 ± 19.3 osteolytic (OL), and 14.7 ± 9.9 bone marrow (BM). The SUV_{max} of (OB) vs. (OL) and (OB) vs. (BM) metastases differed significantly (p ≤ 0.025). A significant negative correlation between HU_{mean} and SUV_{max} (r = −0.23, p < 0.05) was measured [64]. Due to its higher sensitivity ^{18}F-NaF-PET/CT performs better than BS, especially in pretreated patients. Dyrberg E et al. investigated the diagnostic accuracy of ^{68}Ga-PSMA PET/CT in comparison with a superior bone-seeking radiotracer ^{18}F-NaF-PET/CT and WB-MRI for the detection of bone metastases in patients with Pca. The patient-based sensitivity, specificity, overall accuracy were 100%, 100%, 100% for PSMA-PET/CT, 95%, 97%, 96% for ^{18}F-NaF-PET/CT and 80%, 83%, 82% for WB-MRI. The overall accuracy of PSMA-PET/CT was significantly more favorable compared to WB-MRI (p = 0.004), but not to NaF-PET/CT (p = 0.48) [65].

Fig. 9.6 A 76-year-old patient with PCa (Gleason score 4 + 5 and PSA levels of 30 ng/ml). (**a**) BS showed no evidence of metastases. He then underwent ^{68}Ga-PSMA-PET-CT imaging. (**b**) MIP PET images and (**c–d**) axial PET-CT fusion images showed increased uptake in prostate primary (SUVmax: 6) (arrows) and metastases at L4 vertebra (SUV_{max}: 10) with no findings on CT scan (arrow heads)

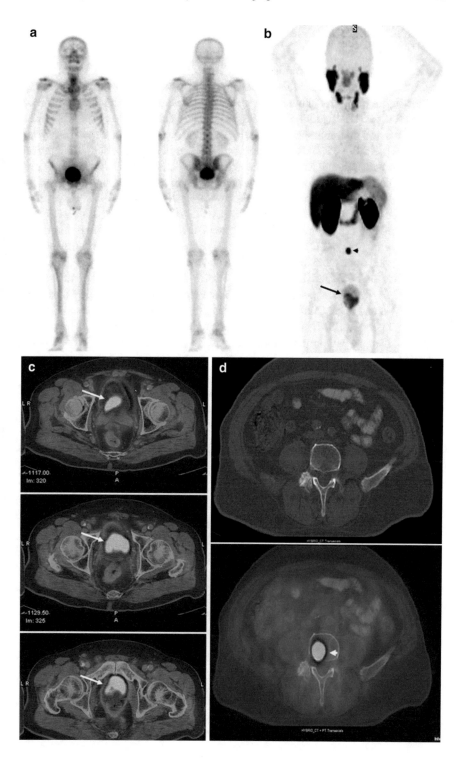

9.5   Recurrent Disease

Between 5 and 20% of men continue to have detectable or persistent PSA after RP. It may result from persistent local disease, pre-existing metastases, or residual benign prostate tissue [66]. Predictors of PSA persistence were higher BMI, higher preoperative PSA, and ISUP grade >3. BCR precedes clinical metastases, and CI modalities like BS and abdominopelvic CT/MRI has low sensitivity in this patient group (<14%) [67]. PSMA PET/CT provides an alternative diagnostic option for recurrent disease and EAU guideline recommends PSMA-PET/ CT if the PSA level is >0.2 ng/ml and if the results will influence subsequent treatment decisions. Several authors studied the value of PSMA-PET in recurrent disease (Fig. 9.7). Natarajan A et al. investigated the performance of ⁶⁸Ga-PSMA PET/CT in patients with BCR after definitive treatment. The median PSA of the positive scans was higher than that of the negative scans (6 vs. 1.7 ng/ml) (p = 0.001). In post-RP group, the detection rates were 23%, 50%, and 82% for PSA <1, 1–2, and >2 ng/ml, respectively. For post-RT, the detection was 86%, 85%, and 95% for PSA 2–5, 5.1–10, and >10 ng/ml, respectively. PSMA-PET/CT showed relapse in prostate/prostatic bed in 26 (27%) patients, nodal metastases in 50 (52%), skeletal metastases in 20 (21%), and other sites in 4 (4%) patients. ⁶⁸Ga-PSMA PET/CT detected nodal metastases in 52 (54%) patients while CT showed pathological nodes only in 27 (28%) patients [68] Sawicki LM

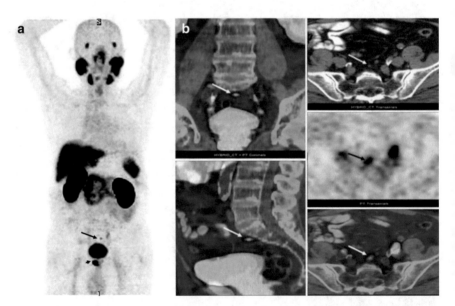

Fig. 9.7 A 78-year-old patient with PCa with recurrence after radiation therapy (Gleason score 4 + 5 and PSA levels of 5 ng/ml) underwent ⁶⁸Ga-PSMA-PET-CT. (**a**) MIP PET images showed, increased uptake in recurrent PCa in prostate (SUV$_{max}$: 6) (arrowhead) and presacral LN (SUVmax: 2) (arrow) (**b**) axial, sagital, coronal PET-CT fusion images showed increased radiotracer uptake in presacral LN with a size of 7 × 3 mm (arrows) which is below the criteria of positivity for CT

et al. compared WB-MRI for detection of BCR in comparison to ^{68}Ga-PSMA PET/CT in Pca patients after RP. ^{68}Ga-PSMA PET/CT detected 56 of 56 lesions (100%) in 20 patients (71.4%), while WB -MRI detected 13 lesions (23.2%) in 11 patients (39.3%). The higher detection rate with ^{68}Ga-PSMA PET/CT was statistically significant on both a per-lesion basis (p < 0.001) and a per-patient basis (p = 0.0167) [69]. Eiber M et al. investigated the detection rate of [68]Ga -PSMA PET/CT in patients with BCR after RP. PSMA-PET/CT detected pathologic findings in 222 (89.5%) patients. The detection rates were 96.8%, 93.0%, 72.7%, and 57.9% for PSA levels of ≥2, 1 to <2, 0.5 to <1, and 0.2 to <0.5 ng/ml, respectively. Whereas detection rates increased with a higher PSA velocity (81.8%, 82.4%, 92.1%, and 100% in <1, 1 to <2, 2 to <5, and ≥5 ng/ml/year, respectively), no significant association could be found for PSA doubling time (82.7%, 96.2%, and 90.7% in >6, 4–6, and <4 month, respectively). ^{68}Ga-PSMA ligand PET (as compared with CT) exclusively provided pathologic findings in 81 (32.7%) patients. In 61 (24.6%) patients, it exclusively identified additional involved regions. In higher Gleason score (≤7 vs. ≥8), detection efficacy was significantly increased (p = 0.0190). No significant difference in detection efficacy was present regarding ADT (p = 0.0783) [70] Ceci F et al. assessed the association between PSA-levels, PSA-kinetics and other factors and ^{68}Ga-PSMA-PET/CT scan in patients with recurrent PCa. PSMA-PET/CT was positive in 52 of 70 patients (74.2%). In 30 patients (42.8%) lesions limited to the pelvis were detected. Distant lesions were observed in 8 of patients (11.4%). Local plus systemic lesions were detected in 14 patients (20%). PSA level (p = 0.017) and PSAdt (p = 0.0001) were significantly different between PET-positive patients (higher PSA level,shorter PSAdt) and PET-negative patients (lower PSA,longer PSAdt). ROC analysis showed that PSAdt 6.5 months and PSA 0.83 ng/ml were optimal cut-off values. ^{68}Ga-PSMA PET/CT was positive in 17 of 20 patients (85%) with PSA < 2 ng/ml and PSAdt < 6.5 months, and in 3 of 16 patients (18.7%) with PSA < 2 ng/ml and PSAdt ≥ 6.5 months [71]. In the age of oligometastatic disease the tumor volume and accurate detection has become more critical, McCarthy M et al. assessed the utility of ^{68}Ga PSMA PET/CT compared with standard imaging, in the determination of oligometastatic disease recurrence and its distribution. In 199 patients with no lesions on restaging CT and BS, 148 patients (74%) demonstrated PSMA-positive lesions, with 113 patients (57%) being oligometastatic. In 39 patients with oligometastatic lesions on restaging CT and BS, 16 patients (41%) were upstaged to polymetastatic. The authors confirms that PSMA PET/CT is significantly more sensitive than standard restaging imaging, and it may be useful in identifying patients for subsequent targeted therapy [72]. ^{68}Ga-PSMA-11, is rapidly excreted into the urinary tract which leads to significant radioactivity in the bladder. Bladder activity may limit detection of local recurrence (LR) of Pca after RP, developing in close proximity to the bladder. Freitag MT et al. analyzed if there is additional value of mpMRI compared to the ^{68}Ga-PSMA-11-PET-component of PET/CT or PET/MRI to detect LR. 18/119 patients (15.1%) were diagnosed with a LR in mpMRI of PET/MRI but only nine were PET-positive in PET/CT and PET/MRI. This mismatch was statistically significant (p = 0.004). The detection of LR using the PET-component was significantly influenced by proximity to the bladder (p = 0.028) [73].

9.6 Clinical Impact

Although PSMA-PET had better detection rates than CI, whether this reflects a major impact on patient management is a matter of clinic and economic debate. Several studies showed the clinical impact of ^{68}Ga-PSMA-PET/CT in different clinical situations. In primary staging of patients with high-risk PCa, Hirmas N et al. showed that ^{68}Ga-PSMA PET/CT had a similar accuracy to MRI in detecting prostate lesions but a higher accuracy for suspicious pelvic LNs (95.2% vs. 80% for MRI and 75% for CT) and extra-pelvic LNs (100% vs. 75%), as well as bone lesions via BS (100% vs. 62.5%). This superiority of ^{68}Ga PSMA-PET/CT changed the management in 11 patients (52%) [74]. In a prospective multicenter study whether ^{68}Ga-PSMA PET/CT imaging affects management intent in patients with primary or recurrent prostate cancer was assessed. Overall, ^{68}Ga-PSMA-PET/CT scanning led to a change in planned management in 51% of patients. The impact was greater in the group of patients with BCR after definitive treatment (62% change) than in patients undergoing primary staging (21% change). Imaging with ^{68}Ga-PSMA-PET/CT revealed unsuspected disease in the prostate bed in 27%, locoregional lymph LNs in 39%, and distant metastatic disease in 16% of patients [75]. Rousseau C et al. in a prospective study (Clinicaltrial: NCT03443609), investigated the impact of ^{68}Ga-PSMA-11 PET-CT on the treatment plan and therapeutic response obtained for patients with PCa presenting a recurrence with a low rising PSA. ^{68}Ga-PSMA-11-positive lesions were detected in 38/52 (73.1%) patients. As a result of the PSMA-PET-CT, therapeutic management changed in 38/52 patients (73.1%). After treatment guided by ^{68}Ga-PSMA-11 PET-CT 10/52 (19.2%) cases had undetectable serum PSA levels and 18/52 (34.6%) patients had a PSA decrease of over 60% [76]. Impact of ^{68}Ga-PSMA-11 PET/CT in PCa patients in early PSA failure (PSA <0.5 ng/ml) after RP was also studied. ^{68}Ga-PSMA-11 PET/CT was found to be positive in 41 of the 119 (34.4%) patients and changed the intended treatment in 36 patients (30.2%). According to the PET/CT results, Salvage-RT was recommended in 70 patients (58.8%), only to the prostate bed in 58 (48.7%) and SBRT in 29 (24.4%). The intended RT planning was modified in 36 (87.8%) of 41 patients [77]. Finally in a systematic review and meta-analysis to evaluate the impact of ^{68}Ga-PSMA PET on management of patients with PCa. The pooled proportion of management changes was 54% by Han S et al. [78] Although the data that was described above showed the high clinical impact of PSMA-PET there is no randomized trial. The recent proPSMA trial is a prospective, multicentre study was organized to study; (1) The diagnostic performance of PSMA-PET compared with CI, (2) Management impact, and (3) Economic benefits if PSMA-PET/CT is incorporated into the management algorithm. The results of this trial will clarify the role of PSMA-PET in the clinical routine [79].

9.6.1 PSMA Guided Surgery

Large proportion of patients with BCR afterdefinitive primary local therapy have nodal recurrence in the pelvic alone and may be still available to local therapy such as RT and/or salvage LN dissection (sLND). sLND, in experienced hands may provide an increase in metastasis-free period and delay ADT. However CT/MRI lack enough sensitivity and accuracy for LN imaging and could not guide surgery. As described previously PSMA-PET is more accurate than CI in LN detection. [68]Ga PSMA-PET could guide the surgeons to the metastatic LNs. However especially in the salvage setting finding of metastatic LNs in a previously treated regions is difficult and outcome of SLND varies. Novel Tc-99m labeled radiotracers may provide intraoperative guidance by using gamma probe and lead to a more accurate resection. Maurer T et al. investigated the feasibility and short-term outcomes of ^{99m}Tc-based PSMA-radioguided surgery (^{99m}Tc-PSMA-RGS) for the removal of recurrent PCa lesions in 31 patients with Pca. On a specimen basis, radioactive rating yielded a sensitivity of 83.6%, a specificity of 100%, and an accuracy of 93.0%. With ^{99m}Tc-PSMA-RGS, all lesions visualized on preoperative ^{68}Ga-PSMA-11 PET could be removed. Moreover, ^{99m}Tc-PSMA-RGS detected additional metastases as small as 3 mm in two patients. A PSA reduction below 0.2 ng/ml was observed in 20 patients. Following salvage surgery, 41.9% of patients remained BCR-free (median follow-up:13.8 months) and 64.5% continued to be treatment free (median follow-up:12.2 months) [80]. Knipper et al. from Martinin-Klinik compared conventional surgical approach (CSA) and PSMA-radioguided surgery in patient groups with similar preoperative characteristics. In 29 patients, the dissection field was based solely ^{68}Ga-PSMA-PET imaging, whereas 13 patients underwent ^{99m}Tc-PSMA-RGS. Final pathology revealed no metastases in nine CSA patients (31%), whereas all visible lesions on preoperative ^{68}Ga-PSMA-PET were removed in patients who underwent RGS. A PSA decline in general, >50% and >90% within 6 weeks was seen in 50%, 29%, and 7% vs. 100%, 92%, and 53% in CSA versus RGS groups, respectively (all p < 0.01) [81]. Several prognostic factors were defined to predict the outcome of patients treated with PSMA-targeted RGS. Significantly longer median BCR free survival was observed in patients with a low preoperative PSA value (p = 0.004, HR: 1.48) and with a single lesion in preoperative PSMA-ligand PET (14.0 vs. 2.5 months, p = 0.002) [82].

9.6.2   PSMA-PET Imaging in Other Urological Cancers

PSMA was expressed in neovasculature of several tumors (Table 9.2). Among these tumors renal cell cancer (RCC) was the most promising tumor to be detected by PSMA-PET (Fig. 9.8). Increased neovascularization and low sensitivity of other tracers like FDG make PSMA-PET an alternative for molecular imaging. Raveennthiran S et al. published a case series of patients who received a ^{68}Ga-PSMA-PET/CT scan for staging or restaging of RCC. In the primary staging of 16 patients 75% showed avid primary lesions, with the majority of clear cell subtype. Management was changed in 43.8% of patients. Restaging scans were performed in 22 patients and ^{68}Ga-PSMA-PET/CT changed management in 40.9% of patients. Management was predominantly changed due to the identification of new sites of suspected metastases, as well as the detection of synchronous primaries that could not be detected by CI [36]. Meyer AR et al. investigated the utility of PSMA-targeted ^{18}F-DCFPyLPET/CT in patients with presumed oligometastatic clear cell RCC in a

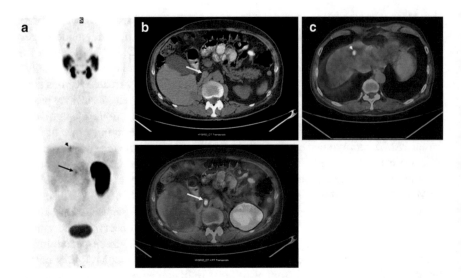

Fig. 9.8 A 55-year-old patient with RCC. The patient underwent ^{68}Ga-PSMA-PET-CT for restaging. (a) MIP PET images (b, c) axial PET-CT fusion images showed increased uptake in recurrent paracaval lesion at nephrectomy site (SUV$_{max}$: 6) (arrows) and in the liver lesion at segment 2 (SUVmax: 4) (arrow head)

clinical trial (ClinicalTrials.gov identifier NCT02687139). Oligometastatic clear cell RCC, defined as $\leq$3 metastatic lesions on CI. The detection rates of CI and ^{18}F-DCFPyL PET/CT for identifying sites of disease were 66.7% and 88.9%, respectively. Of the 21 metastatic lesions detected on CI, 17 (81.0%) had radiotracer uptake. In 4 (28.6%) patients a total of 12 more lesions were identified on ^{18}F-DCFPyL PET/CT than CI. Notably, 3 (21.4%) patients were no longer considered oligometastatic [83]. Although PSMA-PET was effective in RCC the success looks limited to clear cell type. Yin Y et al. investigated the utility of ^{18}F-DCFPyL PET/CT imaging for the detection of sites of disease in patients with metastatic non-clear cell RCC. Only 10 of the 73 lesions (13.7%) were classified as having definitive radiotracer uptake (median SUV$_{max}$=3.25, range=1.2–9.5), so unlike for clear cell RCC, the results of this study indicate that PSMA-based PET is not appropriate for imaging other RCC subtypes [84]. PSMA-PET was also used in imaging of urothelial carcinoma. Three patients with metastatic urothelial carcinoma were imaged ^{18}F-DCFPyL PET/CT allowed for the detection of sites of urothelial carcinoma, albeit with low levels of radiotracer uptake. The relatively low expression of PSMA by urothelial carcinoma likely limits the utility of PSMA-targeted PET imaging of this malignancy [85].

Conclusion PSMA-based imaging has become the imaging modality of choice in patients with Pca. When performed with PET-MRI hybrid devices it can provide an one-stop-shop imaging of Pca. It has high clinical impact and changed management of over 54% of patients predominantly in the recurrence setting. The results of the ongoing clinical trials will further establish the role of PSMA based imaging in the clinical routine.

References

1. Siegel RL, Miller KD, Jemal A. Cancer statistics, 2019. CA Cancer J Clin. 2019;69(1):7–34.
2. Mohler JL, Antonarakis ES, Armstrong AJ, D'Amico AV, Davis BJ, Dorff T, et al. Prostate cancer, version 2.2019, NCCN clinical practice guidelines in oncology. J Natl Compr Cancer Netw. 2019;17(5):479–505.
3. Kasivisvanathan V, Rannikko AS, Borghi M, Panebianco V, Mynderse LA, Vaarala MH, et al. MRI-targeted or standard biopsy for prostate-cancer diagnosis. N Engl J Med. 2018;378(19):1767–77.
4. Rouviere O, Puech P, Renard-Penna R, Claudon M, Roy C, Mege-Lechevallier F, et al. Use of prostate systematic and targeted biopsy on the basis of multiparametric MRI in biopsy-naive patients (MRI-FIRST): a prospective, multicentre, paired diagnostic study. Lancet Oncol. 2019;20(1):100–9.
5. van der Leest M, Cornel E, Israel B, Hendriks R, Padhani AR, Hoogenboom M, et al. Head-to-head comparison of transrectal ultrasound-guided prostate biopsy versus multiparametric prostate resonance imaging with subsequent magnetic resonance-guided biopsy in biopsy-naive men with elevated prostate-specific antigen: a large prospective multicenter clinical study. Eur Urol. 2019;75(4):570–8.
6. von Eyben FE, Picchio M, von Eyben R, Rhee H, Bauman G. (68)Ga-labeled prostate-specific membrane antigen ligand positron emission tomography/computed tomography for prostate cancer: a systematic review and meta-analysis. Eur Urol Focus. 2018;4(5):686–93.
7. Fraum TJ, Ludwig DR, Kim EH, Schroeder P, Hope TA, Ippolito JE. Prostate cancer PET tracers: essentials for the urologist. Can J Urol. 2018;25(4):9371–83.
8. Ghosh A, Heston WD. Tumor target prostate specific membrane antigen (PSMA) and its regulation in prostate cancer. J Cell Biochem. 2004;91(3):528–39.
9. Silver DA, Pellicer I, Fair WR, Heston WD, Cordon-Cardo C. Prostate-specific membrane antigen expression in normal and malignant human tissues. Clin Cancer Res. 1997;3(1):81–5.
10. Krohn T, Verburg FA, Pufe T, Neuhuber W, Vogg A, Heinzel A, et al. [(68)Ga]PSMA-HBED uptake mimicking lymph node metastasis in coeliac ganglia: an important pitfall in clinical practice. Eur J Nucl Med Mol Imaging. 2015;42(2):210–4.
11. Hofman MS, Hicks RJ, Maurer T, Eiber M. Prostate-specific membrane antigen pet: clinical utility in prostate cancer, normal patterns, pearls, and pitfalls. Radiographics. 2018;38(1):200–17.
12. Wright GL Jr, Haley C, Beckett ML, Schellhammer PF. Expression of prostate-specific membrane antigen in normal, benign, and malignant prostate tissues. Urol Oncol. 1995;1(1):18–28.
13. Perner S, Hofer MD, Kim R, Shah RB, Li H, Moller P, et al. Prostate-specific membrane antigen expression as a predictor of prostate cancer progression. Hum Pathol. 2007;38(5):696–701.
14. Evans MJ, Smith-Jones PM, Wongvipat J, Navarro V, Kim S, Bander NH, et al. Noninvasive measurement of androgen receptor signaling with a positron-emitting radiopharmaceutical that targets prostate-specific membrane antigen. Proc Natl Acad Sci U S A. 2011;108(23):9578–82.
15. Minner S, Wittmer C, Graefen M, Salomon G, Steuber T, Haese A, et al. High level PSMA expression is associated with early PSA recurrence in surgically treated prostate cancer. Prostate. 2011;71(3):281–8.
16. Epstein JI, Egevad L, Amin MB, Delahunt B, Srigley JR, Humphrey PA, et al. The 2014 international society of urological pathology (ISUP) consensus conference on gleason grading of prostatic carcinoma: definition of grading patterns and proposal for a new grading system. Am J Surg Pathol. 2016;40(2):244–52.
17. Bakht MK, Derecichei I, Li Y, Ferraiuolo RM, Dunning M, Oh SW, et al. Neuroendocrine differentiation of prostate cancer leads to PSMA suppression. Endocr Relat Cancer. 2018;26(2):131–46.
18. Bronsert P, Reichel K, Ruf J. Loss of PSMA expression in non-neuroendocrine dedifferentiated acinar prostate cancer. Clin Nucl Med. 2018;43(7):526–8.

19. Meller B, Bremmer F, Sahlmann CO, Hijazi S, Bouter C, Trojan L, et al. Alterations in andro-gen deprivation enhanced prostate-specific membrane antigen (PSMA) expression in prostate cancer cells as a target for diagnostics and therapy. EJNMMI Res. 2015;5(1):66.
20. Hope TA, Truillet C, Ehman EC, Afshar-Oromieh A, Aggarwal R, Ryan CJ, et al. 68Ga-PSMA-11 PET imaging of response to androgen receptor inhibition: first human experi-ence. J Nucl Med. 2017;58(1):81–4.
21. Chang SS, Reuter VE, Heston WD, Bander NH, Grauer LS, Gaudin PB. Five different anti-prostate-specific membrane antigen (PSMA) antibodies confirm PSMA expression in tumor-associated neovasculature. Cancer Res. 1999;59(13):3192–8.
22. Salas Fragomeni RA, Amir T, Sheikhbahaei S, Harvey SC, Javadi MS, Solnes LB, et al. Imaging of nonprostate cancers using PSMA-targeted radiotracers: rationale, current state of the field, and a call to arms. J Nucl Med. 2018;59(6):871–7.
23. Sheikhbahaei S, Werner RA, Solnes LB, Pienta KJ, Pomper MG, Gorin MA, et al. Prostate-specific membrane antigen (PSMA)-targeted PET imaging of prostate cancer: an update on important pitfalls. Semin Nucl Med. 2019;49(4):255–70.
24. Dias AH, Bouchelouche K. Prostate-specific membrane antigen PET/CT incidental finding of a schwannoma. Clin Nucl Med. 2018;43(4):267–8.
25. Passah A, Arora S, Damle NA, Tripathi M, Bal C, Subudhi TK, et al. 68Ga-prostate-specific membrane antigen PET/CT in triple-negative breast cancer. Clin Nucl Med. 2018;43(6):460–1.
26. Sathekge M, Lengana T, Modiselle M, Vorster M, Zeevaart J, Maes A, et al. (68)Ga-PSMA-HBED-CC PET imaging in breast carcinoma patients. Eur J Nucl Med Mol Imaging. 2017;44(4):689–94.
27. Bourgeois S, Gykiere P, Goethals L, Everaert H, De Geeter FW. Aspecific uptake of 68GA-PSMA in paget disease of the bone. Clin Nucl Med. 2016;41(11):877–8.
28. Verma P, Malhotra G, Agrawal R, Sonavane S, Meshram V, Asopa RV. Evidence of prostate-specific membrane antigen expression in metastatic differentiated thyroid cancer using 68Ga-PSMA-HBED-CC PET/CT. Clin Nucl Med. 2018;43(8):e265–e8.
29. Castello A, Lopci E. Incidental identification of osteoid osteoma by (68)Ga-PSMA PET/CT. Eur J Nucl Med Mol Imaging. 2018;45(3):509–10.
30. Hangaard L, Jochumsen MR, Vendelbo MH, Bouchelouche K. Metastases from colorectal cancer avid on 68Ga-PSMA PET/CT. Clin Nucl Med. 2017;42(7):532–3.
31. Reale ML, Buttigliero C, Tucci M, Giardino R, Poti C. 68Ga-PSMA uptake in fibrous dyspla-sia. Clin Nucl Med. 2019;44(6):e396–e7.
32. Sasikumar A, Kashyap R, Joy A, Charan Patro K, Bhattacharya P, Reddy Pilaka VK, et al. Utility of 68Ga-PSMA-11 PET/CT in imaging of glioma—a pilot study. Clin Nucl Med. 2018;43(9):e304–e9.
33. Peper JGK, Srbljin S, van der Zant FM, Knol RJJ, Wondergem M. High 18Fluor-DCFPyL uptake in adrenal adenomas. Clin Nucl Med. 2017;42(11):862–4.
34. Perez PM, Flavell RR, Kelley RK, Umetsu S, Behr SC. Heterogeneous uptake of 18F-FDG and 68Ga-PSMA-11 in hepatocellular carcinoma. Clin Nucl Med. 2019;44(3):e133–e5.
35. Bhardwaj H, Stephens M, Bhatt M, Thomas PA. Prostate-specific membrane antigen PET/CT findings for hepatic hemangioma. Clin Nucl Med. 2016;41(12):968–9.
36. Raveenthiran S, Esler R, Yaxley J, Kyle S. The use of (68)Ga-PET/CT PSMA in the stag-ing of primary and suspected recurrent renal cell carcinoma. Eur J Nucl Med Mol Imaging. 2019;46(11):2280–8.
37. Stephens M, Kim DI, Shepherd B, Gustafson S, Thomas P. Intense uptake in amyloidosis of the seminal vesicles on 68Ga-PSMA PET mimicking locally advanced prostate cancer. Clin Nucl Med. 2017;42(2):147–8.
38. Malik D, Kumar R, Mittal BR, Singh H, Bhattacharya A, Sood A, et al. (68)Ga-labelled PSMA (prostate specific membrane antigen) expression in signet-ring cell gastric carcinoma. Eur J Nucl Med Mol Imaging. 2018;45(7):1276–7.
39. Cardinale J, Schafer M, Benesova M, Bauder-Wust U, Leotta K, Eder M, et al. Preclinical evaluation of (18)F-PSMA-1007, a new prostate-specific membrane antigen ligand for pros-tate cancer imaging. J Nucl Med. 2017;58(3):425–31.

40. Rahbar K, Afshar-Oromieh A, Seifert R, Wagner S, Schafers M, Bogemann M, et al. Diagnostic performance of (18)F-PSMA-1007 PET/CT in patients with biochemical recurrent prostate cancer. Eur J Nucl Med Mol Imaging. 2018;45(12):2055–61.
41. Zamboglou C, Schiller F, Fechter T, Wieser G, Jilg CA, Chirindel A, et al. (68)Ga-HBED-CC-PSMA PET/CT versus histopathology in primary localized prostate cancer: a voxel-wise comparison. Theranostics. 2016;6(10):1619–28.
42. Woythal N, Arsenic R, Kempkensteffen C, Miller K, Janssen JC, Huang K, et al. Immunohistochemical validation of PSMA expression measured by (68)Ga-PSMA PET/CT in primary prostate cancer. J Nucl Med. 2018;59(2):238–43.
43. Rowe SP, Pienta KJ, Pomper MG, Gorin MA. PSMA-RADS version 1.0: a step towards standardizing the interpretation and reporting of PSMA-targeted PET imaging studies. Eur Urol. 2018;73(4):485–7.
44. Eiber M, Herrmann K, Calais J, Hadaschik B, Giesel FL, Hartenbach M, et al. Prostate cancer molecular imaging standardized evaluation (PROMISE): proposed miTNM classification for the interpretation of PSMA-ligand PET/CT. J Nucl Med. 2018;59(3):469–78.
45. Uprimny C, Kroiss AS, Decristoforo C, Fritz J, von Guggenberg E, Kendler D, et al. (68)Ga-PSMA-11 PET/CT in primary staging of prostate cancer: PSA and Gleason score predict the intensity of tracer accumulation in the primary tumour. Eur J Nucl Med Mol Imaging. 2017;44(6):941–9.
46. Fendler WP, Schmidt DF, Wenter V, Thierfelder KM, Zach C, Stief C, et al. 68Ga-PSMA PET/CT detects the location and extent of primary prostate cancer. J Nucl Med. 2016;57(11):1720–5.
47. Kalapara AA, Nzenza T, Pan HY, Ballok Z, Ramdave S, O'Sullivan R, et al. Detection and localisation of primary prostate cancer using (68) Ga-PSMA PET/CT compared with mpMRI and radical prostatectomy specimens. BJU Int. 2019;126(1):83–90.
48. Bettermann AS, Zamboglou C, Kiefer S, Jilg CA, Spohn S, Kranz-Rudolph J, et al. [(68)Ga-]PSMA-11 PET/CT and multiparametric MRI for gross tumor volume delineation in a slice by slice analysis with whole mount histopathology as a reference standard—implications for focal radiotherapy planning in primary prostate cancer. Radiother Oncol. 2019;141:214–9.
49. Zhang J, Shao S, Wu P, Liu D, Yang B, Han D, et al. Diagnostic performance of (68)Ga-PSMA PET/CT in the detection of prostate cancer prior to initial biopsy: comparison with cancer-predicting nomograms. Eur J Nucl Med Mol Imaging. 2019;46(4):908–20.
50. von Klot CJ, Merseburger AS, Boker A, Schmuck S, Ross TL, Bengel FM, et al. (68)Ga-PSMA PET/CT imaging predicting intraprostatic tumor extent, extracapsular extension and seminal vesicle invasion prior to radical prostatectomy in patients with prostate cancer. Nucl Med Mol Imaging. 2017;51(4):314–22.
51. Gabriele D, Collura D, Oderda M, Stura I, Fiorito C, Porpiglia F, et al. Is there still a role for computed tomography and bone scintigraphy in prostate cancer staging? An analysis from the EUREKA-1 database. World J Urol. 2016;34(4):517–23.
52. Kiss B, Thoeny HC, Studer UE. Current status of lymph node imaging in bladder and prostate cancer. Urology. 2016;96:1–7.
53. Thoeny HC, Froehlich JM, Triantafyllou M, Huesler J, Bains LJ, Vermathen P, et al. Metastases in normal-sized pelvic lymph nodes: detection with diffusion-weighted MR imaging. Radiology. 2014;273(1):125–35.
54. van Leeuwen PJ, Emmett L, Ho B, Delprado W, Ting F, Nguyen Q, et al. Prospective evaluation of 68Gallium-prostate-specific membrane antigen positron emission tomography/computed tomography for preoperative lymph node staging in prostate cancer. BJU Int. 2017;119(2):209–15.
55. Maurer T, Gschwend JE, Rauscher I, Souvatzoglou M, Haller B, Weirich G, et al. Diagnostic efficacy of (68)Gallium-PSMA positron emission tomography compared to conventional imaging for lymph node staging of 130 consecutive patients with intermediate to high risk prostate cancer. J Urol. 2016;195(5):1436–43.
56. Petersen LJ, Nielsen JB, Langkilde NC, Petersen A, Afshar-Oromieh A, De Souza NM, et al. (68)Ga-PSMA PET/CT compared with MRI/CT and diffusion-weighted MRI for primary

lymph node staging prior to definitive radiotherapy in prostate cancer: a prospective diagnostic test accuracy study. World J Urol. 2019;38(4):939–48.

57. Meyrick DP, Asokendaran M, Skelly LA, Lenzo NP, Henderson A. The role of 68Ga-PSMA-I&T PET/CT in the pretreatment staging of primary prostate cancer. Nucl Med Commun. 2017;38(11):956–63.

58. Thalgott M, Duwel C, Rauscher I, Heck MM, Haller B, Gafita A, et al. One-stop-shop whole-body (68)Ga-PSMA-11 PET/MRI compared with clinical nomograms for preoperative T and N staging of high-risk prostate cancer. J Nucl Med. 2018;59(12):1850–6.

59. Koerber SA, Stach G, Kratochwil C, Haefner MF, Rathke H, Herfarth K, et al. Lymph node involvement in treatment-naive prostate cancer patients—correlation of PSMA-PET/CT imaging and Roach formula in 280 men in the Radiotherapeutic management. J Nucl Med. 2019;61(1):46–50.

60. Shen G, Deng H, Hu S, Jia Z. Comparison of choline-PET/CT, MRI, SPECT, and bone scintigraphy in the diagnosis of bone metastases in patients with prostate cancer: a meta-analysis. Skelet Radiol. 2014;43(11):1503–13.

61. Abuzallouf S, Dayes I, Lukka H. Baseline staging of newly diagnosed prostate cancer: a summary of the literature. J Urol. 2004;171(6 Pt 1):2122–7.

62. Pyka T, Okamoto S, Dahlbender M, Tauber R, Retz M, Heck M, et al. Comparison of bone scintigraphy and (68)Ga-PSMA PET for skeletal staging in prostate cancer. Eur J Nucl Med Mol Imaging. 2016;43(12):2114–21.

63. Tuncel M, Souvatzoglou M, Herrmann K, Stollfuss J, Schuster T, Weirich G, et al. [(11)C]Choline positron emission tomography/computed tomography for staging and restaging of patients with advanced prostate cancer. Nucl Med Biol. 2008;35(6):689–95.

64. Janssen JC, Woythal N, Meissner S, Prasad V, Brenner W, Diederichs G, et al. [(68)Ga]PSMA-HBED-CC uptake in osteolytic, osteoblastic, and bone marrow metastases of prostate cancer patients. Mol Imaging Biol. 2017;19(6):933–43.

65. Dyrberg E, Hendel HW, Huynh THV, Klausen TW, Logager VB, Madsen C, et al. (68)Ga-PSMA-PET/CT in comparison with (18)F-fluoride-PET/CT and whole-body MRI for the detection of bone metastases in patients with prostate cancer: a prospective diagnostic accuracy study. Eur Radiol. 2019;29(3):1221–30.

66. Wiegel T, Bartkowiak D, Bottke D, Thamm R, Hinke A, Stockle M, et al. Prostate-specific antigen persistence after radical prostatectomy as a predictive factor of clinical relapse-free survival and overall survival: 10-year data of the ARO 96-02 trial. Int J Radiat Oncol Biol Phys. 2015;91(2):288–94.

67. Beresford MJ, Gillatt D, Benson RJ, Ajithkumar T. A systematic review of the role of imaging before salvage radiotherapy for post-prostatectomy biochemical recurrence. Clin Oncol (R Coll Radiol). 2010;22(1):46–55.

68. Natarajan A, Agrawal A, Murthy V, Bakshi G, Joshi A, Purandare N, et al. Initial experience of Ga-68 prostate-specific membrane antigen positron emission tomography/computed tomography imaging in evaluation of biochemical recurrence in prostate cancer patients. World J Nucl Med. 2019;18(3):244–50.

69. Sawicki LM, Kirchner J, Buddensieck C, Antke C, Ullrich T, Schimmoller L, et al. Prospective comparison of whole-body MRI and (68)Ga-PSMA PET/CT for the detection of biochemical recurrence of prostate cancer after radical prostatectomy. Eur J Nucl Med Mol Imaging. 2019;46(7):1542–50.

70. Eiber M, Maurer T, Souvatzoglou M, Beer AJ, Ruffani A, Haller B, et al. Evaluation of hybrid (6)(8)Ga-PSMA Ligand PET/CT in 248 patients with biochemical recurrence after radical prostatectomy. J Nucl Med. 2015;56(5):668–74.

71. Ceci F, Uprimny C, Nilica B, Geraldo L, Kendler D, Kroiss A, et al. (68)Ga-PSMA PET/CT for restaging recurrent prostate cancer: which factors are associated with PET/CT detection rate? Eur J Nucl Med Mol Imaging. 2015;42(8):1284–94.

72. McCarthy M, Francis R, Tang C, Watts J, Campbell A. A multicenter prospective clinical trial of (68)Gallium PSMA HBED-CC PET-CT restaging in biochemically relapsed prostate

carcinoma: oligometastatic rate and distribution compared with standard imaging. Int J Radiat Oncol Biol Phys. 2019;104(4):801–8.
73. Freitag MT, Radtke JP, Afshar-Oromieh A, Roethke MC, Hadaschik BA, Gleave M, et al. Local recurrence of prostate cancer after radical prostatectomy is at risk to be missed in (68) Ga-PSMA-11-PET of PET/CT and PET/MRI: comparison with mpMRI integrated in simultaneous PET/MRI. Eur J Nucl Med Mol Imaging. 2017;44(5):776–87.
74. Hirmas N, Al-Ibraheem A, Herrmann K, Alsharif A, Muhsin H, Khader J, et al. [(68)Ga]PSMA PET/CT improves initial staging and management plan of patients with high-risk prostate cancer. Mol Imaging Biol. 2019;21(3):574–81.
75. Roach PJ, Francis R, Emmett L, Hsiao E, Kneebone A, Hruby G, et al. The impact of (68) Ga-PSMA PET/CT on management intent in prostate cancer: results of an Australian prospective multicenter study. J Nucl Med. 2018;59(1):82–8.
76. Rousseau C, Le Thiec M, Ferrer L, Rusu D, Rauscher A, Maucherat B, et al. Preliminary results of a (68) Ga-PSMA PET/CT prospective study in prostate cancer patients with occult recurrence: diagnostic performance and impact on therapeutic decision-making. Prostate. 2019;79(13):1514–22.
77. Farolfi A, Ceci F, Castellucci P, Graziani T, Siepe G, Lambertini A, et al. (68)Ga-PSMA-11 PET/CT in prostate cancer patients with biochemical recurrence after radical prostatectomy and PSA <0.5 ng/ml. Efficacy and impact on treatment strategy. Eur J Nucl Med Mol Imaging. 2019;46(1):11–9.
78. Han S, Woo S, Kim YJ, Suh CH. Impact of (68)Ga-PSMA PET on the management of patients with prostate cancer: a systematic review and meta-analysis. Eur Urol. 2018;74(2):179–90.
79. Hofman MS, Murphy DG, Williams SG, Nzenza T, Herschtal A, Lourenco RA, et al. A prospective randomized multicentre study of the impact of gallium-68 prostate-specific membrane antigen (PSMA) PET/CT imaging for staging high-risk prostate cancer prior to curative-intent surgery or radiotherapy (proPSMA study): clinical trial protocol. BJU Int. 2018;122(5):783–93.
80. Maurer T, Robu S, Schottelius M, Schwamborn K, Rauscher I, van den Berg NS, et al. (99m) Technetium-based prostate-specific membrane antigen-radioguided surgery in recurrent prostate cancer. Eur Urol. 2019;75(4):659–66.
81. Knipper S, Tilki D, Mansholt J, Berliner C, Bernreuther C, Steuber T, et al. Metastases-yield and prostate-specific antigen kinetics following salvage lymph node dissection for prostate cancer: a comparison between conventional surgical approach and prostate-specific membrane antigen-radioguided surgery. Eur Urol Focus. 2019;5(1):50–3.
82. Horn T, Kronke M, Rauscher I, Haller B, Robu S, Wester HJ, et al. Single lesion on prostate-specific membrane antigen-ligand positron emission tomography and low prostate-specific antigen are prognostic factors for a favorable biochemical response to prostate-specific membrane antigen-targeted radioguided surgery in recurrent prostate cancer. Eur Urol. 2019;76(4):517–23.
83. Meyer AR, Carducci MA, Denmeade SR, Markowski MC, Pomper MG, Pierorazio PM, et al. Improved identification of patients with oligometastatic clear cell renal cell carcinoma with PSMA-targeted (18)F-DCFPyL PET/CT. Ann Nucl Med. 2019;33(8):617–23.
84. Yin Y, Campbell SP, Markowski MC, Pierorazio PM, Pomper MG, Allaf ME, et al. Inconsistent detection of sites of metastatic non-clear cell renal cell carcinoma with PSMA-targeted [(18)F]DCFPyL PET/CT. Mol Imaging Biol. 2019;21(3):567–73.
85. Campbell SP, Baras AS, Ball MW, Kates M, Hahn NM, Bivalacqua TJ, et al. Low levels of PSMA expression limit the utility of (18)F-DCFPyL PET/CT for imaging urothelial carcinoma. Ann Nucl Med. 2018;32(1):69–74.

Part III
Latest Visualization and Surgical Planning Tools

Chapter 10
Introduction and Taxonomy

Giovanni E. Cacciamani, Daniele Amparore, and Domenico Veneziano

10.1 Introduction

In the era of management of uro-oncological diseases with "precision surgery", a great revolution has been done in the field of image guidance. New scenarios are opening every day, thanks to the new technological advances that allow urologist to abandon the concept of the "one for anyone" in favour to the "patient tailored fit" treatments. New technologies that are becoming day-by day part of our daily practice need a correct denomination, in order to identify the best tool for each patient [1].

10.2 3D Rendering in Urology

"*3D rendering* is a digital synthesis of a computer-aided design (*CAD*) model that can be visualized on screen and is rotatable and zoomable upon user's preference. It is often interactive and allows removal of some portions of the model for optimized visualization" [1]. With the magnification of 3D vision allowed by the introduction of robotic technology, the need for an upgrade of the standard bi-dimensional

---

G. E. Cacciamani
Department of Urology, Catherine and Joseph Aresty, USC Institute of Urology, Keck School of Medicine, USC/Norris Comprehensive Cancer Center, Los Angeles, CA, USA

Department of Radiology, University of Southern California, Los Angeles, CA, USA

D. Amparore
Division of Urology, Department of Oncology, School of Medicine, San Luigi Hospital, University of Turin, Orbassano, Turin, Italy

D. Veneziano (✉)
Grande Ospedale Metropolitano, Reggio Calabria, Italy

© Springer Nature Switzerland AG 2021
E. Huri, D. Veneziano (eds.), *Anatomy for Urologic Surgeons in the Digital Era*,
https://doi.org/10.1007/978-3-030-59479-4_10

imaging brought to the development of new technological advances, such as 3D models automatically rendered via radiological software [2]. The availability of consultable three-dimensional models of the organs to operate, allowed the surgeon to modulate each surgery specifically for the patient. This new tool found application in different scenarios, from surgical planning to intraoperative assistance and patients counselling. Kidney and prostate cancer have been the most widely investigated urological diseases for this field of research, given their well-depictable margins that allow easier tracking by the software.

In order to improve the quality of rendered 3D models, a standardization in the field of three-dimensional reconstruction has been recently published. Thanks to the teamwork among urologist, radiologist and the new figure of the bio-engineer, together with the use of new dedicated professional software, "high-definition" reconstructions have been developed, named hyper-accuracy 3D virtual models (HA3D) [3]. Technically, the new generation 3D virtual models are obtained from standard CT-scan or mp-MRI (for kidney and prostate HA3D virtual models respectively). The images in DICOM format are processed using a set of different software authorized for medical use. At first, the four-phase CT-scan images are evaluated by the bio-engineer using a DICOM viewer. The first segmentation process is performed semi-automatically (similarly to the old rendering process). The three-dimensional reconstructions are then refined by the biomedical engineer under the supervision of an experienced urologist, using a contour-based method. For the kidney, the refining of the bi-dimensional enhanced four-phases CT images is focused on the renal vasculature up to the segmental intrarenal vessels (both arterial and venous), collecting system, kidney shape, and tumour features. For the prostate, the virtual reconstruction involves the prostate gland, the urethra and the urethral sphincter, the neurovascular bundles (NVBs), and the tumour, as identified by the different mp-MRI sequences. After embedding those different datasets, the virtual reconstructions are converted into a mathematical HA3D model, a transcription code for the visualization of the HA3D reconstruction in an interactive 3D-PDF format, which makes each single structure removable. This allows the understanding of the relationships among the tumour and the other components of the organ. Looking at the experiences already published in Literature on this topic, 3D virtual models have been tested in many different settings. The aid given by the 3D virtual models in easing the decision-making process by the surgeon during the preoperative planning is reported by different experiences. Irrespectively from the technique of virtual reconstruction used, the advantages given by the availability of a three-dimensional image of the organ to treat, allows the surgeon to avoid the building-in-mind process necessary to understand the spatial distribution of the target structures. This different perspective in evaluating the relationships among each single part of the organ to treat, can favour a change of the surgical strategy (i.e. the clamping strategy during robotic partial nephrectomy) but also the surgical indication (i.e. from radical to partial approach in case of complex renal tumours) [3].

Notwithstanding the improvements given by 3D virtual models in comparison with the standard bi-dimensional imaging, their consultation is often performed on common 2D flat supports, with limitations regarding the fine perception of the space depth and of some details enhanced by 3D view. To overcome these limitations, their visualization is nowadays performable also via holograms in the real-world environment (mixed reality). The Literature experiences on this topic are still anecdotal, especially for robotics, but underline the potential improvements for the surgeon in perceiving details of the structures of interest, while increasing surgical planning quality [4]. Concerning the intraoperative assistance of the 3D virtual models, only few experiences are currently available; notwithstanding the small number of papers published in Literature, there is unanimous opinion in recognizing their aid to the surgeon during the intervention both in kidney and prostate oncologic surgery. The most explored field of research is their application in cognitive procedures, during whom the 3D virtual model can be consulted "on demand" via laptops or tablets. The availability of a 3D virtual reconstruction of the organ undergoing surgery, allows to have a comprehensive understanding of the anatomy, thus enabling a more detailed planning. This can be easily understandable by thinking to the identification of the vascular anatomy of the kidney: during the renal pedicle dissection, with the aid given by 3D imaging, it is possible to perform a remote navigation and identify the direction of the segmental vessels, in order to set a selective clamping [3]. Moreover, such technology finds a role in prostate cancer surgery: during the NVBs management, the availability of a 3D virtual model showing the area of suspicious capsular involvement by the tumour, allows to modulate the depth of bundles' dissection [5].

10.3 3D Printing in Urology

"*3D printing*, also called additive manufacturing, is a process that builds a physical object by adding material layer-by-layer, starting from a CAD model" [1]. 3D-printing deeply impacted medicine in the last decade. It has been used to pattern cells, create prototypes, replicate tissues or organs, to create surgical replicas for planning, counselling and training and finally to build medical prosthetics and in numerous other biomedical applications [6]. Numerous types of technologies have been created in order to enable the production of 3D objects with different printable materials, ranging from different types of polymers, ceramics, wax, metals to human cells [7]. It has been shown that patients counselling, surgical planning and training have been impacted by 3D-prinitng. 3D-printed anatomical models for surgical planning have a wide array of applications in the hospital inpatient setting and have been demonstrated to be a game-changer in the field of surgical simulation. Especially in urology, simulation-based training is being progressively used for trainees in order to reduce steepest learning curves for the acquisition of surgical skills and 3D-printing represents unique tool for the direct "printing" of organ structures making possible a standardization of the training. Moreover, several studies have shown that 3D-printing of anatomical models can be used by Urologist to create a more accurate and tactile picture, to support in preoperative planning and surgical education [8]. Drawbacks of this technology are represented by the high costs and long timing in manufacturing [6].

10.4   Extended Reality in Urology

The videogaming field opened way in the last decade to a series of different con-sumer tools to allow immersion in a different environment. This possibility started to be experimentally applied to surgery as well, in order to enhance planning or to allow better understanding of a procedure with educational purpose. We are talking about the so-called Extended Reality technologies, including Virtual Reality (VR), Augmented Reality (AR) and Mixed Reality (MR).

"*Virtual reality (VR)*: creates a digital environment that replaces the user's real-world environment. It relies on a visor to provide an immersive experience to the user" [1].

After early testing in the field of entertainment with poor success, the conver-gence and *demonetization* of technologies like high-definition screens, motion and position sensors and advanced graphic boards allowed the development of low-cost, yet highly performing visors, like the Oculus Rift (Oculus VR, Menlo Park, California, U.S) or the HTC Vive (HTC, Taoyuan, Taiwan). With prices ranging down to around USD250 the Oculus Go allows today to enjoy the full experience of VR in any environment, thus bringing three-dimensional CAD visualization to another level, for everyone. In Urology the use of VR systems is still limited, prob-ably due to the poor knowledge about these latest products available and is mostly applied to training. As an example, Intuitive Surgical (Sunnyvale, California, United States) is using VR within its Backpack trainer on the Da Vinci platforms, to simu-late training environments, while companies like VirtaMed (Schlieren, Swiss), Surgical Science (Göteborg, Sweden) and Medical-X (Rotterdam, the Netherlands) are using this technology for their surgical simulators, but without any support for VR visors. At last, some limited evidence exists about other potential applications of 3D virtual models, like education/training and patient counselling. Literature suggests that three-dimensional imaging could be helpful in the surgical strategy comprehension and learning by young urologists, as well as in enhancing the dia-logue with patients, giving them a direct perception of the disease and its treatment, but their role is still under scrutiny [9].

"*Augmented Reality (AR)* overlays digitally-created content into the user's real-world environment. Visors, smartphones or tablets provide a spatial registration that may enable geometric persistence concerning placement and orientation within the real world [1]".

AR applications are well established in the computing and gaming world, and are now entering the surgical mainstream too. Being the AR technology based on the concept of image alignment and/or superimposition, it is considerable for sure a fruitful field of research, but it is burdened at the same time by a high technical complexity that limits its development.

In fact, together with the availability of a platform to perform the overlay, a tracking of the surgical instruments, as well as the tracking of any motion of the targeted organs and surrounding anatomies, is necessary. The wide use of Intuitive Da Vinci systems with 3D visors embedded in their console, allowed to easily run early testing of AR applied to the operative field. Some feasibility studies have been attempted for both robotic partial nephrectomy and radical prostatectomy [10, 11]. All the studies performed were focused on the capability of such technology in organ/tumour targeting. Notwithstanding the technologies developed for obtaining the AR surgery differed study by study, all demonstrated at least a rudimental efficacy in driving the surgeon for the identification of the structures of interest. If we consider the importance of millimetric guidance in order to avoid unwanted complication, it is easy to understand how this can still be today a huge limitation to the widespread of such a technology. However, being the AR setting the current most attractive field of application of the 3D virtual models, great technical steps forward have been made in the last few years, refining the first prototypes. The next goal is to demonstrate, together with the feasibility, their clinical applications.

"*Hologram*: is a representation of a CAD model that appears to be three-dimensional to the naked eye, with no need for a supplementary headset. It can be visible by different users at the same time and from different angles with proper spatial registration" [1]. Holograms are an evolution of AR, as they don't require any visor, as previously stated. They can be today created thanks to specifically engineered displays, which can even provide touch feedback to the user via ultrasonic air blast (touchable holograms) [12]. Even if this technology has no application in Urology yet, it might be useful to perform surgical planning along the procedure, without any physical display to be touched by the surgeon and with the possibility to discuss the plan together with the rest of the surgical team, in real-time.

"*Mixed reality (MR)*: an experience that seamlessly blends the user's real-world environment and digitally-created content, where both environments can coexist and interact with each other. MR anchors digital objects to real-world objects and enables interaction with them. To produce it, a visor with environmental scanning is needed" [1]. This advancement of AR didn't yet find any real application in Urology up to now. Such an interactive system is today enabled by very few, expensive devices and no software has been until now developed in order to benefit of this tool in our field. The direct interaction with a virtual environment might allow anyway to perform emergency simulation and to perform team training, involving interaction with other team members and the surrounding objects.

10.5 Radiomics in Urology

Radiomics is an evolving field of quantitative imaging with a variety of applications in clinical oncology, where delivers a comprehensive noninvasive characterization of the whole tumor, using a panel of quantifiable cancer metrics: the radiomics signature (RS). RS are extracted from medical images including computed tomography (CT), positron emission tomography (PET), magnetic resonance imaging (MRI), and ultrasonography (US). Radiomics uses computerized feature analysis methods for extracting subvisual characteristics at the imaging for characterizing disease appearance and behavior on radiographic images. Radiomics represent a powerful tool that applies Artificial intelligence (AI) and deep learning models to defining tissues with more accuracy [13]. They have been used in prostate, kidney and bladder to predict the actual pathology and aggressiveness of tumors, predict the stage, and the response to therapy [14]. Prostate cancer (PCa) patients could take full advantage of radiomics. Multiparametric MRI (mpMRI) are extensively used in the diagnosis of PCa. However the role of mpMRI is confined to staging and is affected by several pitfalls [15] and inter reader variability [16]. Recent applications of radiomics have shown advantages compared with conventional methods in PCa detection and characterization [17]. The application of radiomics could enable the quantification of intra-lesion heterogeneity by extracting a feature from imaging data with a possible impact on cancer detection accuracy, treatment efficacy and patients' outcomes and risk stratification [18, 19]. Promising applications of radiomics (associated or not to machine learning) in the management of bladder cancer have been reported. Radiomics could potentially serve in bladder cancer detection, staging, grading, and response to therapy [14].

10.6 Conclusions

We are observing in this decade the rise of several new technologies aimed to a better comprehension of clinical cases. Most of them are still in a research phase, with low reliability and limits mostly related to the lack of a proper commercialization of dedicated tools. Given the unprecedented potential of such technologies, we can easily expect that the analysis of pre-operatory images will anyway undergo profound changes in the next few years, until the moment we will ask ourselves "how could we even rely on a RAW CT scan?". Case-study is going to change, and it will be a real disruption.

References

1. Veneziano D, Amparore D, Cacciamani G, et al. Climbing over the barriers of current imaging technology in urology. Eur Urol. 2020;77(2):142–3.
2. Bertolo R, Fiori C, Piramide F, et al. Assessment of the relationship between renal volume and renal function after minimally-invasive partial nephrectomy: the role of computed tomography and nuclear renal scan. Minerva Urol Nefrol. 2018;70(5):509–17.
3. Porpiglia F, Fiori C, Checcucci E, Amparore D, Bertolo R. Hyperaccuracy three-dimensional reconstruction is able to maximize the efficacy of selective clamping during robot-assisted partial nephrectomy for complex renal masses. Eur Urol. 2018;74(5):651–60.
4. Bertolo R, Checcucci E, Amparore D, et al. Current status of three-dimensional laparoscopy in urology: an ESUT systematic review and cumulative analysis. J Endourol. 2018;32(11):1021–7.
5. Checcucci E, Amparore D, De Luca S, Autorino R, Fiori C, Porpiglia F. Precision prostate cancer surgery: an overview of new technologies and techniques. Minerva Urol Nefrol. 2019;71(5):487–501.

6. Cacciamani GE, Okhunov Z, Meneses AD, et al. Impact of three-dimensional printing in urology: state of the art and future perspectives. A systematic review by ESUT-YAUWP group. Eur Urol. 2019;76(2):209–21.
7. Schubert C, van Langeveld MC, Donoso LA. Innovations in 3D printing: a 3D overview from optics to organs. Br J Ophthalmol. 2014;98(2):159–61.
8. Hoang D, Perrault D, Stevanovic M, Ghiassi A. Surgical applications of three-dimensional printing: a review of the current literature & how to get started. Ann Transl Med. 2016;4(23):456.
9. Porpiglia F, Bertolo R, Checcucci E, et al. Development and validation of 3D printed virtual models for robot-assisted radical prostatectomy and partial nephrectomy: urologists' and patients' perception. World J Urol. 2018;36(2):201–7.
10. Porpiglia F, Amparore D, Checcucci E, et al. Current use of three-dimensional model technology in urology: a road map for personalised surgical planning. Eur Urol Focus. 2018;4(5):652–6.
11. Porpiglia F, Checcucci E, Amparore D, et al. Three-dimensional elastic augmented-reality robot-assisted radical prostatectomy using hyperaccuracy three-dimensional reconstruction technology: a step further in the identification of capsular involvement. Eur Urol. 2019;76(4):505–14.
12. Russon M. Touchable 3D holograms in daylight now possible using superfast femtosecond lasers. International Business Times UK. Retrieved 2016-02-12, from https://www.ibtimes.co.uk/touchable-3d-holograms-daylight-now-possible-using-superfast-femtosecond-lasers-1508599
13. Koçak B, Durmaz EŞ, Ateş E, Kılıçkesmez Ö. Radiomics with artificial intelligence: a practical guide for beginners. Diagn Interv Radiol. 2019;25(6):485–95.
14. Cacciamani E, Nassiri N, et al. Radiomics and bladder cancer: current status. Bladder Cancer. 2020;6(3):343–62.
15. Panebianco V, Giganti F, Kitzing YX, et al. An update of pitfalls in prostate mpMRI: a practical approach through the lens of PI-RADS v. 2 guidelines. Insights Imaging. 2018;9(1):87–101.
16. Sonn GA, Fan RE, Ghanouni P, et al. Prostate magnetic resonance imaging interpretation varies substantially across radiologists. Eur Urol Focus. 2019;5(4):592–9.
17. Sun Y, Reynolds HM, Parameswaran B, et al. Multiparametric MRI and radiomics in prostate cancer: a review. Australas Phys Eng Sci Med. 2019;42(1):3–25.
18. Varghese B, Chen F, Hwang D, et al. Objective risk stratification of prostate cancer using machine learning and radiomics applied to multiparametric magnetic resonance images. Sci Rep. 2019;9(1):1570.
19. Cuocolo R, Cipullo MB, Stanzione A, et al. Machine learning applications in prostate cancer magnetic resonance imaging. Eur Radiol Exp. 2019;3(1):35.

Chapter 11
Augmented Reality

Enrico Checcucci, Daniele Amparore, Paolo Verri, Sabrina De Cillis, Federico Piramide, Matteo Manfredi, Cristian Fiori, and Francesco Porpiglia

11.1 Introduction

Technology is nowadays constantly evolving, trying to fulfill the need to reach the best surgical planning and oncological outcome. In order to improve the efficacy and quality of surgical procedures, a "tailored" planning and dedicated instruments should be used [1].

3D virtual reconstructions of 2D cross-sectional imaging can help the surgeon to plan thoroughly the surgical act and to deeply understand the surgical anatomy [2].

At current times, thanks to dedicated software and to the constant collaboration between urologists and bioengineers, 3D hyper-accurate models can be created [3], offering a new way of understanding surgical anatomy and intra-operative approach to the organ [4, 5].

An additional chance offered by these systems is to overlay virtual 3D-models over the surgical fields, guiding the surgeon during minimally invasive procedures. Thanks to this technology, augmented-reality (AR) surgery can be actually performed [6].

The overlap of digitally created images over the real-world environment can be defined as "augmented-reality" (AR) [7].

Some basic steps are needed, in order correctly perform an AR procedure.

Firstly, 3D surgical models must be created. Secondly, the real anatomy must be carefully evaluated and 3D reconstructions must be overlapped. Finally, the surgical system must be set correctly in order to perform an accurate tracking of the surgical instruments, target organs and surrounding anatomy [8, 9].

E. Checcucci · D. Amparore · P. Verri · S. De Cillis · F. Piramide · M. Manfredi · C. Fiori
F. Porpiglia (✉)
Department of Urology, San Luigi Gonzaga Hospital, University of Turin,
Orbassano, Turin, Italy
e-mail: cristian.fiori@unito.it

© Springer Nature Switzerland AG 2021
E. Huri, D. Veneziano (eds.), *Anatomy for Urologic Surgeons in the Digital Era*,
https://doi.org/10.1007/978-3-030-59479-4_11

The aim of this chapter is to review and analyse the preliminary application and potential advance or benefits of AR in urologic surgery.

11.2 Augmented Reality in Prostate Cancer

There are currently few preliminary experiences focusing on AR-laparoscopic surgery for prostate cancer, showing the different advantages of this technology. Ukimura et al. used real-time transrectal ultrasonography during laparoscopic radical prostatectomy with the aim to improve oncological and functional outcomes, having an enhanced anatomical prospective [9, 10]. Recently, Simpfendörfer and colleagues created an AR navigation system in order to increase intraoperative anatomical accuracy, leading the surgeon towards a more precise procedure [11].

Cohen et al. were AR pioneers, presenting the first AR robot-assisted radical prostatectomy (RARP) in 2010 using 3D models created from mpMRI images. The outcomes of this experimenting technique were relevant, since the authors concluded that this AR procedure could help to improve the learning curve, functional and oncological outcomes [12].

Thompson et al. [13] in 2013 designed an intraoperative image-guided system and used it during robot-assisted radical prostatectomy: during the procedure, unprocessed T2 images were directly overlapped to the intraoperative anatomy. The system was initially used on cadaveric specimen and afterwards on a total of 13 patients.

Porpiglia et al. tried to overlap 3D rendered images of the prostate to the intraoperative field using an integrated software in the Da Vince console, performing an AR assisted RARP [14]. Intrafascial nerve-sparing technique was performed in 16 patients with cT2 prostate cancer while standard nerve sparing technique and selective biopsies of the operative field (suspect of extra capsular extension) were performed in 14 patients with cT3 tumors. Positive surgical margins rate was 30% and no positive surgical margin was found in pT2 neoplasms. AR guided selective biopsies confirmed extra-prostatic extension in 11/14 (78%) biopsies. Prostate specimens were scanned, revealing a mismatch between the 3D model and the real prostate from 1 to 5mm.

This work was recently updated by the same team [15]. Eleven cases, thanks to preoperative mpMRI, were classified as cT2 while 19 cases as cT3. In all cases, after performing a pathological examination, the location of the index lesion perfectly matched the 3D reconstruction overlapped to the real anatomy during the intervention (Fig. 11.1). 15 out of 19 (79%) cases, which were classified as cT3 thanks to preoperative MRI, had a confirmed pT3a stage. Among these patients, 11/15 (73.3%) had neoplastic cells adjacent to the extra-capsular extension area, in the neurovascular bundles.

Conclusion assessed that this technology, when handled by expert surgeons, can reach high success rates, with particular efficacy during the key steps of the procedure [16].

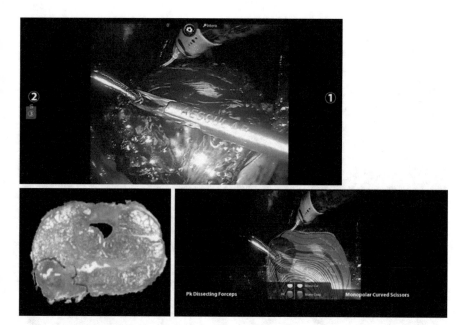

Fig. 11.1 After prostate removal, the 3D rigid virtual model was overlapped to in-vivo anatomy. The metallic clip placed at the level of the index lesion, as indicated by the 3D model, correctly identified the underlying tumour

All these techniques, however, imply the use of rigid 3D models. These rigid and static structures don't represent accurately the actual anatomy. Biological tissues are subject to constant deformations during the procedure in particular during the nerve-sparing phase, when the surgeon mobilizes the prostate with robotic arms during the exertion phase.

In this scenario, new "deformable" 3D reconstructions were designed thanks to the application of nonlinear parametric variables, namely "bend" and "stretch", in order to approximate the deformation of the target organ, performing a 3D elastic AR assisted RARP [17]. The "bend" deformer used the Y axis as the main deformation axis in both directions, while the "stretch" deformer used the Y axis alone. These two deformers proved to be very accurate in estimating prostate deformations during surgery. Despite the prostate traction exercised by the robotic arms, the 3D elastic overlapping system determined, during the dynamic nerve-sparing phase, the correct identification of the lesion in 100% of the cases (Fig. 11.2).

11.3 Augmented Reality in Kidney Cancer

Concerning renal cancer, despite the increasing number of works published, only exploratory clinical studies have focused on AR applied on partial nephrectomy [18].

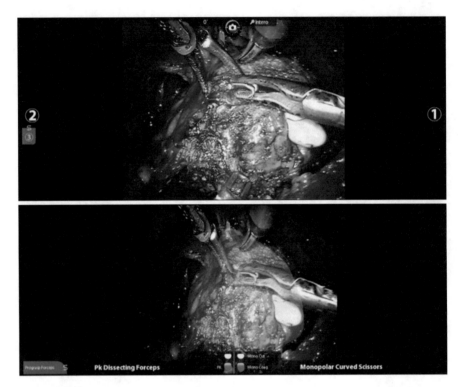

Fig. 11.2 During the nerve-sparing phase the Elastic Augmented Reality models correctly identified the tumour location

In 2009 Su et al. [19] developed a markerless intraoperatory tracking system based on preoperatory CT images, performing an AR real-time stereo-endoscopic robot-assisted nephron sparing procedure. After the initial procedures, essential for the system calibration, the 3D-to-3D registration was performed, observing an accuracy between the superimposed images and the real surgical field of only of 1 mm.

Nostrati et al. [20] developed an alternative technique to localize, during an endoscopic procedure, visible and hidden structures. During challenging robotic nephron-sparing procedures, they performed the procedure helped by vascular pulsation cues registered by dedicated instruments, determining a 45% accuracy improvement, compared to standard methods [21].

In 2018, Wake et al. published a video article, describing step by step the creation of 3D printed and AR kidney models, using Unity® software, used during robotic nephron sparing surgery. These models were successively deployed to Microsoft's HoloLens® system. 3D models and AR were used preoperatively and intraoperatively to assist the surgeon. Conclusions assessed that the use of AR 3D models is safe, feasible and it influenced the decision of the surgeon, not determining significant changes in the procedure's outcome [22].

In 2017 Singla et al. [23] proposed an AR guidance system, using ultrasonography for the lesion tracking during robotic nephron-sparing procedures' simulations. The registered error was around 1 mm and the authors could consequently assess that this system can significantly reduce the excised peritumoral healthy tissue during surgery (30.6 vs. 17.5 cm³).

A pioneering experience was published by Porpiglia et al. [4], who merged hyper-accuracy models (HA3D™) with Da Vince software using Tile-Pro®. Concerning selective ischemia, AR guidance proved to be as valid as the cognitive guidance and offered the surgeon the chance to stay constantly focused on the surgical field (Fig. 11.3).

This preliminary experience, similarly to RARP performed for prostate cancer, implied the use of rigid 3D virtual models, unable to simulate intraoperative tissue deformations.

The same group, afterwards, collaborating with engineers of *Politecnico* of Turin, developed an evolved software, introducing elastic AR (Fig. 11.4).

This system was particularly useful during the identification of hidden, endophytic tumours, also when they were located in the posterior face of the kidney. During the procedure, in order to demonstrate the overlapping accuracy, endoscopic ultrasonography was used and consequently showed the perfect match between the virtual model and the lesion [24].

AR impact on surgical learning methods was also studied: Kobayashi et al. [25] developed a software allowing to overlap and synchronize endoscopic images with

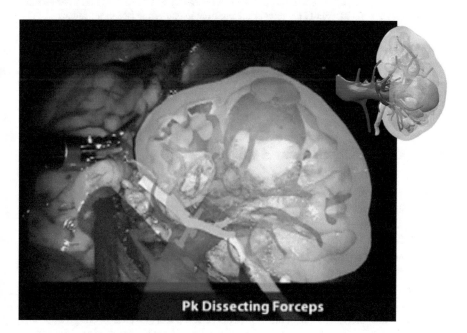

Fig. 11.3 The 3D model overlapped to the kidney allowed to visualize the kidney arteries and veins, also the intraparenchymal one. Moreover, the endophytic lesion was showed

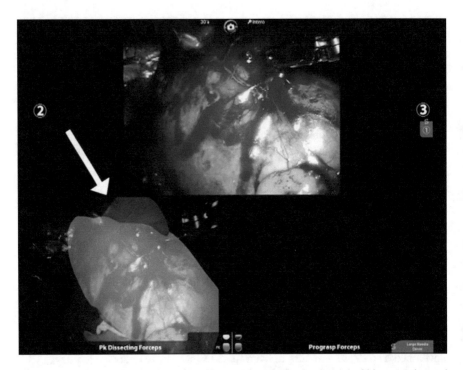

Fig. 11.4 The 3D Elastic Augmented Reality model correctly simulated the kidney rotation and deformation allowing to identify the tumour arising from the posterior face of the kidney

3D models during robotic NSS. Using this method, skills of two expert surgeons were evaluated: in particular, great attention was headed to the identification and dissection of renal artery. Results showed how the number of inefficient motions (i.e. "insert", "pull" and "rotate") was significantly reduced.

11.4 Others Preliminary Application

Kidney and prostate cancer surgery still remain the main application fields of AR technology: nevertheless, some preliminary experiences have been made in non-oncological surgery.

Renal stone surgery, in particular, represents the most fascinating urological application, since it implies a careful preoperative planning and a precise percutaneous puncture.

Choosing the best access location and performing a correct caliceal puncture is probably the most important step during percutaneous nephrolithotomy (PCNL). This procedure has the steepest learning curve, since it requires a thorough anatomical knowledge and needs an optimal access to the upper urinary tract in order to remove all the stones and to reduce complication rate.

In the later years, AR technology has been used in *ex vivo* settings to plan and guide the needle trajectory. Preoperative CT or MRI images, 3D models and intraoperative ultrasonographic images were merged together to perform the puncture: this system proved to be effective and very accurate [26].

Rassweiler et al. [27, 28] described the first experiences with AR-percutaneous puncture, overlaying 3D models on intraoperative images using a tablet camera.

Registration is based on fiducial markers and camera calibration. This phantom study assessed a decrease in puncture time and radiation exposure for urology trainees, compared to other non-AR techniques (fluoroscopy and US).

In 2019 Akand et al. [29] experimented a new technique which used a dedicated software (performing mathematical calculations), 3D modelling and AR technology to perform percutaneous puncture during PCNL, presenting the first results in two different *ex-vivo* models. Two different experiments, in two different models, were performed twice: the first model was a stone placed in gel cushion, the second was a bovine kidney placed into a chicken. A correct puncture was performed in every model, during every attempt. The accuracy of the puncture was evaluated by feeling crepitations on the stone's surface and observing, via CT scan, the touch of the needle tip with the stone.

Rassweiler-Seyfried [30] recently published the first human experience with an iPad-assisted percutaneous puncture. Match paired analysis was performed, comparing the accuracy and efficacy of AR system to standard procedure in 22 patients per group (Fig. 11.5).

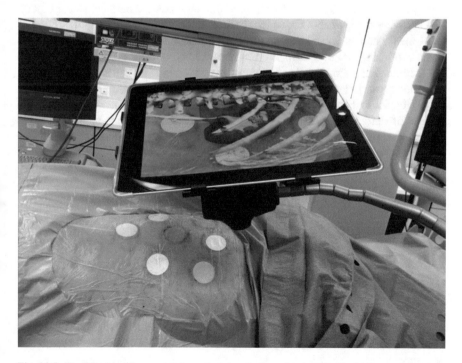

Fig. 11.5 The 3D virtual image overlapped via i-pad allowed to localize the kidney and the stone in order to guide the percutaneous puncture. Courtesy of Dr. Marie-Claire Rassweiler-Seyfried

A significative difference was found radiation exposure time ($p < 0.01$ in advantage of the standard technique) and puncture time ($p = 0.01$). There was no significant difference in puncturing attempts ($p = 0.45$).

11.5 Limits and Future Perspective

At current times, AR still remains a newborn and emerging technology with consequent limitations that need to be overcome [31]. Recording intraoperative movements and simulating tissue deformations still represent the two main challenges.

Different recording settings are available (such as manual, surface based, fiducial based and 3D-CT stereoscopic) but up to now there are technical limitations which make a precise real-time tissue tracking a challenge [32].

To overcome this limit, two main approaches have been proposed. The first implies the application of endoscopic landmarks which can be detected by the AR system in order to perfectly overlap the images [19, 20]. The second strategy, more challenging and expensive, involves a markerless approach based on machine learning algorithms.

Tissue deformation is maybe the hardest challenge: biomechanical models are under development and the laboratory results are still complex and unfit for clinical practice.

Payan et al. [33] have recently reported that less than ten biomechanical modelling software are available for surgical practice, emphasising how computation of real-time (or at least interactive) models is the most complex challenge to be faced. Some promising projects have been proposed [34], but fast computation of non-linear finite element models is still an unsolved problem.

In this scenario Porpiglia et al. [17, 35] introduced 3D-elastic AR robotic procedures, thanks to HA3D™ reconstructions and to the application of a non-linear parametric deformer [36]. With this technology, it was possible to approximate the deformation of the target organ, offering the surgeon a good image overlap in the crucial phase of the procedure, given the organ deformation.

Future technology, with the access to artificial intelligence [37], will offer the chance to process more complex data, allowing to accurately simulate real-time tissue dynamics and deformation for every organ [38].

11.6 Conclusions

In an even more tailored surgery era, the image guided surgery plays a fundamental role. Among the different technology available, the Augmented-Reality gives the possibility to enhance the in-vivo anatomy images with the overlapping of the 3D virtual models, increasing surgeons' perception of the disease and patients' anatomy.

Up to now we scratch the surface of this new technology, however the clinical applications seem to be promising, with a potential real benefit for the patients.

References

1. Autorino R, Porpiglia F, Dasgupta P, Rassweiler J, Catto JW, Hampton LJ, Lima E, Mirone V, Derweesh IH, Debruyne FMJ. Precision surgery and genitourinary cancers. Eur J Surg Oncol. 2017;43:893–908.
2. Porpiglia F, Amparore D, Checcucci E, Autorino R, Manfredi M, Iannizzi G, Fiori C, for ESUT Research Group. Current use of three-dimensional model technology in urology: a road map for personalised surgical planning. Eur Urol Focus. 2018;4:652–6.
3. Porpiglia F, Bertolo R, Checcucci E, et al. Development and validation of 3D printed virtual models for robot-assisted radical prostatectomy and partial nephrectomy: urologists' and patients' perception. World J Urol. 2018;36:201–7.
4. Porpiglia F, Fiori C, Checcucci E, Amparore D, Bertolo R. Hyperaccuracy three-dimensional reconstruction is able to maximize the efficacy of selective clamping during robot-assisted partial nephrectomy for complex renal masses. Eur Urol. 2018;74:651–60.
5. Porpiglia F, Manfredi M, Bertolo R, Mele F, Amparore D, Garrou D, Checcucci E, Alleva G, Niculescu GR, Piana A, Toso S. Does 3D prostate mp-MRI reconstruction for cognitive robot assisted radical prostatectomy affect oncological outcomes? Eur Urol Suppl. 2017;16:61.
6. Yoon JW, Chen RE, Kim EJ, et al. Augmented reality for the surgeon: systematic review. Int J Med Robot Comput Assist Surg. 2018;14:e19141.
7. Veneziano D, Amparore D, Cacciamani G, Porpiglia F, Uro-technology, SoMe Working Group of the Young Academic Urologists Working Party of the European Association of Urology, European Section of Uro-technology. Climbing over the barriers of current imaging technology in urology. Eur Urol. 2019;77(2):142–3. https://doi.org/10.1016/j.eururo.2019.09.016.
8. Ukimura O, Gill IS. Augmented reality for computer- assisted image-guided minimally invasive urology. In: Ukimura O, Gill IS, editors. Contemporary interventional ultrasonography in urology. London: Springer; 2009. p. 179–84.
9. Ukimura O, Gill IS, Desai MM, et al. Real-time transrectal ultrasonography during laparoscopic radical prostatectomy. J Urol. 2004;172:112–8.
10. Ukimura O, Magi-Galluzzi C, Gill IS. Real-time transrectal ultrasound guidance during laparoscopic radical prostatectomy: impact on surgical margins. J Urol. 2006;175:1304–10.
11. Simpfendörfer T, Baumhauer M, Müller M, Gutt CN, Meinzer H-P, Rassweiler JJ, Guven S, Teber D. Augmented reality visualization during laparoscopic radical prostatectomy. J Endourol. 2011;25:1841–5.
12. Cohen D, Mayer E, Chen D, Anstee A, Vale J, Yang GZ, et al. Augmented reality image guidance in minimally invasive prostatectomy. In: Madabhushi A, Dowling J, Yan P, Fenster A, Abolmaesumi P, Hata N, editors. Prostate cancer imaging. Computer-aided diagnosis, prognosis, and intervention. Prostate cancer imaging. Lecture notes in computer science, vol. 6367. Berlin: Springer; 2010. p. 101–10.
13. Thompson S, Penney G, Billia M, Challacombe B, Hawkes D, Dasgupta P. Design and evaluation of an image-guidance system for robot-assisted radical prostatectomy. BJU Int. 2013;111:1081–90.
14. Porpiglia F, Fiori C, Checcucci E, Amparore D, Bertolo R. Augmented reality robot-assisted radical prostatectomy: preliminary experience. Urology. 2018;115:184.
15. Porpiglia F, Checcucci E, Amparore D, et al. Augmented-reality robot-assisted radical prostatectomy using hyper-accuracy three-dimensional reconstruction (HA3D™) technology: a radiological and pathological study. BJU Int. 2019;123:834–45.

16. Porpiglia F, Bertolo R, Amparore D, Checcucci E, Artibani W, Dasgupta P, Montorsi F, Tewari A, Fiori C, ESUT. Augmented reality during robot-assisted radical prostatectomy: expert robotic surgeons' on-the-spot insights after live surgery. Minerva Urol Nefrol. 2018;70:226–9.
17. Porpiglia F, Checcucci E, Amparore D, et al. Three-dimensional elastic augmented-reality robot-assisted radical prostatectomy using hyperaccuracy three-dimensional reconstruction technology: a step further in the identification of capsular involvement. Eur Urol. 2019;76:505–14.
18. Checcucci E, De Cillis S, Porpiglia F. 3D-printed models and virtual reality as new tools for image-guided robot-assisted nephron-sparing surgery: a systematic review of the newest evidences. Curr Opin Urol. 2019;30(1):55–64.
19. Su L-M, Vagvolgyi BP, Agarwal R, Reiley CE, Taylor RH, Hager GD. Augmented reality during robot-assisted laparoscopic partial nephrectomy: toward real-time 3D-CT to stereoscopic video registration. Urology. 2009;73:896–900.
20. Nosrati MS, Abugharbieh R, Peyrat J-M, Abinahed J, Al-Alao O, Al-Ansari A, Hamarneh G. Simultaneous multi-structure segmentation and 3D nonrigid pose estimation in image-guided robotic surgery. IEEE Trans Med Imaging. 2016;35:1–12.
21. Amir-Khalili A, Peyrat J-M, Abinahed J, Al-Alao O, Al-Ansari A, Hamarneh G, Abugharbieh R. Auto localization and segmentation of occluded vessels in robot-assisted partial nephrectomy. Med Image Comput Comput Assist Interv. 2014;17:407–14.
22. Wake N, Bjurlin MA, Rostami P, Chandarana H, Huang WC. Three-dimensional printing and augmented reality: enhanced precision for robotic assisted partial nephrectomy. Urology. 2018;116:227–8.
23. Singla R, Edgcumbe P, Pratt P, Nguan C, Rohling R. Intraoperative ultrasound-based augmented reality guidance for laparoscopic surgery. Healthc Technol Lett. 2017;4(5):204–9.
24. Porpiglia F, Checcucci E, Amparore D, et al. Three-dimensional augmented reality transperitoneal robot assisted partial nephrectomy (3d ar-rapn): a new tool to identify the hidden tumours. Eur Urol Suppl. 2018;6:e2690.
25. Kobayashi S, Cho B, Huaulmé A, Tatsugami K, Honda H, Jannin P, Hashizumea M, Eto M. Assessment of surgical skills by using surgical navigation in robot-assisted partial nephrectomy. Int J Comput Assist Radiol Surg. 2019;14:1449–59.
26. Detmer FJ, Hettig J, Schindele D, Schostak M, Hansen C. Virtual and augmented reality systems for renal interventions: a systematic review. IEEE Rev Biomed Eng. 2017;10:78–94.
27. Rassweiler JJ, Müller M, Fangerau M, Klein J, Goezen AS, Pereira P, Meinzer H-P, Teber D. iPad-assisted percutaneous access to the kidney using marker-based navigation: initial clinical experience. Eur Urol. 2012;61:628–31.
28. Müller M, Rassweiler M-C, Klein J, Seitel A, Gondan M, Baumhauer M, Teber D, Rassweiler JJ, Meinzer H-P, Maier-Hein L. Mobile augmented reality for computer-assisted percutaneous nephrolithotomy. Int J Comput Assist Radiol Surg. 2013;8:663–75.
29. Akand M, Civcik L, Buyukaslan A, Altintas E, Kocer E, Koplay M, Erdogru T. Feasibility of a novel technique using 3-dimensional modeling and augmented reality for access during percutaneous nephrolithotomy in two different ex-vivo models. Int Urol Nephrol. 2019;51:17–25.
30. Rassweiler-Seyfried M-C, Rassweiler JJ, Weiss C, Müller M, Meinzer HP, Maier-Hein L, Klein JT. iPad-assisted percutaneous nephrolithotomy (PCNL): a matched pair analysis compared to standard PCNL. World J Urol. 2019;38(2):447–53. https://doi.org/10.1007/s00345-019-02801-y.
31. Checcucci E, Amparore D, Fiori C, et al. 3D imaging applications for robotic urologic surgery: an ESUT YAUWP review. World J Urol. 2019;38(4):869–81. https://doi.org/10.1007/s00345-019-02922-4.
32. Hughes-Hallett A, Mayer EK, Marcus HJ, Cundy TP, Pratt PJ, Darzi AW, Vale JA. Augmented reality partial nephrectomy: examining the current status and future perspectives. Urology. 2014;83:266–73.
33. Payan Y. Soft tissue biomechanical modeling for computer assisted surgery. New York: Springer; 2012. https://doi.org/10.1007/978-3-642-29014-5.

34. González D, Cueto E, Chinesta F. Computational patient avatars for surgery planning. Ann Biomed Eng. 2016;44:35–45.
35. Porpiglia F, Checcucci E, Amparore D, Piramide F, Piazzolla P, Bellin A, Fiori C. 3D elastic augmented reality robot-assisted partial nephrectomy for central and posterior renal masses: a new tool for a better resection of the tumor. Eur Urol Suppl. 2019;18:e2276.
36. Amparore D, Checcucci E, Gribaudo M, et al. Non-linear-optimization using SQP for 3D deformable prostate model pose estimation in minimally invasive surgery. In: Advances in intelligent systems and computing, vol. 943. New York: Springer; 2020. p. 477–96.
37. Checcucci E, Autorino R, Cacciamangi GE, et al. Artificial intelligence and neural networks in urology: current clinical applications. Minerva Urolo Nefrol. 2019;72(1):49–57.
38. Haouchine N, Dequidt J, Berger M-O, Cotin S. Deformation-based augmented reality for hepatic surgery. Stud Health Technol Inform. 2013;184:182–8.

Chapter 12
Virtual Reality and Animation

Musa Batuhan Yolcu, Emre Huri, and Senol Emre

12.1 Introduction

Digital technologies are developing rapidly today and while new technologies are emerging, they are also called disruptive technologies because they destroyed the previous technologies. Visual technologies, which are a part of these, keep up with this speed. These are Virtual Reality (VR), Augmented Reality (AR) and Mixed Reality (MR). One of the reasons for the emergence of visual technologies was that when transferring the content, the technologies at that time were insufficient. After the development of Virtual Reality technology, the formats of the contents also evolved to this. Among these, 3D Models and Animations are at the forefront.

The use of these technologies in the field of health extends from education level to clinical practice. There are academic studies on the use of these technologies in medical education [1]. This section includes the importance of immersive technologies. There are many changes and developments from virtual reality devices to produced content. Thus, the interconnectedness of Virtual Reality and Animation concepts is a field that can be examined.

M. B. Yolcu (✉)
Cerrahpasa Medical Faculty, Istanbul University-Cerrahpasa, Istanbul, Turkey
e-mail: musabatuhan.yolcu@ogr.iu.edu.tr

E. Huri
Department of Urology, Hacettepe University, Ankara, Turkey

S. Emre
Cerrahpasa Medical Faculty, Department of Pediatric Surgery, Istanbul University-Cerrahpasa, Istanbul, Turkey

© Springer Nature Switzerland AG 2021
E. Huri, D. Veneziano (eds.), *Anatomy for Urologic Surgeons in the Digital Era*,
https://doi.org/10.1007/978-3-030-59479-4_12

12.2 What Is Virtual Reality (VR)?

This definition, which is one of the first examples of definitions made with different sentences for years, explains the limits of technology well. It contains three-dimensional (3D), stereoscopic, head-tracked displays, hand/body tracking and binaural sound content in a simulated environment rather than real environment. VR is an immersive, multisensory experience [2].

VR and Animation are complementary elements. Experiencing 3D Animations can be made possible thanks to VR [3]. It is also necessary to mention other technologies that basically have similar purposes to VR. Some of these are Augmented Reality (AR) and Mixed Reality (MR). These technologies require different devices but use similar technical infrastructures [4]. For example, while AR can be used for mobile devices such as mobile phones and tablets, advanced MR glasses are required for MR [5].

In fact, the technology called MR combines the interactivity in VR and the ability to experience virtual environments and objects in the real environment as in AR (Fig. 12.1). If we include 360° videos and hologram in all these visual technologies, it is possible to gather them all under the title of Augmented Virtuality (AV) [6].

So how can these technologies be developed and offer such an experience on people, let's explain.

12.3 What Are Basics of VR?

VR consists of two bases. These are Engineering and Reverse Engineering. The Engineering section includes the Software and Hardware section of VR. Reverse Engineering part consists of human physiology and human perception (Fig. 12.2) [7].

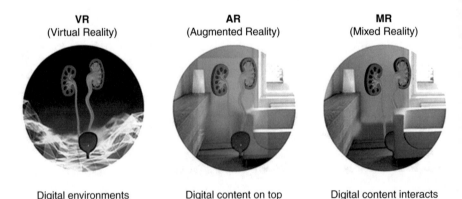

| VR (Virtual Reality) | AR (Augmented Reality) | MR (Mixed Reality) |

Digital environments that shut out the real world.

Digital content on top of your real world.

Digital content interacts with your real world.

Fig. 12.1 Views of VR, AR and MR technologies

Fig. 12.2 Engineering and reverse engineering in VR

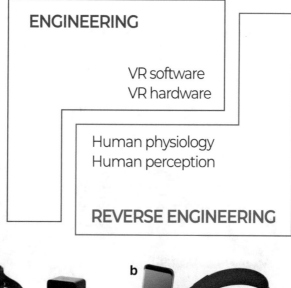

ENGINEERING

VR software
VR hardware

Human physiology
Human perception

REVERSE ENGINEERING

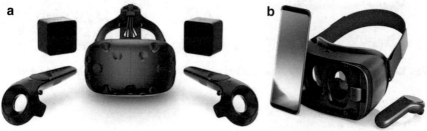

Fig. 12.3 (a) Virtual Reality System. (b) VR glasses that can be used by wearing a mobile phone in front of it

Hardware and software come to the forefront to examine VR technical subheadings. Today, VR Headsets are undoubtedly one of the equipment, specially developed for VR. Although there are many different versions of these headsets, their working principles are similar. VR Headsets generally consist of screens and lens (Fig. 12.3) [8]. In some portable VR headsets, this screen feature can also be provided with external devices such as mobile phones [9].

Although there is a large field of work for developers on the software side, it increases even more with the increase in investments in this sector. The software section is also divided into subtitles. These can be simplified as the creation and interactive content. As a user, the data received from the movements and behaviors made by people are stimulated via VR Headset and transferred to the user again (Fig. 12.4) [10].

These movements and data received and transmitted can be provided with many different technological equipment. This equipment is appeals to people's sense organs which are the organ of vision, Tactile, Olfactory, Taste, Auditory Organs [11]. Studies are continuing for the integration of some sense organs into VR headsets. These pieces of VR Headsets are developed day by day.

Fig. 12.4 Interaction
diagram between
organization and VR
Headsets

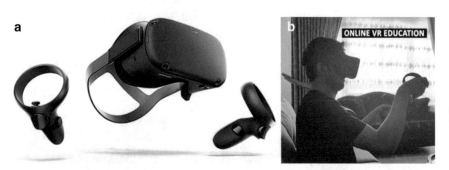

Fig. 12.4 Interaction diagram between organization and VR Headsets

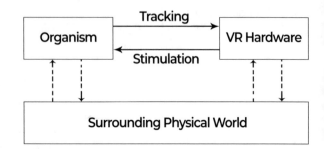

Fig. 12.5 (**a**) Oculus Quest VR Headset. (**b**) Online VR Student Education in Medical Faculty

12.4   VR Headsets

Let's examine a device that is both portable and at a level that many people can reach and use. One of the most up-to-date released devices at the time of this content is Oculus Quest (Fig. 12.5) [12]. Among the features of this device is the fact that it is portable. Despite working with a mobile processor, it can identify your hand in mesh form in 3D with the software on it.

In this way, you are able to move your hand synchronously in the virtual environment. While you are in a virtual environment with VR Headset, it allows you to break from the real environment easily with the internal speakers on the device. At the same time, it is possible to make an application that works with your voice command with the built-in microphone on it [13].

To illustrate this, it is possible for a surgical assistant to have an interactive experience in VR with only voice commands without the need for any other controller during the operation [14]. Some features mentioned here can also be found in other similar devices. Devices that can appeal to more than one sense organ are becoming more common nowadays thanks to haptic devices [15]. It is possible that we will see future additions to these devices that may appeal to our other sense organs.

12.5   Animations in VR

We can use these technologies when you want to create a virtual copy of our real world or situations that cannot exist. When switching from 2D Animations to 3D Animations, we need to switch from PC screens or projection devices to VR-AR devices. We need 3D environments to use the feature of 3D effectively. If we explain with an example, drawing or photographing an anatomical structure to be used for educational purposes will be able to give us information from a single angle frame in 2D.

In order to get more information from the visuals, photographs or illustrations drawn from more than one angle may be required. Video's started to be used, which recorded 24 frames in 1 s. 24 frames represent 24 photos. This concept is defined as Fps (frames per second) relative to the frame rate viewed in 1 s. These videos can also be composed of hundreds of photographs recorded or they can be obtained by combining hundreds of drawings. With this method, 2D animations and videos are made by bringing the drawings and visuals created on the computer consecutively. Today, 24 fps and 60 fps are used frequently while making video and animation (Fig. 12.6). In this way, it is possible to receive many visual information in a short time while watching a single video or animation.

Nowadays, it is tried to increase the transfer power of information with better methods than videos and animations. Having work done, it becomes possible to make what can be done repeatable in reality or to eliminate negative scenarios in a virtual environment where they cannot be actually done. Therefore, content that can be considered as 3D Video is needed. The most important technical source of 3D Content is 3D Animations. However, it is not convenient to experience these 3D animations on 2D screens. Different devices are needed for this [16].

The first examples of these devices are VR Headsets which Virtual Reality (VR) content can be used. The first versions available to the user were wired and connected to the computer. This system needed a VR headset and a high processing computer. Today, there are still professional devices that continue with this system (Fig. 12.7) [17].

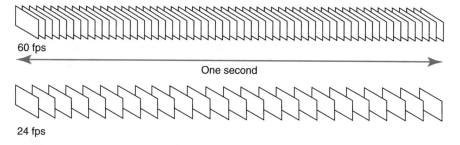

Fig. 12.6 The number of frames captured in 1 s with 24 fps and 60 fps

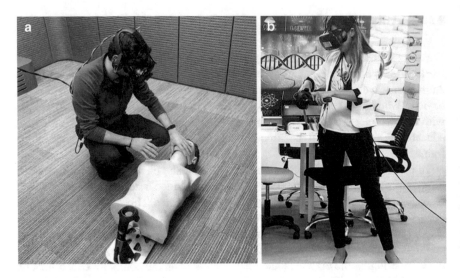

Fig. 12.7 (**a**) Using HTC Vive VR glasses on first aid training in healthcare. (**b**) Experiencing open heart surgery in a virtual environment

12.6 How to Create 3D Content in Medicine?

When talking about VR content, 3D models and animations come first. 3D models are required to transfer real world assets to a virtual environment or to create imaginary virtual environments. 3D Models can be obtained in different ways. If the content you want to develop is unique to you, it may be necessary to model 3D models from scratch.

It is necessary to explain with an example, a disease-specific model has been developed in pediatric urology. For this, you need to model the anatomical organ structures and deformations you want by using one of the 3D modeling programs on the computer. This method gives you the possibility of originality and freedom on the model. 3D models developed with this method can only be used in educational simulations (Fig. 12.8) [18].

When you want to study a case in the clinic, you will need to use the patient's own visual data, such as Computed Tomography (CT) or Magnetic Resonance Imaging (MRI). For this method, there are many computer applications that are specific in different fields. Through these applications, soft tissues and other structures on the radiological image can be modeled in 3D by separating them from each other. This process is called segmentation (Fig. 12.9). Although some advanced software can do this semi-automatic process, unfortunately, a system that can perform this process fully automatic in many areas is not common yet. In general, it is possible to arrange the 3D model with different 3D model editing programs obtained with this method. Surgery planning on 3D models instead of 2D radiological images can provide advantages in terms of time and success. From the studies on this field, it seems promising.

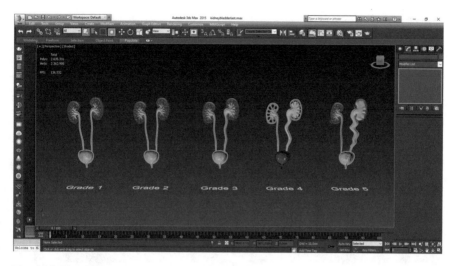

Fig. 12.8 Five different Vesicoureteric Reflux (VUR) models on computer environment with Autodesk 3dsMax according to classification

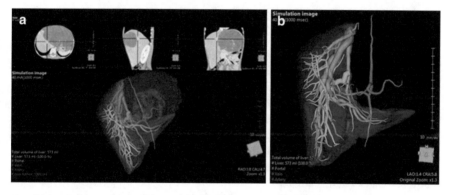

Fig. 12.9 (a) Segmented tumor structure in the liver of an anonymous patient data. (b) Tumor structure isolated from the liver

If we continue the example of the operation, it should be ensured that the movements are simulated and interactive so that these 3D models can simulate the reality. It can be modeled in 3D by scanning an operating room or operation (Fig. 12.10). At this point, the behavior and positions of 3D models in the virtual environment can be transformed into 3D animation through many different programs on the computer. The animations created include the flow of an event.

For example, each stage of an operation can be prepared as a 3D animation for a virtual environment.

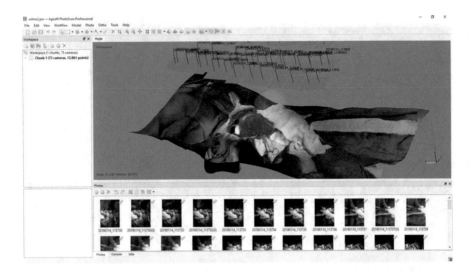

Fig. 12.10 Photographs of an anonymous Wilms' tumor and surgical environment are processed in Agisoft PhotoScan Professional in 3D

12.7 How to Create VR Content?

With the increasing use of VR, portable versions of devices began to become widespread [19]. After the development of VR devices, the need for appropriate content in the device started to increase. Big companies tend to develop their infrastructures rather than entering the development race here. This is a good approach that paves the way for the development of such technologies today. Thanks to this, developers from all over the world began to develop VR-AR content similar to developing a mobile application or a game. VR and AR are very similar to each other as application development stages [20]. Let's examine the development process through a study carried out in this context.

In this study conducted in the field of Istanbul University-Cerrahpasa, Cerrahpasa Medical Faculty, Department of Pediatric Surgery, Division of Pediatric Urology, an AR application that can be used on mobile devices has been developed using AR technology. Vesicoureteral Reflux (VUR), one of the congenital anomalies, is selected for the sample study. Under the leadership of physicians with clinical experience, five types of VUR disease are modeled on the computer with the Autodesk 3dsMax, 3D modeling software. The models are transferred to the Unity program, a game development platform (Fig. 12.11) [21].

Google ARCore infrastructure is used and interactive features such as move, rotate and scale are added to the models. From the production of 3D models in this study to the development of a mobile application on a platform, it is similar to VR. Then, device-specific interactions (such as voice commands) are added to the software by using infrastructures developed by VR devices' brands. It is published in brands' online stores and offered for free or for a fee.

Fig. 12.11 View of Vesicoureteric Reflux
(VUR) 3D model on AR mobile application

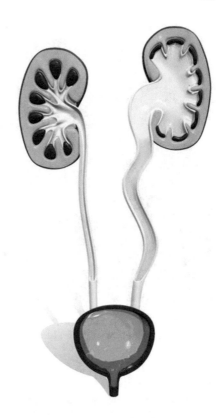

12.8   What Are These Immersive Technologies?

There are basic VR applications in medicine, but studies on specific areas have not become widespread yet. This development of VR is followed by Augmented Reality (AR) technology. For AR, you can use your own mobile phone or tablet (providing minimum requirements and updates) [22]. There are some advantages and disadvantages compared to VR. While AR can provide ease of use without the need for another device in your environment, it cannot offer you a high experience like VR. Mixed Reality (MR) devices have been developed by blending two technologies to meet this need. These devices allow you to capture the VR experience in terms of interactivity and interaction while in the real environment where you are like AR.

12.9   Current Virtual Reality in Medicine

"The daVinci® Surgical System has evolved since the original version was released in 2000 at the time of FDA approval. According to the 2012 Intuitive Surgical Annual Report, there were 2585 da Vinci® Surgical Systems installed worldwide,

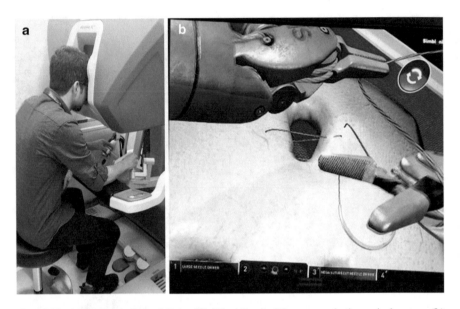

Fig. 12.12 (**a**) Surgeon's Control Unit of Da Vinci Surgical System, a robotic surgical system. (**b**) Screen while suturing to soft tissue like skin with controls

including 1878 in the U.S., 416 in Europe, and 291 in the rest of the world. The growth in overall 2013—procedure volume was driven by the growth in U.S. general surgery procedures, U.S. gynecologic procedures, and urology procedures outside of the USA [23]." Studies show that developed VR contents in robotic surgery can be used in surgical assistant training (Fig. 12.12) [24]. It shows that as the quality of VR content increases, it may enter our lives more in the future.

Thanks to these VR contents, it is possible to reduce the possibility of a surgical assistant or a surgeon who focuses on the preoperative case to make a mistake with a practical method [25]. At the same time, simulation versions of rare cases can be created and practiced repeatedly. One of the best examples of an interactive virtual reality application is simulations in robotic surgery. With these applications, it is possible to direct surgical instruments with your haptic controllers while you are in a virtual environment with glasses with VR [26]. The truthfulness of the experience here can increase the success during the operation on the patient in practice.

12.10 Future of Immersive Technologies

According to the Gartner reports, VR technology, which is one of the new developing technologies, has passed the Hype Cycle in 2017 (Fig. 12.13). AR is followed immediately after. In 2018 reports, VR completed the cycle and experienced new diffraction along with AR, enabling MR technology to progress in this cycle (Fig. 12.14). In 2019, VR, AR and MR technologies all seem to have completed this

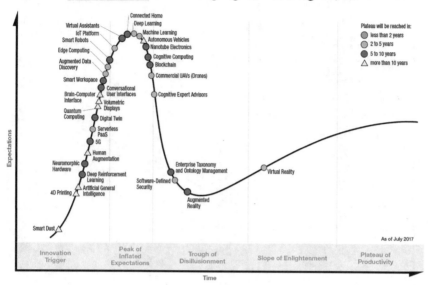

Fig. 12.13 Hype cycle chart according to 2017 Gartner report

cycle (Fig. 12.15). This means that they have passed through the developing technology phase and become a mature technology. In the upcoming reports of this year,
the sub-diffractions of these immersive technologies will probably enter or complete this cycle.

12.11   Effective Usage of Virtual Reality

Both the increase in investments and the number of developers can be predicted for
the proven VR Technology. This increasingly cheap technology can be used in many
different areas from healthcare to primary care, from education to patient information. With VR technology, many problems existing in the clinic will be solved over
time. In the coming years, even if the technology is not on the manufacturer or
developer side, it will be necessary to be able to use and consume it in the profession.

So how can these devices start to spread in this way? Some of the most important
factors that ensure these are miniaturized electronics and fit comfort. The rapid
development and spread of VR headsets also supports this situation. They are making wearable systems more feasible [15].

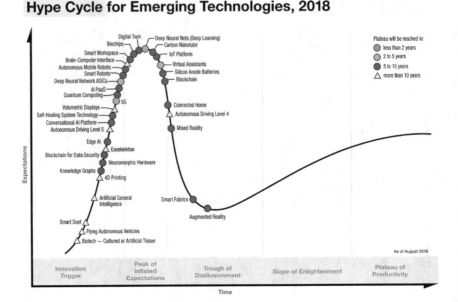

Fig. 12.14 Hype cycle chart according to 2018 Gartner report

Thus, the availability of VR technology in the field of health has increased. Especially, healthcare use of wearable devices provides novel methods for monitoring and potentially enhancing users' health [27]. The use of VR in the field of health is very important. This technology, which is becoming widespread in the field of medicine, can be used for different fields from cell culture studies to operations, medical student education to surgical assistant training (Fig. 12.16).

12.12 Virtual Reality in Urology

Surgical education has usually been based on the Halstedian methodology of "see one, do one, teach one". This methodology depends on the volume of patients as well as the access them. The field of surgery covers a wide range of complicated procedures. Teaching or learning with the Halstedian method is a challenge due to the increased public awareness of patient safety [28]. Three different VR simulators were produced in the project of MedTRain3Dmodsim as VR cystoscopy, VR retrograde intrarenal surgery and VR laparoscopic nephrectomy. Tatar et al. reported that surgical complications could be decreased if more 3D medical surgical models were used within surgical training. The learning curve of surgical anatomy could be

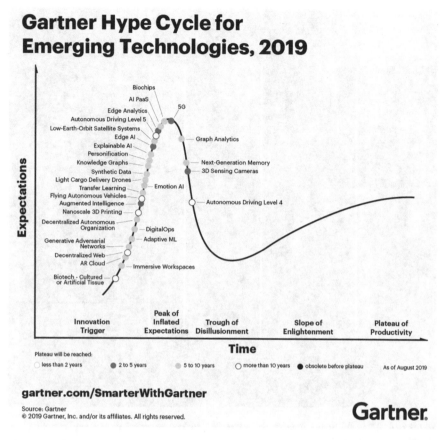

Fig. 12.15 Hype cycle chart according to 2019 Gartner report

improved with these models depicting correct anatomical plans, proper surgical planning, and increased visualization of solid organ anatomy [28]. Jimenez et al. stressed the importance of VR approaches for image-guided surgery have demonstrated potential in the field of urology by supporting guidance for various disorders. Increased number of pre and intraoperative imaging modalities can be used to create detailed surgical route maps [29]. However, use of 3D virtual reality for surgical planning is another major section in digital urologic surgery. Shirk et al. stated that use of a 3-dimensional, virtual reality model when performing robotic partial nephrectomy improved important surgical outcome parameters with lower operative time (141 min vs. 201 min, P < 0.0001), clamp time (13.2 min vs. 17.4 min, P = 0.0274), and estimated blood loss (134 cc vs. 259 cc, P = 0.0233) [30].

According to the MedTRAin3DModsim team's experience of developing virtual simulators; production of 3D model with using patient-specific CT reconstructed is crucial to maintain similar anatomic shape, size and applicable physical simulators. Medical 3D simulation technology has developed exciting new solutions and possibilities for medical diagnosis and practice. A common 3D model was used to

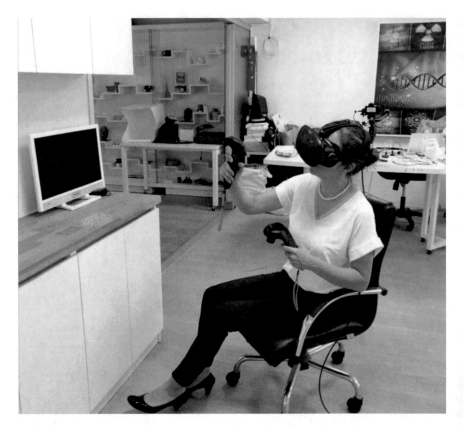

Fig. 12.16 TETLab, which focuses on VR studies in Turkey, develops VR applications about surgery and cell culture studies

generate steps for both static bio models and physical simulators. The processes began with CT or MRI data, from patients or cadavers, which were generated from DICOM files. These were then imported into software programs, where the anatomy was segmented to create the desired anatomic structures. The data was further modified and repaired, wherever needed, with the Autodesk 3dsMax and Z-brush 3D model editing tool. The texturing process was performed using Adobe Photoshop CC to express a realistic anatomical texture. Next, polygonal mesh (stereolithography, STL) files were generated for 3D Printing (3DP) or Virtual Reality. That data can be used for generating a virtual reality model or a printed model.

12.13 Conclusion

With the decrease in the price of VR devices and their widespread usage, we cannot ignore the possibility that everyone can have VR devices as well as mobile phones. Therefore, it seems that we will be able to use VR technology, VR headsets and animated content more in the future.

The field of health is among the most important areas in which innovations should be applied. Physicians will be able to decide how to integrate the new technologies developed as the benefit of the patient is prioritized in medicine. Because of this situation, it is necessary to show how these technologies work and how they can be used with scientific methods. The most important points in these technologies are the possibilities and the content created by the developed devices. With the multidisciplinary approach in the content development process, it is possible to benefit for everyone according to their competence. Hence, scientific studies can be done on this by analyzing the sections where these visual technologies can be useful.

Acknowledgement   The authors of this chapter would like to thank Prof. Sinan Celayir, MD for sharing their academic studies in VR and AR in Pediatric Surgery.

References

1. Yolcu MB, Emre S, Celayir S. Use of augmented reality in medicine and pediatric surgery. J Turk Assoc Pediatr Surg Soc Pediatr Urol Turk. 2018;32(3):89–92. https://doi.org/10.5222/jtaps.2018.089.
2. Gigante M. Virtual reality: definitions, history and applications. In: Virtual reality systems. London: Academic Press; 1993. p. 3–14.
3. Waters R, Anderson D, Barrus J, Brogan D, Casey M, McKeown S, Nitta T, Sterns I, Yerazunis W. Diamond park and spline: social virtual reality with 3D animation, spoken interaction, and runtime extendability. Presence Teleop Virt Environ. 1997;6:461–81.
4. Welch WH, TeKolste RD, Chung H, Cheng H. Methods and system for creating focal planes in virtual and augmented reality. United States Patent. No: US 2015/0346495 A1 dated 12.3.2015; 2015.
5. Tepper OM, Rudy HL, Lefkowitz A, Weimer KA, Marks SM, Stern CS, Garfein ES. Mixed reality with hololens. Plast Reconstr Surg. 2017;140(5):1066–70.
6. Nielsen CW, Anderson MO, McKay MD, Wadsworth DC, Boyce JR, Hruska RC, Koudelka JA, Whetten J, Bruemmer DJ. Methods and systems relating to an augmented virtuality environment. United States Patent. No: US 8,732,592 B2 dated 5.20.2014; 2014.
7. LaValle SM. Virtual reality. Finland: Cambridge University Press; 2019. p. 5–8.
8. Luckey P, Trexler BI, England G, McCauley J. Virtual reality headset. United States Patent. No: USD701.206S dated 3.18.2014; 2014.
9. Hillmann C. Comparing the Gear VR, Oculus Go, and Oculus Quest. In: Unreal for mobile and standalone VR. New York: Apress; 2019. p. 141–67. https://doi.org/10.1007/978-1-4842-4360-2_5.
10. LaValle SM. Virtual reality. Finland: Cambridge University Press; 2019. p. 40–65.
11. LaValle SM. Virtual reality. Finland: Cambridge University Press; 2019. p. 373–95.
12. Huang Y, Shakya S, Odeleye T. Comparing the functionality between virtual reality and mixed reality for architecture and construction uses. J Civil Eng Archit. 2019; https://doi.org/10.17265/1934-7359/2019.07.001.
13. Facebook Technologies, LLC. Oculus Quest features; 2020. https://www.oculus.com/quest/features. Accessed 11 Apr 2020.
14. Ferracani A, Faustino M, Giannini G, Landucci L, Del Bimbo A. Natural experiences in museums through virtual reality and voice commands. Proceedings of the 2017 ACM on Multimedia Conference—MM '17. 2017. https://doi.org/10.1145/3123266.3127916
15. Stoppa M, Chiolerio A. Wearable electronics and smart textiles: a critical review. Sensors. 2014;14(7):11957–92.

16. Masia B, Wetzstein G, Aliaga C, Raskar R, Gutierrez D. Display adaptive 3D content remapping. Comput Graph. 2013;37:983–96.
17. Moro C, Štromberga Z, Stirling A. Virtualisation devices for student learning: comparison between desktop-based (Oculus Rift) and mobile-based (Gear VR) virtual reality in medical and health science education. Australas J Educ Technol. 2017;33(6) https://doi.org/10.14742/ajet.3840.
18. Emre S, Yolcu M, Celayir S. Three dimensional printers and pediatric surgery. Turk Assoc Pediatr Surg. 2015;29(3):77–82. https://doi.org/10.5222/jtaps.2015.077.
19. Jung T, tom Dieck MC, Rauschnabel PA, editors. Augmented reality and virtual reality. Cham: Springer; 2020. https://doi.org/10.1007/978-3-030-37869-1.
20. Glover J. Complete virtual reality and augmented reality development with unity: leverage the power of unity and become a pro at creating mixed reality applications. 1st ed. Birmingham: Packt; 2019.
21. Yolcu MB, Ovunc SS, Emre S, Mammadov E, Celayir S. Hybrid book supported by augmented reality in pediatric surgery. 37th National Pediatric Surgery Congress, 15–19 Oct 2019, Video Presentation, Ankara; 2019.
22. Shumaker R, Lackey S, editors. Virtual, augmented and mixed reality. Designing and developing virtual and augmented environments. Lecture notes in computer science. Cham: Springer; 2014. https://doi.org/10.1007/978-3-319-07458-0.
23. Intuitive Surgical Inc. Annual report 2012; 2013. http://www.annualreports.com/Company/intuitive-surgical-inc. Accessed 11 Apr 2020.
24. Kenney PA, Wszolek MF, Gould JJ, Libertino JA, Moinzadeh A. Face, content, and construct validity of dV-trainer, a novel virtual reality simulator for robotic surgery. Urology. 2009;73(6):1288–92.
25. Gallagher AG, Ritter EM, Champion H, Higgins G, Fried MP, Moses G, Satava RM. Virtual reality simulation for the operating room. Ann Surg. 2005;241(2):364–72. https://doi.org/10.1097/01.sla.0000151982.85062.80.
26. Choi KS, Soo S, Chung FL. A virtual training simulator for learning cataract surgery with phacoemulsification. Comput Biol Med. 2009;39(11):1020–31. https://doi.org/10.1016/j.compbiomed.2009.08.003.
27. Chai PR, Wu RY, Ranney ML, Porter PS, Babu KM, Boyer EW. The virtual toxicology service: wearable head-mounted devices for medical toxicology. J Med Toxicol. 2014;10(4):382–7.
28. Tatar İ, Huri E, Selçuk İ, Moon YL, Paoluzzi A, Skolarikos A. Review of the effect of 3D medical printing and virtual reality on urology training with 'MedTRain3DModsim' Erasmus + European Union Project. Turk J Med Sci. 2019;49(5):1257–70.
29. Del Pozo JG, Rodríguez Monsalve M, Carballido Rodríguez J, Castillón VI. Virtual reality and intracorporeal navigation in urology. Esp Urol. 2019;72(8):867–81.
30. Shirk JD, Kwan L, Saigal C. The use of 3-dimensional, virtual reality models for surgical planning of robotic partial nephrectomy. Urology. 2019;125:92–7.

Chapter 13
Three-Dimensional Medical Printing in Urology

Mehmet Ezer and Emre Huri

13.1 Introduction

Three-dimensional (3D) printers are devices that make 3D designs prepared in computer-aided design (CAD) programs into real 3D objects using various materials. Additive manufacturing (AM) is another name frequently used in the literature for 3D printer technology. It was the first known step in 3D printers to polymerize a photosensitive resin by ultraviolet light for the first time in 1986 by Charles W. Hull [1]. In their early years, they used it widely in architecture, automotive, and aerospace industries. It created a technological revolution by giving engineers, architects, and designers a chance to transform a model they designed in a fully virtual environment into a real three-dimensional object. Although the photosensitive resin was originally used for production; many new materials, from ceramics to various polymers, from metal types to wax and even human cells, can be used in production with new technological developments [2]. Today, 3D printers have become an accessible technological product with the developing technological infrastructure, where individual users can make their own installations and create their own 3D models and products.

In the absence of medical imaging techniques, information about the patient's body was limited only by physical examination. The anatomical conditions of the sick organs were an enigma, and perhaps their real condition had a chance to be detected only intraoperatively. When German physicist Wilhelm Conrad Roentgen announced that he discovered X-rays with his article "Ober eine neue Art von Strahlen" on December 28, 1895; one of the first big steps was taken for medical imaging [3]. Following this big step, X-ray radiographs became the most important

M. Ezer (✉)
Department of Urology, School of Medicine, Kafkas University, Kars, Turkey

E. Huri
Department of Urology, Hacettepe University, Ankara, Turkey

imaging method in the field of medicine used for a long time. With the advancing technology, new imaging techniques such as computed tomography (CT), Ultrasonography (US) and magnetic resonance imaging (MRI) have led to revolutionary results in diagnostic algorithms. The ability of clinicians to use cross-sectional imaging when trying to diagnose patients has enabled the organs to be evaluated in detail, thereby making it easier to diagnose correctly. Although the cross-sectional imaging methods provide much more anatomical details than classical radiographs, it may be inadequate to enable us to understand the interrelationships of organs and tissues that are making important neighborhoods with each other in a 3D space. The unique contribution of 3D modeling in the field of medical imaging helps exactly to illuminate this "blind spot".

Awareness of the use of 3D printers in the medical field has been on the agenda in the last few decades [4]. In general, it is noticed that this new technology, which has led to groundbreaking results in the sectors it has been used to date, can be used in many fields of medicine. For each patient, 3D models can be created for surgical planning, and these 3D models can be used both to inform the patient and to understand the treatment process. At the same time, using these models, education can be given in the field of medicine, or research assistants who are undergoing surgical training can be given the chance to undergo surgical training without the risk of harming the patient. With this novel technology, customized medical equipment and prosthesis can be produced for the patient.

In this book section, it is aimed to review the applications of 3D printer technology in the field of urology, to evaluate its potential benefits and limitations, and to evaluate our future expectations.

13.2 How 3D Printing Is Work?

13.2.1 Creation of 3D Models

In order to print in 3D printers, a 3D model ready to be printed must be prepared first. Although the 3D modeling process is described in detail in a separate chapter in this textbook; it is deemed necessary to give a brief information about the process in this chapter. With an overall perspective, the production of organs from a real patient or a cadaver as a 3D model involves a process consisting of multiple stages (Fig. 13.1). The cross-sectional views of the patient, which is obtained in DICOM format in 2D, are converted to 3D with the help of CAD programs. The artifacts that occur when converting to 3D are taken to an edit and repair process to obtain a more realistic model. At the end of all these processes, a 3D model is created in ".stl" format suitable for printing on a 3D printer. The format called "the Standard Tessellation Language" or "Standard Triangle Language" abbreviated as STL is the standard software format used by CAD programs. Only the surface anatomy is defined to consist of small triangles, with no color or pattern in the STL format.

Fig. 13.1 Production steps of a 3D printing model

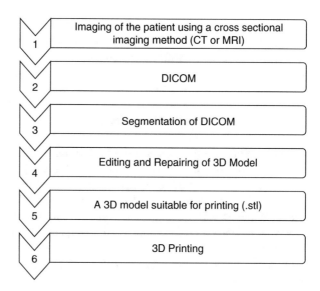

1 Imaging of the patient using a cross sectional imaging method (CT or MRI)

2 DICOM

3 Segmentation of DICOM

4 Editing and Repairing of 3D Model

5 A 3D model suitable for printing (.stl)

6 3D Printing

Unlike other common formats, OBJ contains color or pattern information different from STL format, while PLY format can contain additional data such as transparency [5]. After the 3D models are ready to be printed, the printing phase can be started by selecting the appropriate 3D printer, which differs according to the intended use and the type of material desired to be printed.

13.2.2 3D Printing Technology

In the introduction part of this chapter, we have stated that there are many different 3D printer technologies and many materials from resin to various metals can be used as printing material. A brief summary of 3D printing technologies is important to higher perceive the present and potential applications of 3D printing technologies in the medical field. Although the technological options we have are very diverse, four basic 3D printing technologies are used more. These can be listed as fused deposition modeling (FDM), inkjet printing, powder-based printing, and stereolithography (SLA) [6].

13.2.2.1 Fused Deposition Modeling

FDM technology is the most widely used and low-cost 3D printing technology today [7]. The FDM method is one of the subtypes of extrusion-based printing technology. It works on the principle of heating and melting a thermoplastic filament to form three-dimensional layers [8]. Overlapping layers create a 3D model when the writing phase is complete. An important limitation of FDM technology is that it can be printed using only one color, except for models that allow double filament to be used. Also, when the printing phase is completed, the layer marks forming the model can be selected with the naked eye when viewed from the outer surface of the model.

13.2.2.2 Inkjet Printing (Material Jetting)

Inkjet-based (or droplet-based) printing technology occurs by placing the droplets on top of each other in a form that creates a 3D model [7]. An interesting and prominent feature in these printing technologies is the ability to print by combining scaffolds with live cells or using bioinks containing living cells. Inkjet-based technologies are the common names for subgroups such as multijet modeling (MJM), wax deposition modeling (WDM), binder jetting (BJ), and laser-induced forward transfer (LIFT) [9–11].

In MMJ, liquid acrylic polymers are layered on a building platform using a print head with one or more nozzles. Cured by exposure to UV lamps after layering. Melted wax is also used to provide a support structure with acrylic polymer to ensure structural durability during the process. The wax around the 3D model is cleaned with the melting process after printing [7].

In WDM technology, wax is first melted and deposited on a building platform layer by layer through a print head. The melted wax cools down on this platform to become solid and takes its final shape [7].

In the technology called BJ, a 3D model is created by connecting an adhesive substance sprayed from the print head and various powder materials such as ceramics, metals and polymers. Therefore, BJ technology can be considered as a kind of powder based technology [12].

Since laser light is used in LIFT technology, it does not require a printhead [13]. After the laser absorbent layer is covered with ink material, the laser light focuses on this layer and turns the metal into gas-plasma state. The vapor pocket formed at this time, extracts a droplet from the ink material. This technology, which was used only for metals when it was first used, has recently been used for cell-laden hydrogels.

13.2.2.3 Powder-Based Printing

Although the source of energy used and the types of powder materials differ, the logic in all of the powder-based 3D printer technologies relies on heating to ensure the integrity of the powder materials. Selective laser sintering (SLS), direct metal laser sintering (DMLS), selective laser melting (SLM) and electron beam melting (EBM) can be classified under the heading of powder based printing technologies [14].

Although there are technological similarities between the sintering process and the melting process, there are some important differences in terms of the resulting product. In the sintering process, the resulting material has a porous internal structure and a rough surface, since the powders are not completely melted. In the melting process, the powders are completely melted and combined so that a higher density and more solid 3D printing can be obtained [15].

In SLS, SLM and DMLS methods, laser beams directed with the help of mirrors are used for heating. Although SLS and DMLS methods are roughly similar technologies, a wide variety of materials can be used for printing in the SLS method, while only metal material can be used in DMSL.

In EBM technology, high energy electron beam is used through electromagnetic coils. For this system to work, a vacuumed working environment is required, and the cost increases compared to other powder-based printers.

13.2.2.4 Vat Polymerization-Based Printing

In the technology called vat photopolymerization printing, light waves focus on a wat which is filled with a UV-sensitive resin material. The focused ultraviolet light hardens one layer at a time, forming layers in a row [7]. Vat Polymerization-based Printing technology includes stereolithography (SLA), direct or digital light processing (DLP) and continuous directlight processing/continuous liquid interface production (CDLP/CLIP).

The first 3D printer technique found by Charles W. Hull in 1986 was a SLA method [1]. In SLA technique, an ultraviolet (UV) light sensitive resin is polymerized with UV and converted into a solid state. It is the most commonly used 3D printer technology in the surgical planning stage today because it gives very close results to the reality [16].

The DLP method is very similar to the SLA, but uses a shallower resin container. It provides the opportunity to print faster because it uses a digital light projector that is under the resin container and cures the entire layer at once [17].

In addition to DLP method in CDLP (or CLIP) method, the build plate moves in the Z-direction continuously [7]. This additional feature allows the printing time to be shortened thoroughly.

13.3 Using of 3D Medical Printing in Urology

13.3.1 Pre- and Intraoperative Surgical Planning

An important issue in which three-dimensional medical technologies can be beneficial is the pre-surgical planning stage. The data obtained by the patient's imaging methods can be made three-dimensional in the virtual environment, and the neighborhoods of the tissues and organs and the anatomical location of the structure to be intervened can be evaluated in detail before surgery, and a more realistic assessment opportunity can be obtained while planning in the preoperative period.

Surgical treatment of kidney stone diseases is one of the urological study areas where technology is developing rapidly. In addition to the developed laser systems, ultrasonic lithotripters and flexible instruments, the use of 3D technologies seems to increase this development rate.

In 2017 Ghazi et al. kidney including the pelvicaliceal system and relevant adjacent structure models were created using polyvinyl alcohol hydrogels and three-dimensional-printed injection molds [18]. All steps of a percutaneous nephrolithotomy (PCNL) were simulated including percutaneous renal access, nephroscopy, and lithotripsy steps. Five experts with >100 caseload and 10 novices with a previous <20 caseload from both urology (performing the full procedure) and interventional radiology (performing access only) departments completed the simulation. Face and content validity were calculated using model ratings for similarity to the real procedure and usefulness as a training tool. The similarity and conformity of the prepared models to the real procedure were evaluated by the participants as very successful.

Atalay et al. used 3D replicated models which has been previously created with usage of preoperative images of five patients during pre-operative training [19]. The trainees had progression with a range of 60–88% in understanding of calyceal localizations and determination of axcess side. More, the same authors informed the patients preoperatively with their pre-printed models [20]. Surveys were fulfilled by patients and the results relieved that there an increase of patient knowledge of stone localization, kidney anatomy and possible complications during the procedures by aid of informative printed models.

Models obtained with 3D printer technology can be used by offering in vitro work environment for different studies besides preoperative planning, medical education and patient information. Antonelli et al. described usage of a polythene sac ''The PercSac'' in order to prevent migration of stone fragments during the PCNL procedure performed on 3D printed kidney models [21].

In 2019, Xu et al. evaluated the effectiveness of usage of 3D printed models for optimal calyx selection and stone free rate among staghorn stones [22]. According to their results, 3D printed models may be used to achieve better stone free rates with most suitable axcess side selection during PCNL procedures among patients with staghorn stones [22]. Similarly at same year Bianchi et al. evaluated the improvement of axcess sides during PCNL with aid of 3D kidney models [23]. According to their evaluation of 3D-guided approach on PCNL of a 25 × 15 mm left kidney stone, the preoperative planning of the puncture with better knowledge of the renal anatomy and may be helpful to reduce operative time and improve the learning curve [23]. Canat et al. also declared that stone volume calculation using CT based 3D-reconstructed algorithm improves the accuracy of stone volume estimation and this measurement is superior to ellipsoid formula [24].

Besides from PCNL as considering the ureteroscopic lithotripsy Kuroda et al. demonstrated a case of allograft ureteral stone which has been treated with antegrade approach with usage of a 3D printed model to determine the ideal approach [25]. Due to the anatomical difficulty regarding the patients allograft kidney, they had prepared a 3D image and model for selecting the best percutaneous approach [25].

The "partial nephrectomy" procedure, also called nephron-sparing surgery, is the primary treatment for small kidnet masses with suspected renal cancer. Factors such as the location of the mass on the kidney, the depth of invasion closely affect the parameters such as the duration of surgery, the amount of bleeding, the possibility of complications. One of the most common uses of 3D modeling in the field of urology is the preoperative planning of the surgeries of the masses detected on the kidney. In a study carried out by Smektala et al. in Poland, patient images were processed, mold modeling was made, casting molds were created, and silicone replicas were produced through these molds, in which five cases planned to undergo laparoscopic partial nephrectomy surgery with suspicion of renal carcinoma [26]. The models obtained in this low cost study were first used for surgical planning before partial nephrectomy, and in the later period, they were used in laparoscopic surgery training.

Wake et al. created personalized replicated kidneys through 3D printers in the preoperative period, by processing the MRI of a series of 10 cases with a nephrometry score between 6 and 10 [27]. Three surgeons whom have been experienced in the field of urooncology completed a questionnaire about their surgical approach plans without replica models first and then with replica models [27]. It was interesting in the results of the research is that the transperitoneal or retroperitoneal surgical approach plans made without seeing the model change at a rate of 30–50% after the model is seen [27]. 3D replicas of the mass to be surgically caused serious changes in the decision of the surgeons making plans by looking at MRI.

Westerman et al; In a study comparing the use of 3D printer material replicated kidneys when performing surgical planning with the use of CAD programs for surgical planning in cases of challenging nephron-sparing surgery, they obtained data indicating that models produced using a 3D printer provide more successful surgical planning [28].

Golab et al. performed preoperative planning with cardiovascular surgery via a 3D model of a renal cancer case with a thrombus extending to the right atrium where multidisciplinary approach is required during surgery [29]. So, the 3D models produced specifically for the patient can facilitate joint preoperative planning in complex cases where teams with different specialties will enter together.

An interesting study was performed considering the 3D printing assisted laparoscopic cryoablation of small renal tumors [30]. The 3D reconstruction was used to mimic cryoablation procedure. The results showed that the 3D printing technology assisted laparoscopic cryoablation is a feasible method to treat renal tumors, which maybe a better way to preserve nephrons, especially for those elderly and/or comorbid patients [30].

There also exists different interesting cases of renal tumors which has been successfully treated surgically with help of 3D printing technology. As an example, Mercader et al. reported the aid of 3D printed modelling during the surgical planning of a patient with horseshoe kidney [31].

According to a study that evaluating the 3D printed modelling on laparoscopic partial nephrectomy(LPN), 3D models supplied a shorter ischemia time but longer surgery waiting time [32]. The patients with RENAL score ≥8, the 3D-LPN group had significantly shorter warm ischemic time and less intraoperative blood loss than the traditional LPN group. Intra- and postoperative hospital complication rates were similar for 3D-LPN and traditional LPN groups (8.7% vs. 13.7%) [32]. Similarly, Kyung et al. also evaluated the application of 3D printed kidney models during partial nephrectomy to predict surgical outcomes [33]. The translation of 2D images of CT or MRI data to a 3D model helps surgeons improvements regarding tumor localization [34].

Moreover, recent studies also investigated 3D printed models among bladder, prostate and retroperitoneal tumors in urology [35–37]. Laparoscopic radical cystectomy with an introcorporeal neobladder is one of challenging cases in urooncology. Bejrananda et al. described the patients Y pouch neobladder in a 3D printed model during the follow-up in order to help the patient to understand the morphology and neobladder capacity after the initial surgery [35]. In order to improve the validation considering the prostate cancer diagnosis and treatment plan, Rutkowski et al. suggested a MRI-based cancer lesion analysis with 3D printed patient specific prostate cutting guides [36]. According to their study 10 patients with prostate cancer were evaluated with Prostate Specific Membrane Antigen (PSMA) Positron Emission Tomography (PET)/MRI both before and after chemohormonal treatment. Post-treatment images were used to design patient-specific prostate cutting guides that were used to create uniform thickness sections of surgically removed prostates. So that The prostate cutting guides were used to successfully section the prostate for histopathogical evaluation and slice-by-slice MRI comparison [36]. Effectiveness of 3D printing modelling to plan a retroperitonel tumor was investigated among 24 surgeons [37]. Regarding a single case all the surgeons were asked to compare the CT and 3D models. Especially junior surgeons declared that the 3D models provide greater help for preoperative planning and confidence building than using CT in resection of retroperitoneal tumor [37].

Besides urooncology and endourology there are special subgroups of urological interventions where 3D printing models may also take place. Renal transplantation is one of the urological study areas where the use of 3D printers is applied. In a study conducted in 2015, the donor kidney and the pelvic cavity of the recipient patient were rendered in 3D by imaging the patients before the renal transplantation, and printed as replica models [38]. During the study, it was aimed to decrease the vascular clamp time and bleeding amount in the intraoperative period by evaluating the pelvic vascular structures and their neighbors, the pelvic location and location of the kidney to be transplanted, and the vascular lengths required for anastomosis [38]. Urethral injury is an important problem among patients with pelvic fractures. Posterior urethral anastomosis during urethroplasty may be a challenging intervention. Joshi et al. conducted a study consisted of 3D printed models composed of pelvic fracture patients with urethral injuries [39]. A total of 10 models were printed which were obtained by 3D CT images. According to their results 3D printing can be applied to pelvic fracture urethral injury to understand the anatomy of the posterior urethra and its relations with peri neighbouring important anatomical structures [39]. Even, individualized 3D printed extravascular titanium stents have been shown to be used as a minimally invasive treatment option among patients with nutcracker syndrome [40].

13.3.2   Education and Training

The "primum non nocere", namely the "do not harm first" principle of the Ionian Physician Hippocrates, who is known as the founding father of medicine, is a basic principle that is taught to every physician candidate who is preparing to embark on his career. The methodology used in classical medicine education is based on the "see, do, teach" algorithm of William Stewart Halsted, who is accepted as the founder of modern surgery. In an education system based on Halsted methodology, it will run parallel with the number of patients with access to education and experience that the person can obtain. It is also obvious that using the human body, which is the main object of the medical education process, as training material in processes with potential for harm, will create ethical, moral and legal problems due to the indispensable and indisputable importance of human life. Cadavers have been used as the most important educational tools of medical education for many years in order to overcome various problems caused by the trainings given on the patient's body. However, difficulties in cadaver supply, limitations such as not being able to observe physiological changes in a living organism and religious prejudices brought new searches [41]. Although various animal models used in medical education make important contributions to education, education remains far from the targeted quality due to the physiological and anatomical differences between the living body used as educational material and the human body. All these limitations and difficulties in medical education require the use of applications such as simulation, augmented reality and virtual reality in the medical education process.

In 2019, Tatar et al. published an important review considering the importance and validity of 3D medical printing and virtual reality on urology training with 'MedTRain3DModsim' Erasmus + European Union Project [42]. At the same year Guliev et al. evaluated the use of a 3D printed segmented collapsible model of pelvicalyceal system during urology training [43]. According to their study the determination of the anterior and posterior calyces of the upper group was improved by 61% and 69%, the difference in the determination of the calyces of the middle group was 60% and 51%, and the answers regarding the number of the anterior and posterior calyces of the lower group became better by 67% and 74%, respectively ($p < 0.001$). The ability to select the optimal calyx for the primary and the second access became better by 60% and 55%, respectively ($p < 0.001$) [43].

There exists an increase in the usage of ultrasound guidance during recent years on both endoscopic and percutaneous interventions. Aro et al. developed 3D printed kidney models especially ultrasound-compatible ones in order to be used during training [44]. Day by day there is an increasing interest and studies go on. Recently, Melynk et al. published a technical report that indicates the usage of perfused hydrogel kidney model created using 3D printed injection moldings for RAPN simulation and training [45]. Anatomically correct, tumor-laden kidney models were created from 3D-printed casts designed from a patient's CT scan and injected with poly-vinyl alcohol (PVA). A variety of testing methods quantified Young's modulus in addition to comparing the functional effects of bleeding and suturing among fresh porcine kidneys and various formulations of PVA kidneys. It was the first study that utilize extensive material testing analyses to determine the mechanical and functional properties of a perfused, inanimate simulation platform for RAPN, fabricated using a combination of image segmentation, 3D printing and PVA casting [45].

The predominant use of 3D printers in the area of prostate diseases is the diagnosis and treatment of prostate cancer. There are studies in the literature that support the combination of multiparametric prostate MRI (mpMRG) and 3D prostate model to increase the success rates in the diagnosis of prostate adenocarcinoma. In a study conducted by Wang et al. Published in 2015, all of the 16 patients with suspected prostate cancer had 3.0 Tesla mpMRG, and STL files obtained from the processed images were created in 3D with prostate models. Cognitive fusion prostate biopsy was performed on patients by evaluating mpMRG and 3D prostate models together. When evaluating the results, the researchers stated that they performed higher rates of prostate cancer detection compared to cognitive fusion biopsies in the current literature and argued that the combination of mpMRG and 3D model will increase the diagnostic value of prostate biopsy [46].

If the dorsolateral neurovascular bundles cannot be distinguished and preserved during radical prostatectomy, which is the gold standard treatment of non-metastatic prostate adenocarcinoma, erectile dysfunction may develop permanently in the postoperative period [47]. Intraoperative discrimination of dorsolateral neurovascular bundles is a problem that forces surgeons. In a study conducted by Jomoto et al. In a combination of magnetic resonance angiography and patient-specific 3D prostate models, the use of the 3D prostate model made it easier to find neurovascular bundles intraoperatively, thus facilitating radical prostatectomy with a nerve-sparing technique [48].

Apart from urological surgery, there are several studies in the literature that demonstrate the advantages of custom made 3D prostate models during the application of different treatment modalities such as cryotherapy, HIFU (High Intensity Focused Ultrasound) and brachytherapy used in the treatment of prostate cancer [49, 50].

As we take a look to very recent studies, Choi et al. described a phantom model for simulation and quantitative evaluation of transurethral resection of the prostate [51]. The phantom mirrors the anatomy and haptic properties of the gland and permits quantitative evaluation of important surgical performance indicators. Mixtures of soft materials are engineered to mimic the physical properties of the human tissue, including the mechanical strength, the electrical and thermal conductivity, and the appearance under an endoscope. Electrocautery resection of the phantom closely resembles the procedure on human tissue. Quantitative criteria for performance assessment are established and evaluated by automated image analysis. According to their results surgery on the phantom was accepted to be useful for medical training [51].

Witthaus et al. incorporated and validated the clinically relevant performance metrics of simulation (CRPMS) in to a novel full-immersion simulation platform for nerve-sparing robot-assisted radical prostatectomy (NS-RARP) utilizing 3D printing and hydrogel technology [52]. Anatomically accurate models of the human pelvis, bladder, prostate, urethra, neurovascular bundle (NVB) and relevant adjacent structures were created from patient MRI by injecting polyvinyl alcohol (PVA) hydrogels into three-dimensionally printed injection molds. The steps of NS-RARP were simulated: bladder neck dissection; seminal vesicle mobilization; NVB dissection; and urethrovesical anastomosis (UVA). Five experts (caseload >500) and nine novices (caseload <50) completed the simulation. Force applied to the NVB during the dissection was quantified by a novel tension wire sensor system fabricated into the NVB. Post-simulation margin status (assessed by induction of chemiluminescent reaction with fluorescent dye mixed into the prostate PVA) and UVA weather tightness (via a standard 180-mL leak test) were also assessed. Objective scoring, using Global Evaluative Assessment of Robotic Skills (GEARS) and Robotic Anastomosis Competency Evaluation (RACE), was performed by two blinded surgeons. GEARS scores were correlated with forces applied to the NVB, and RACE scores were correlated with UVA leak rates. The correlation of validated objective metrics (GEARS and RACE) with our CRPMS suggests their application as a novel method for real-time assessment and feedback during robotic surgery training [52].

In another study, in a patient who tried to preserve the functions of adrenal hormone secretion in the long term by performing partial adrenalectomy on one side and partial adrenalectomy on the other side, a case presentation was performed preoperatively, the 3D adrenal gland model was produced, and the adrenal gland volume to be used in the patient was calculated and used as a guide during surgery [53]. In a study conducted by Cheung et al. In 2014, a simulator for pediatric pyeloplasty surgery was created with a 3D model produced using silicone material from a model created by processing images of a pediatric patient with ureteropevic junction stenosis with CAD programs [54].

As considered for andrology training Pinto et al. described an artificial model composed of two vas deferens made with silicone tubes, covered by a White resin, measuring 10 cm in length and internal and external diameters of 0.5 and 1.5 mm, respectively [55]. The holder of the ducts is made by a small box developed with polylactic acid, using a 3D print [55].

13.3.3 Patient Counseling

Today, with the developing technology, patients can easily access most information about their diseases. However, many patients do not have the level of knowledge to understand the current state of the disease, to evaluate different treatment methods that can be applied together with their physician and to decide what is appropriate for their condition. Materials embedded thanks to 3D printer technology can also help clinicians inform patients.

13.3.4   Other 3D Printers Applications in Urology

Del Junco and colleagues made flow dynamics measurements using double j stents (DJS) produced using a 3D printer and a saline solution in a pig model [56]. In another study conducted in 2015, Park and his friends made pressure measurements with DJS produced with a 3D printer that showed anti-reflux feature thanks to the polymeric valves [57]. More, Russo et al. described the new perspectives of 3D printing in andrology [58].

13.4   Future Aspects of 3D Medical Printing in Urology

The area where 3D printer technology is expected to cause the biggest changes in medicine may be the field of tissue engineering. The rabbit urethra, produced by Zhang et al. using organic materials and living cells, can be considered as a step closer to the point that human beings dream of producing living tissues and organs in the laboratory environment and transplanting them to patients [59].

Kim et al. published a very important study that considering the structure establishment of 3D cell culture printing model for bladder cancer [60]. They constructed a 3D cell scaffold using gelatin methacryloyl (GelMA) and compared cell survival in 3D and 2D cell cultures. 3D cell cultures showed higher cancer cell proliferation rates than 2D cell cultures, and the 3D cell culture environment showed higher cell-to-cell interactions through the secretion of E-cadherin and N-cadherin. The effects of drugs for bladder cancer such as rapamycin and BCG showed that the effect in the 2D cell culture environment was more exaggerated than that in the 3D cell culture environment. They fabricated 3D scaffolds with bladder cancer cells using a 3D bio printer, and the 3D scaffolds were similar to bladder cancer tissue [60]. So the technique can be used to create a cancer cell-like environment for a drug screening platform.

13.5   Conclusions

When the current technology is evaluated, it is an indisputable fact that training with models obtained with 3D printers cannot replace the clinical training given on a real case. However, the use of this new technological application in the education of less experienced people, especially at the beginning of the training curve; Reducing the possible complications that may be encountered due to inexperience at the beginning of the training process may be beneficial in terms of increasing patient safety. The use of 3D printed models produced with the help of 3D technologies during preoperative evaluation in many diseases provides a better evaluation of anatomical structures, increases surgical success rates and, reduces complication rates. 3D printing models are among the most powerful assistants who strengthen the hand of physicians in informing patients and their relatives about the disease and treatment processes. In the future, it is thought that 3D printer technologies will be used more widely in the field of medicine with decreasing costs and increasing prevalence.

References

1. Hull CW. Apparatus for production of three-dimensional objects by stereolithography. Google Patents; 1986.
2. Schubert C, van Langeveld MC, Donoso LA. Innovations in 3D printing: a 3D overview from optics to organs. Br J Ophthalmol. 2014;98(2):159–61.
3. Babic RR, Stankovic Babic G, Babic SR, Babic NR. 120 YEARS SINCE THE DISCOVERY OF X-RAYS. Med Pregl. 2016;69(9–10):323–30.
4. Cacciamani GE, Okhunov Z, Meneses AD, Rodriguez-Socarras ME, Rivas JG, Porpiglia F, et al. Impact of three-dimensional printing in urology: state of the art and future perspectives. A systematic review by ESUT-YAUWP Group. Eur Urol. 2019;76(2):209–21.
5. Parikh N, Sharma P. Three-dimensional printing in urology: history, current applications, and future directions. Urology. 2018;121:3–10.
6. Chen MY, Skewes J, Desselle M, Wong C, Woodruff MA, Dasgupta P, et al. Current applications of three-dimensional printing in urology. BJU Int. 2020;125(1):17–27.
7. Liaw CY, Guvendiren M. Current and emerging applications of 3D printing in medicine. Biofabrication. 2017;9(2):024102.
8. Wong KV, Hernandez A. A review of additive manufacturing. Int Scholarly Res Notices. 2012;2012
9. Upcraft S, Fletcher R. The rapid prototyping technologies. Assem Autom. 2003;23(4):318–30.
10. Do A-V, Khorsand B, Geary SM, Salem AK. 3D printing of scaffolds for tissue regeneration applications. Adv Healthcare Mater. 2015;4(12):1742–62.
11. Ozbolat IT. Scaffold-based or scaffold-free bioprinting: competing or complementing approaches? J Nanotechnol Eng Med. 2015;6(2).
12. Sachs EM, Haggerty JS, Cima MJ, Williams PA. Three-dimensional printing techniques. Google Patents; 1994.
13. Malda J, Visser J, Melchels FP, Jüngst T, Hennink WE, Dhert WJ, et al. 25th anniversary article: engineering hydrogels for biofabrication. Adv Mater (Deerfield Beach, Fl). 2013;25(36):5011–28.
14. Shirazi SFS, Gharehkhani S, Mehrali M, Yarmand H, Metselaar HSC, Adib Kadri N, et al. A review on powder-based additive manufacturing for tissue engineering: selective laser sintering and inkjet 3D printing. Sci Technol Adv Mater. 2015;16(3):033502.
15. Kruth J-P, Mercelis P, Van Vaerenbergh J, Froyen L, Rombouts M. Binding mechanisms in selective laser sintering and selective laser melting. Rapid Prototyp J. 2005;11(1):26–36.
16. Kim GB, Lee S, Kim H, Yang DH, Kim Y-H, Kyung YS, et al. Three-dimensional printing: basic principles and applications in medicine and radiology. Korean J Radiol. 2016;17(2):182–97.
17. Billiet T, Vandenhaute M, Schelfhout J, Van Vlierberghe S, Dubruel P. A review of trends and limitations in hydrogel-rapid prototyping for tissue engineering. Biomaterials. 2012;33(26):6020–41.
18. Ghazi A, Campbell T, Melnyk R, Feng C, Andrusco A, Stone J, et al. Validation of a full-immersion simulation platform for percutaneous nephrolithotomy using three-dimensional printing technology. J Endourol. 2017;31(12):1314–20.
19. Atalay HA, Ulker V, Alkan I, Canat HL, Ozkuvanci U, Altunrende F. Impact of three-dimensional printed pelvicaliceal system models on residents' understanding of pelvicaliceal

system anatomy before percutaneous nephrolithotripsy surgery: a pilot study. J Endourol. 2016;30(10):1132–7.

20. Atalay HA, Canat HL, Ulker V, Alkan I, Ozkuvanci U, Altunrende F. Impact of personalized three-dimensional – 3D-printed pelvicalyceal system models on patient information in percutaneous nephrolithotripsy surgery: a pilot study. Int Braz J Urol. 2017;43(3):470–5.

21. Antonelli JA, Beardsley H, Faddegon S, Morgan MS, Gahan JC, Pearle MS, et al. A novel device to prevent stone fragment migration during percutaneous lithotripsy: results from an in vitro kidney model. J Endourol. 2016;30(11):1239–43.

22. Xu Y, Yuan Y, Cai Y, Li X, Wan S, Xu G. Use 3D printing technology to enhance stone free rate in single tract percutaneous nephrolithotomy for the treatment of staghorn stones. Urolithiasis. 2019;

23. Bianchi L, Schiavina R, Barbaresi U, Angiolini A, Pultrone CV, Manferrari F, et al. 3D Reconstruction and physical renal model to improve percutaneous punture during PNL. Int Braz J Urol. 2019;45(6):1281–2.

24. Canat L, Atalay HA, Degirmentepe RB, Bayraktarli R, Aykan S, Cakir SS, et al. Stone volume measuring methods: should the CT based three-dimensional-reconstructed algorithm be proposed as the gold standard? What did the three-dimensional printed models show us? Arch Esp Urol. 2019;72(6):596–601.

25. Kuroda S, Kawahara T, Teranishi J, Mochizuki T, Ito H, Uemura H. A case of allograft ureteral stone successfully treated with antegrade ureteroscopic lithotripsy: use of a 3D-printed model to determine the ideal approach. Urolithiasis. 2019;47(5):467–71.

26. Smektala T, Golab A, Krolikowski M, Slojewski M. Low cost silicone renal replicas for surgical training – technical note. Arch Esp Urol. 2016;69(7):434–6.

27. Wake N, Rude T, Kang SK, Stifelman MD, Borin JF, Sodickson DK, et al. 3D printed renal cancer models derived from MRI data: application in pre-surgical planning. Abdominal Radiol (New York). 2017;42(5):1501–9.

28. Westerman ME, Matsumoto JM, Morris JM, Leibovich BC. Three-dimensional printing for renal cancer and surgical planning. Eur Urol Focus. 2016;2(6):574–6.

29. Golab A, Slojewski M, Brykczynski M, Lukowiak M, Boehlke M, Matias D, et al. Three-dimensional printing as an interdisciplinary communication tool: preparing for removal of a giant renal tumor and atrium neoplastic mass. Heart Surg Forum. 2016;19(4):E185–6.

30. Jian C, Shuai Z, Mingji Y, Kan L, Zhizhong L, Weiqing H, et al. Evaluation of three-dimensional printing assisted laparoscopic cryoablation of small renal tumors: a preliminary report. Urol J. 2020;

31. Mercader C, Vilaseca A, Moreno JL, Lopez A, Sebastia MC, Nicolau C, et al. Role of the three-dimensional printing technology incomplex laparoscopic renal surgery: a renal tumor in a horseshoe kidney. Int Braz J Urol. 2019;45(6):1129–35.

32. Fan Y, Wong RHL, Lee AP. Three-dimensional printing in structural heart disease and intervention. Ann Transl Med. 2019;7(20):579.

33. Kyung YS, Kim N, Jeong IG, Hong JH, Kim CS. Application of 3-D printed kidney model in partial nephrectomy for predicting surgical outcomes: a feasibility study. Clin Genitourin Cancer. 2019;17(5):e878–e84.

34. Wake N, Wysock JS, Bjurlin MA, Chandarana H, Huang WC. "Pin the tumor on the kidney": an evaluation of how surgeons translate CT and MRI data to 3D models. Urology. 2019;131:255–61.

35. Bejrananda T, Liawrungrueang W. Successful transitional cell carcinoma of bladder underwent laparoscopic radical cystectomy with orthotopic intracorporeal Y pouch neobladder using a 3D digital printing model for surgical post op pouch evaluation. Urol Case Rep. 2020;31:101190.

36. Rutkowski DR, Wells SA, Johnson B, Huang W, Jarrard DF, Lang JM, et al. Mri-based cancer lesion analysis with 3d printed patient specific prostate cutting guides. Am J Clin Exp Urol. 2019;7(4):215–22.

37. Sun G, Ding B, Yu G, Chen L, Wang Z, Wang S, et al. Three-dimensional printing – assisted planning for complete and safe resection of retroperitoneal tumor. J Xray Sci Technol. 2020;28(3):471–80.

38. Kusaka M, Sugimoto M, Fukami N, Sasaki H, Takenaka M, Anraku T, et al. Initial experience with a tailor-made simulation and navigation program using a 3-D printer model of kidney transplantation surgery. Transplant Proc. 2015;47(3):596–9.
39. Joshi PM, Kulkarni SB. 3D printing of pelvic fracture urethral injuries-fusion of technology and urethroplasty. Turk J Urol. 2020;46(1):76–9.
40. Wang H, Guo YT, Jiao Y, He DL, Wu B, Yuan LJ, et al. A minimally invasive alternative for the treatment of nutcracker syndrome using individualized three-dimensional printed extravascular titanium stents. Chin Med J. 2019;132(12):1454–60.
41. Hasan T. Is dissection humane? J Med Ethics Hist Med. 2011;4:4.
42. Tatar I, Huri E, Selcuk I, Moon YL, Paoluzzi A, Skolarikos A. Review of the effect of 3D medical printing and virtual reality on urology training with 'MedTRain3DModsim' Erasmus + European Union Project. Turk J Med Sci. 2019;49(5):1257–70.
43. Guliev B, Komyakov B, Talyshinskii A. The use of the three-dimensional printed segmented collapsible model of the pelvicalyceal system to improve residents' learning curve. Turk J Urol. 2020;46(3):226–30.
44. Aro T, Lim S, Petrisor D, Koo K, Matlaga B, Stoianovici D. Personalized renal collecting system mockup for procedural training under ultrasound guidance. J Endourol. 2020;34(5):619–23.
45. Melnyk R, Ezzat B, Belfast E, Saba P, Farooq S, Campbell T, et al. Mechanical and functional validation of a perfused, robot-assisted partial nephrectomy simulation platform using a combination of 3D printing and hydrogel casting. World J Urol. 2020;38(7):1631–41.
46. Wang Y, Gao X, Yang Q, Wang H, Shi T, Chang Y, et al. Three-dimensional printing technique assisted cognitive fusion in targeted prostate biopsy. Asian J Urol. 2015;2(4):214–9.
47. Nguyen LN, Head L, Witiuk K, Punjani N, Mallick R, Cnossen S, et al. The risks and benefits of cavernous neurovascular bundle sparing during radical prostatectomy: a systematic review and meta-analysis. J Urol. 2017;198(4):760–9.
48. Jomoto W, Tanooka M, Doi H, Kikuci K, Mitsuie C, Yamada Y, et al. Development of a three-dimensional surgical navigation system with magnetic resonance angiography and a three-dimensional printer for robot-assisted radical prostatectomy. Cureus. 2018;10(1):e2018-e.
49. Wendler JJ, Klink F, Seifert S, Fischbach F, Jandrig B, Porsch M, et al. Irreversible electroporation of prostate cancer: patient-specific pretreatment simulation by electric field measurement in a 3D bioprinted textured prostate cancer model to achieve optimal electroporation parameters for image-guided focal ablation. Cardiovasc Intervent Radiol. 2016;39(11):1668–71.
50. Wang J, Zhang F, Guo J, Chai S, Zheng G, Zhang K, et al. Expert consensus workshop report: Guideline for three-dimensional printing template-assisted computed tomography-guided 125I seeds interstitial implantation brachytherapy. J Cancer Res Ther. 2017;13(4):607.
51. Choi E, Adams F, Palagi S, Gengenbacher A, Schlager D, Muller PF, et al. A high-fidelity phantom for the simulation and quantitative evaluation of transurethral resection of the prostate. Ann Biomed Eng. 2020;48(1):437–46.
52. Witthaus MW, Farooq S, Melnyk R, Campbell T, Saba P, Mathews E, et al. Incorporation and validation of clinically relevant performance metrics of simulation (CRPMS) into a novel full-immersion simulation platform for nerve-sparing robot-assisted radical prostatectomy (NS-RARP) utilizing three-dimensional printing and hydrogel casting technology. BJU Int. 2020;125(2):322–32.
53. Srougi V, Rocha BA, Tanno FY, Almeida MQ, Baroni RH, Mendonca BB, et al. The use of three-dimensional printers for partial adrenalectomy: estimating the resection limits. Urology. 2016;90:217–20.
54. Cheung CL, Looi T, Lendvay TS, Drake JM, Farhat WA. Use of 3-dimensional printing technology and silicone modeling in surgical simulation: development and face validation in pediatric laparoscopic pyeloplasty. J Surgic Educ. 2014;71(5):762–7.
55. Pinto L, de Barros CAV, de Lima AB, Dos Santos DR, de Bacelar HPH. Portable model for vasectomy reversal training. Int Braz J Urol. 2019;45(5):1013–9.
56. del Junco M, Yoon R, Okhunov Z, Abedi G, Hwang C, Dolan B, et al. Comparison of flow characteristics of novel three-dimensional printed ureteral stents versus standard ureteral stents in a porcine model. J Endourol. 2015;29(9):1065–9.

57. Chang-Ju P, Hyeon-Woo K, Sangdo J, Seungwan S, Yangkyu P, Sang MH, et al. Anti-reflux ureteral stent with polymeric flap valve using three-dimensional printing: an in vitro study. J Endourol. 2015;29(8):933–8.
58. Russo GI, Di Mauro M, Cimino S. Use of 3D printing in andrological surgery: what are the new perspectives. Int J Impot Res. 2019;
59. Zhang K, Fu Q, Yoo J, Chen X, Chandra P, Mo X, et al. 3D bioprinting of urethra with PCL/PLCL blend and dual autologous cells in fibrin hydrogel: an in vitro evaluation of biomimetic mechanical property and cell growth environment. Acta Biomater. 2017;50:154–64.
60. Kim MJ, Chi BH, Yoo JJ, Ju YM, Whang YM, Chang IH. Structure establishment of three-dimensional (3D) cell culture printing model for bladder cancer. PLoS One. 2019;14(10):e0223689.

Chapter 14
Synthetic Models

Ahmed Ghazi, R. Devotini, and Domenico Veneziano

14.1 Introduction

Surgical simulation development, as described several times in literature [1–3], is a process that follows very strict steps with the final goal of replicating (simulating) a real procedure for training and assessment purposes. The most engaging step of the process is undoubtedly the design and production of the simulator itself, being it digital or physical. In the physical domain, in a field where standardization is the main rule, synthetic models may fit perfectly the needs of a novel protocol, but require very specific knowledge to be designed and built. Indeed, not only a new synthetic simulator has to maintain fidelity to the real thing, but also has to embed assessment tools, has to be easy to produce and replicate and its cost needs be kept as low as possible, in order to provide maximum distribution. The actors needed to succeed in such a generation process include clinicians, researchers, psychometricians, engineers, and even artists.

Clinician He acts as the expert in the group and provides information regarding the real procedure to be simulated. He needs to have a deep knowledge on every single aspect of the procedure, including anatomical details.

A. Ghazi
Department of Urology, University of Rochester Medical Center, Rochester, NY, USA

Simulation Innovation Laboratory, Department of Urology, University of Rochester, Rochester, NY, USA

R. Devotini
Department of Vascular Surgery, Grande Ospedale Metropolitano, Reggio Calabria, Italy

D. Veneziano (✉)
Grande Ospedale Metropolitano, Reggio Calabria, Italy
e-mail: info@domenicoveneziano.it

© Springer Nature Switzerland AG 2021
E. Huri, D. Veneziano (eds.), *Anatomy for Urologic Surgeons in the Digital Era*,
https://doi.org/10.1007/978-3-030-59479-4_14

Researcher He is in charge of interrogating the clinician to collect all the data that might be useful for the process. The interrogation phase is formally called Cognitive Task Analysis (CTA) and is constitutes the solid base of the development.

Psychometrician He analyses the CTA and, in close collaboration with the clinician and the researcher, translates the collected data into metrics, in order to objectively measure the outcomes of the simulation.

Engineer Based on the metrics and the assessment requirements, he develops the systems that will allow objective measurement. These include both hardware (sensors, displays) and software. He may also help to suggest modifications to be applied to the prototype to allow a wiser planning of the production phase.

Artist Several different artists may be included in the team. 3D designers are critical to create CAD (Computer-aided drafting) models for rigid parts, for example supports or housings for electronic parts. Prop artists work at the same time on the build of physical soft parts, which may also embed the electronics or the metric tools previously designed.

Given the huge availability of literature on the topic of simulation development and its clinical process, this chapter will focus mainly on the design and development of the physical part: the real core of the simulator.

14.2   History of Prosthetic Makeup and Synthetic Models

The use of synthetic materials to develop medical teaching models brings us back to the eighteenth century, when the first crude fabric dolls were assembled by a pioneering French midwife, Angelique Marguerite Le Boursier du Courday, to "simulate" obstetrical maneuvers. By the time a conflict arose between male and female practitioners, as men were starting to call themselves surgeons and to assert their roles in medicine and health, including childbirth that was usually taken care by midwives. Courday fought to support women in this period of time, until the moment she started to personally teach midwifery all over rural France. Between 1760 and 1783, Coudray created what she called "the machine" (Fig. 14.1), a life-size obstetrical manikin that could also include some real human bones in the torso. The machine was including many relevant anatomic structures and was so accurate that the Academy of Surgery approved it as a suitable model for childbirth practice. The best evolution of Coudray's machine are today the Cardiopulmonary resuscitation (CPR) manikins. Not only they provide realistic aesthetics, but also guarantee high educational value, thanks to the electronics embedded. In 1940 Asmund S. Laerdal founded in Norway a children's publishing and toy company. Thanks to the introduction of soft plastics, Laerdal started to produce the doll Anne, named "Toy of the Year", with sleeping eyes and natural hair. Given this experience, the company was

Fig. 14.1 "The machine"
created by Courday

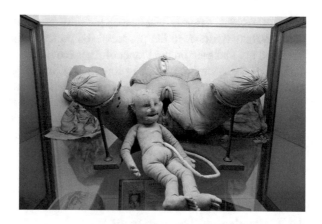

approached by the Norwegian Civil Defence to design natural looking imitation
wounds for military training. Soon after in 1960, in collaboration with the anaesthe-
siologist Dr. Peter Safar, the world's first patient simulator was produced. It was
named Resusci Anne, as a citation of the toy that was inspiring it, and was just the
beginning of a great CPR manikin legacy. CPR manikins where resembling the
physical properties of a real patient, like weight, height or thoracic expansion, while
the inner body was filled up with sensors and mechanical parts. A similar concept
was afterwards applied to dummies for crash tests, which were using several sensors
for data collection during collisions, taking the place of previously used cadavers
and animals. While the use of soft plastic allowed the early productions of training
full-body manikins, the development of realistic organs for surgical training might
find its roots in one of the most fascinating aspects of Hollywood productions: special effects. Given a distinction between *mechanical effects* and *optical effects*, in
this case the first ones are those we are referring to. While optical effects include
anything that is just visual (created photographically or computer-generated),
mechanical effects (also called *practical* or *physical* effects) are usually accomplished during the live-action shooting. This includes the use of mechanized props,
scenery, scale models, animatronics, pyrotechnics and atmospheric effects. For
example, prosthetic makeup can be used to make an actor look like a non-human
creature. The first actor to use special effects makeup was Lon Chaney, who created
his own looks for The Hunchback of Notre Dame, Phantom of the Opera and many
other films in the 1920s. The ability of makeup artists to create prosthetics increased
greatly in the 1930s with the introduction of foam latex. Latex was much easier to
use than the previously used wax, as it could be applied thinly and did not crack. In
1931 the sci-fi horror Frankenstein by James Whale was using an "out of kit" (thus
non-reusable) prosthetics, an adaptation of theatrical special effects. In these years
the field was revolutionised by John Chambers, an American make-up artist and
veteran makeup expert in television and film. During World War II he worked as a
medical technician and found employment by repairing faces and building prosthetic limbs for wounded veterans. By that time, the link between special effects and
medicine started to become clear and allowed several patients to live better despite

their deformities. After the war he took his skills to work at NBC, to work in makeup and prosthetics. Between his products, the famous pointy ears of Spock for Star Trek and the make-up on the Planet of Apes movie.

Due to the complex physical properties of intra-abdominal structures, artistic skills, matched with evidence based educational contents and deep anatomical knowledge, allow today the development of hyper realistic models to allow rehearsing actual surgical procedures. Back in time they were looking at surgery as if it was an art. Today we know that science and art are not anymore synonyms, but one can be definitely functional to the other to push forward the modern concept of patient safety.

14.3   Technical Background

The process of creating a prosthetic appliance for movie SFX begins with the individual: lifecasting is the process of creating a mold from a body part, to be used as a base for sculpting a prosthetic. The early lifecast molds were made from prosthetic alginate, that has been replaced by skin-safe silicon rubber. The negative mold (also called female mold), after being reinforced with plaster or fiberglass bandages, can be eventually used to make a "positive mold" (also called male mold). The two molds are different because while the male mold is covered by the preferred material, the female mold is used to pour in the material chosen. The positive in handy for movie production in order to create masks or appliances for special effects. Materials used for prosthetics are usually latex, gelatin, silicone or similar materials.

When it comes to human organs, lifecasting is obviously not possible, despite 1:1 realism being here particularly important. That's why DICOM images become the new base for surgical-training model production. After the acquisition of a CT scan, the 3D images can be used to manually sculpt an organ made by clay (Fig. 14.2a), thus following the "old-school" technique. In this case a negative mold (Fig. 14.2b) is afterwards derived from the clay model and then used to pour in the chosen material for the final product (Fig. 14.2c).

In order to achieve even more detail, a digital process can be followed instead of the described old procedure. After having selected the DICOM sequence, a single organ is isolated from the rest of the body and "cleaned" by a 3D artist. The highly-detailed CAD model is now ready for the development of a mold, that is digitally created for 3D printing. During the casting phase, additional technical tools can be embedded in the model, to match the surgical training requirements. Different materials can be used to create inner body organs:

14.3.1   Hydrogel

A study group at the Simulation Innovation Laboratory at the University of Rochester Medical Center have combined 3D printing with polymer casting

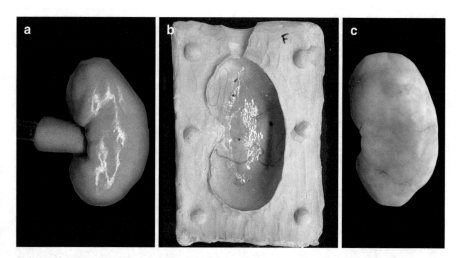

Fig. 14.2 "Old school" casting technique (courtesy of INTECH S.R.L.). (**a**) Clay model. (**b**) Concrete mold prepped for casting. (**c**) Silicon model

technology to develop full-procedural simulation platforms for minimally invasive partial nephrectomy (MIPN) [4] and radical prostatectomy [5]. The process entails perfecting two broad facets: geometry and material properties.

Polyvinyl Alcohol (PVA) is a biocompatible and inexpensive hydrogel that can be adapted to mimic human tissue properties in the fabrication process [6]. By varying the PVA concentration and number of processing (freeze/thaw) cycles that form polymeric bonds, it can reproduce the variable mechanical properties of different tissues such as tissue parenchyma, blood vessels, tumors and fat. The desired concentration is obtained by heating commercially available PVA powder and varying amounts of water. The result is relatively vicious gel that is shelf stable and costs under $1 per liter. PVA's phase change property is also critical for the fabrication process: the induction of cross-links through successive freeze/thaw cycles polymerizes it from an injectable gel into a progressively stiffer solid, texture that upholds its shape. To configure this PVA hydrogel into the geometry of an organ specific anatomy, a combination of additive and subtractive methods is utilized.

As an example, during the experiment published by Ghazi et al. [4], the fabrication of a kidney model started by importing DICOM files from a C.T. scan with a renal tumour suitable for a MIPN into Mimics 20.0 (Mimics, Materialise, Belgium). Segmentation was completed for each component of the kidney including: parenchyma, tumor, inferior vena cava with renal vein, abdominal aorta with renal artery, and urinary drainage system. Most structures were isolated with the thresholding and region growing tools. Multiple slice edit was used to increase the accuracy of the segmentation for non-contrasted structures. Each component is then converted to a 3D mesh (Fig. 14.3a) and imported into 3-matic 12.0 (Mimics, Materialise, Belgium) to form a computer aided design (CAD) model of the patient's anatomy. Each structure was wrapped and corrections were applied following

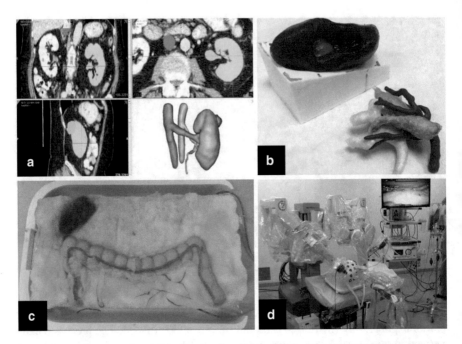

Fig. 14.3 Fabrication of the perfused hydrogel model for Robot-assisted Partial Nephrectomy. (**a**) Segmentation of patient CT scan. (**b**) 3D printed injection casts with hollow vasculature and urinary system prior to registration into the kidney cast. (**c**) Simulation platform for RAPN; including Kidney (containing renal hilar vessels, PCS and tumors), major abdominal vessels, perinephric fat, posterior abdominal muscles, spleen and overlying bowel. (**d**) Simulation with the daVinci Xi robot docked

recommendations from the *fix wizard* included in the software. The parts were smoothed using a combination applying a first order Laplacian function and local smoothing tool to remove artefacts from the segmentation. To incorporate the functionality of the model in terms of bleeding and urine leakage, the hilar structures (arterial, venous and calyx urinary systems) were printed to create a hollow, watertight vascular and urinary system. These structures along with the prefabricated tumor were then registered into the kidney mold and surrounded by PVA hydrogel, to mimic the mechanical properties of living kidney tissue (Fig. 14.3b). Guided by studies demonstrating that porcine kidneys can be utilized as human surrogates [7], fresh porcine kidney specimens have been tested, using a series of mechanical trials (unconfined uniaxial compression, indentation and elastography testing) and functional tests (designed to test bleeding and suturing). The published results demonstrated that PVA kidneys, fabricated using 7% PVA at three freeze-thaw cycles, is the formula that most closely approximates the mechanical and functional properties of fresh living kidney tissue [8]. To establish a procedural simulation platform, the kidney phantom and other PVA structures (retroperitoneal fat and muscle, a

partial colon segment, spleen, and anterior abdominal wall) were assembled in anatomic orientation and subjected to final processing for organ cohesion (Fig. 14.3c).
Artificial blood was perfused through the model's vasculature to simulate bleeding
and the model is placed in a box trainer where the daVinci robot can be docked
(Fig. 14.3d). Using the robotic platform all steps of a robotic partial nephrectomy
can be performed including; preoperative CT review (Fig. 14.4a), dissection of the
renal hilum (Fig. 14.4b), intraoperative intraoperative ultrasound imaging
(Fig. 14.4c), perfused tumor resection (Fig. 14.4d), and repair of the calyceal and
parenchymal defects (Fig. 14.4e). Following fabrication, the models are stored in a
vacuum sealed bag to remove any excess moisture and prevent dryness of the PVA
components. The models remain viable up to 90 days from fabrication however it is
recommended to be utilized within 30 days of fabrication to maintain their realistic
mechanical properties based on unpublished data from our laboratory demonstrated
that there is minimal change in the mechanical properties of the models (delta of
0.03 in Youngs modulus) following 30 days of storage.

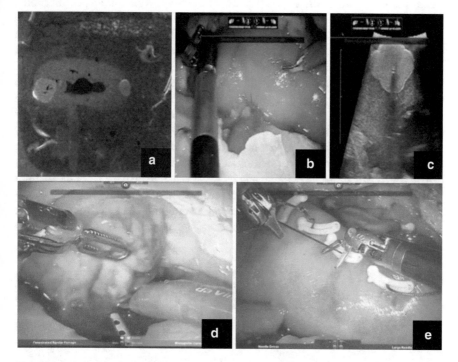

Fig. 14.4 Validation of the simulation platform for Robot-assisted Partial Nephrectomy. (**a**) CT
imaging of the model for preoperative review and surgical planning. (**b**) Preoperative planning on
hydrogel model. (**c**) Intraoperative ultrasound of the simulated tumor (Left) with probe on model
after dissection of Gerotas fascia (Right). (**d**) Simulated excision of tumor with functional bleeding. (**e**) Simulated closure of the parenchymal defect, demonstrating sliding clip renorrhaphy after
tumor resection

14.3.2   Silicon

After the creation of a mold, a valid alternative to hydrogel is silicon. Silicon comes in different pre-arranged densities, usually in A+B parts to be mixed in a lab with pre-determined mixing rates, together with drops of the desired color. Curing time depends on the density of the selected silicon and usually harder ones have a faster curing than the softer ones. While with hydrogel freeze/thaw cycles allow to alter consistency, *deadener* or *hardener* fluids can be added to the mix in order to soften or harden the selected silicon. *Thinner* fluid can be used to produce thin layers of material, while a *retarder* can be mixed to slow down curing time, thus allowing the casting of more complex molds. In some cases, catalysts may be required to start the curing process. *Mold-release* spray is applied to the inner face of the molds to ease even more the detachment.

Soft silicon could tear under the traction of a suture. A thin mesh can be placed in the outer layers of the model to increase its strength, when it is expected to apply stitches or strong tractions. This is the case of the Major Vessel Injury repair model [9], today used on a regular base for intermediate urological laparoscopic skills acquisition. Handling silicon requires high precision and expertise: different organ tissue properties can be achieved with different recipes, by mixing the right amount of the different products described.

Just like for the previously described process, also in this case 3D CAD design software (Fig. 14.5a) is used to create a mold and 3D print it (Fig. 14.5b). The design has the goal to create pieces that can be easily dismounted, to allow proper detach of the silicon model (Fig. 14.5b, c). The use of transparent resin for mold printing can aid color check, while also avoiding unwanted air bubbles, even along the casting process. After the extraction of the model from the mold, further layers can be added to achieve more detail and increase visual realism (Fig. 14.6a–c), until "hyper-realistic" results are reached. Apart from its high flexibility in terms of density and visual configurations, one of the most important characteristics of silicon is its retention of physical properties over time. Indeed, silicon model maintains its

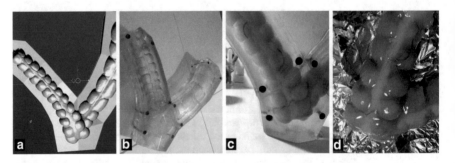

Fig. 14.5 From 3D CAD modeling to the final silicon product (courtesy of INTECH S.R.L.). (**a**) CAD model design of the mold. (**b**) 3D printed resin mold. (**c**) Silicon model inside the mold. (**d**) Final hyper-realistic silicon model

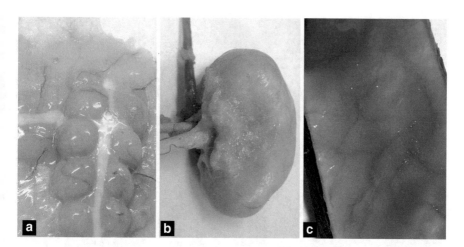

Fig. 14.6 Hyper-realistic silicon models after external detailing (courtesy of INTECH S.R.L.). (**a**) Colon model. (**b**) Kidney model. (**c**) Abdominal wall details

characteristics for years, which is crucial for storage purposes. Silicon models might also be reusable, if properly designed. The use of interchangeable parts, together with the lasting properties, make silicon very suitable for high-volume production and distribution, despite being slightly inferior to hydrogel regarding tissue fidelity.

14.3.3 Latex

Another valid alternative to the aforementioned materials is latex, already largely used in the medical environment for its mechanical properties. Between the most common latex products we can mention surgical gloves, balloons, bandages, just to name a few. In the surgical simulation field, rubber latex is often used to create low or high-fidelity vascular structures. Pre-vulcanized rubber latex is a natural resin that hardens at ambient temperature to form a stable rubber. This material is extremely handy and easy to use: after the having built a mold (Fig. 14.7a), the fluid rubber is applied over it by brush with multiple coats (Fig. 14.7b). Alternatively, the mold can be dipped inside a tray filled up with rubber fluid, as it happens for the serial production of latex gloves. Curing of the product depends on the thickness of the layer and on the environmental temperature. Evaporation is indeed simplified in case high temperature is applied (for e.g.: with a hairdryer or with a heating machine), which considerably lowers the time of the whole process. Once dried, the model can be easily detached from the mold without any mold-release product (Fig. 14.7c, d). Several models can be produced starting from a single 3D mold. Previously formed rubber latex vascular structures can be jointed or welded by

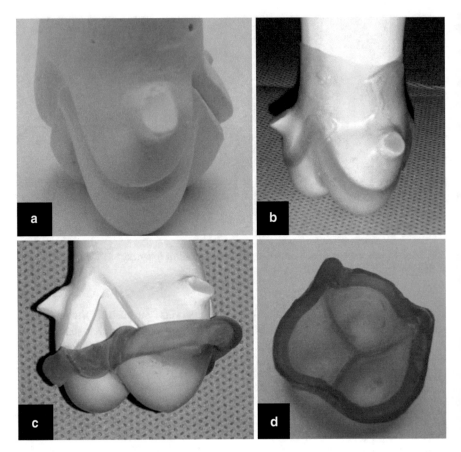

Fig. 14.7 From the mold to the final latex product. (**a**) The mold. (**b**) Latex is applied by brush. (**c**) The model is removed from the mold. (**d**) Final model

applying a few drops of latex to the connection points (Fig. 14.8). Between the main physical characteristics of latex, is its elasticity and strength. Latex models can be stretched and pressurized and that's why this material is optimal for conduits or vessels in general. Thanks to the possibility of creating strong models with very thin layers of material, this option is feasible also when transmitting pulsations is between the requirements of the simulator. Latex is also stable to atmospheric degradation and has an excellent resistance to stitching with surgical sutures. Tridimensional fine details are well respected, while coloring is limited up to 5% the total weight of material casted, if full elasticity is needed. Higher quantities of pigments may allow higher aesthetic fidelity, but could alter the final physical properties.

It is very important to point out that latex and silicon are not fully compatible with each other: while latex naturally vulcanizes and cures over a layer of silicon mold-release spray, curing of silicon components is not regularly happening over a latex layer, if not previously sealed. This step becomes critical if both latex and silicon materials are needed in order to fulfill the simulation requirements.

Fig. 14.8 Additional parts
are jointed to a latex model

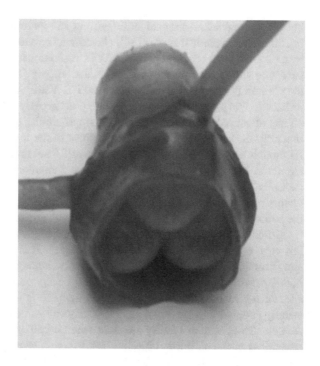

14.4 Comparison with Different Simulation Systems

In a complex field like the surgical education one, synthetic models need to be compared with the other available training systems. Choosing the one to use depends on goals of the training session and which skills need to be achieved by the participant. Arranging a training session for endoscopy, laparoscopy of robotic surgery is also requiring different simulators, which makes the choice even more difficult. As such, surgical education is struggling for example to identify the ideal skills training platform for robotic surgery [10]. Historically, cadavers and animals have been considered as the gold standards for realistic full procedural simulation, but their high cost, regulated availability, risks of transferable diseases, and potential ethical concerns limit their widespread use [11]. Additionally, such animal or cadaveric models also lack specific pathology (e.g. renal tumor) that may be advantageous in order to achieve advanced surgical proficiency [12].

The use of cadavers represents the only truly anatomical simulator with the highest possible fidelity available to practice entire operations. To combine accurate human anatomy with physiological and circulatory conditions, human cadavers have been artificially perfused to replicate the real-life parameters of dissection with haemostasis leading to an approximate cost of $1000/cadaver [13]. Qualitative data from a study in which 26 learners participated in a surgical skills acquisition curriculum demonstrated that using perfused cadavers improved acquisition of new knowledge, enhanced surgical skill learning and increased confidence in performing the skill in a clinical setting [14]. Nevertheless, these attempts have been limited by a positive viral profile, the difficulty of vascular access and/or clearing the vascular tree due to previous vascular or cardiac surgery [15]. Moreover, cadavers lack the possibility of objective data collection. The history of crash test dummies brings us back to this problem, as cadavers were used in early times to understand the real effects of car collisions on humans. The impossibility of collecting actual information after the impact, lead to the development of the first *dummies*. Today's Hybrid III models are equipped with an average of 21 sensors, to measure accelerations along the impact, which make them today not anymore replaceable by old-school cadavers. The latest development of more electronically advanced and realistic simulators might have the same effect in the surgical training environment, leading to the point where cadavers and animals might look equally obsolete.

Virtual Reality training systems have been facing a relevant improvement in the last year, especially in relation to robotic surgery. This is mostly related to human-simulator interfaces, that may not be effective enough when tactile feedback is highly expected by the surgeon in training (for e.g.: in laparoscopy). On the opposite, during robotic training, the interface adopted is just the same console that is usually coupled to a Da-Vinci Robot, or anyway something designed to mimic it. Advantages of Virtual Reality are clear when it comes to replicability of the task, reusability of the platform, objective assessment. Development costs are anyway a big downside of VR, as well as physics realism. Collisions, lights, fluid dynamics are not easy to calculate in a virtual environment and this is all up to the graphic/physics engines and how they are programmed. Programming a videogame may involve tens to hundreds of people, with large investments required. Despite being robotic training the most suitable for this technology, the advent of novel robotic systems might create new issues in terms of standardization. Companies like Intuitive (Sunnyvale, CA, USA) have already implemented their own training software, provided as a backpack computing unit together with the Da Vinci console. Different robotic surgery brands are meanwhile developing their own simulation software, which might create confusion when it comes to finding the referral training system to adopt for international official certifications.

The ideal simulator should be indeed usable on any surgical platform and provide the same objective metrics, while still ensuring reusability and standardization at a relatively low price. In consideration of what has just been said, synthetic models, which might look outdated when compared to some digital systems, might demonstrate their higher overall efficiency. Perfused anatomical hydrogel models, which replicate the mechanical (tissue characteristics) and functional attributes (urine and blood) of a renal system immersed in accurate anatomical surroundings, may help resolve some of the main aforementioned issues with cadaveric models. These models, just like the silicon or latex ones, can replicate a standardized or patient-specific anatomy, thus allowing several different operative options, and can be monitored thanks to embedded sensors, if needed. Moreover, synthetic materials provide high adoptability as they avoid religious, location and storage issues.

14.5 Costs of Synthetic Model Development

Another great advantage of synthetic materials is their development and production cost, as opposed to other organic or digital options. Indeed, cadavers require the use of dedicated environments, just like animals, which ale need to be raised up in specific farms until they reach the correct size to undergo the surgical session. Right after, they are suppressed, thus allowing to take advantage of the expense just for a single time. VR simulators, as already described, require high investments for software development, as well as for the production of the physical peripheral. Development of synthetic models, including the design and 3D printing of the mold, is definitely cheaper, with costs ranging from 500 € to 4000 € for products with different complexity (including early design and prototyping). Materials used are also particularly cheap: the PVA partial nephrectomy procedural model costs $143 in material, $260 in personnel and $182 in consumables per participant trial, thereby facilitating widespread use and individualized training. Regarding silicons, a 10 kg bin of Platsil gel 10 (Polytek Development Corp., Easton, PA, USA), one of the most used silicon products for training model development, can be easily found online for purchase at 200 € and allows production of hundreds of small training models. In this case specialized manufacturing might rise up the costs, which result to be anyway low enough to maintain a reasonable selling price. Limitations are in this case connected to the expertise required to handle the materials, which can be overcome with proper training of the workers involved. Pre-vulcanized latex can be also found on the market for very affordable prices, with a 25 l bin costing around 160 €. Although this doesn't consider the startup cost of a daVinci robot and instruments, the non-biohazardous nature of synthetic models negates the need for a dedicated teaching robot, wet-lab facilities, and associated setup and running costs. Furthermore, the absence of an infection risk, customizable pathology, and the ability to simulate complications such as bleeding and collateral organ damage provide a significantly favorable economic evaluation compared to similar procedural models.

14.6 Future Perspectives

Simulation training in this context has been based on the concept of skills generalization where the trainees learn fundamental skills (e.g. instrument handling, suturing etc.) that are crucial for their early development. However, evidence examining the role of simulation in reducing errors for practicing clinicians is lacking. Skill transfer refers to a training modality that directly emulates the task to be performed in vivo and requires simulations that focus on optimizing the preparation of practicing physicians immediately before the actual intervention for an individual patient (patient-specific simulation). Patient-specific rehearsals would allow practicing surgeons to practice, plan, and address potential problems related to a specific patient's case, thus optimizing the real intervention.

The Simulation innovation laboratory have refined their process to develop a patient-specific simulation platform for kidney cancer surgery using a combination of image segmentation, 3D printing and hydrogel molding to fabricate patient-specific models suitable for surgical rehearsals directly prior to the live procedure. Preliminary data has demonstrated an improvement in patient outcomes as a result of this intervention [16].

As previously stated, between the great advantages of synthetic models, is the possibility of embedding hidden technology to make them "phygital". This neologism matches together the words physical (analogic) and digital, to produce a unique result that allows the tactile feedback of a real product, together with the feasibility of electronic measurements. Companies like INTECH (Innovative Training Technologies, Milan, Italy) are actually developing training systems that allow the visual tracking of synthetic models, thus collecting data while producing objective assessment. Meanwhile, hydrogel models are already allowing patient specific production of 1:1 surgical scenario, which can provide the surgeon an actual testing of the procedure, even before touching the corresponding patient for the first time. Training systems like these might change completely what we call today surgical training, as they might not only provide us large scale information on how surgeons are preparing their practice, but also give them more tools to increase the safety of their patients. Visual tracking systems will indeed enable "smart-teaching" even without physical tutors and will collect data about the re-certification of surgeons, generating as a side-effect potential radical changes in the field of health insurance. A doctor might be requested to remotely re-certify his skills on a smart training box, or even to simulate the full procedure of the day after, on a hydrogel model created on-the-fly. The convergence of novel materials, scientific evidence and artificial intelligence is pushing forward a field that has been under-evaluated for decades, while finally providing invaluable tools to surgeons. Within few years they will be able to get trained in a standardized way, wherever they want, at any time and with possibility to track and certify their improvements, even on patient-specific scenarios.

References

1. Veneziano D, Hananel D. The Smith's textbook of endourology, Chapter 75. 4th ed. Wiley; 2019.
2. Veneziano D, et al. Development methodology of the novel endoscopic stone treatment step 1 training/assessment curriculum: an international collaborative work by European Association of Urology Sections. J Endourol. 2017;31(9)
3. Salmon P, Stanton N, Gibbon A, Jenkins D, Walker G. Cognitive task analysis. In: Human factors methods and sports science; 2009.
4. Ghazi A, et al. Validation of a full-immersion simulation platform for percutaneous nephrolithotomy using three-dimensional printing technology. J Endourol. 2017;
5. Witthaus MW, et al. Incorporation and validation of clinically relevant performance metrics of simulation (CRPMS) into a novel full-immersion simulation platform for nerve-sparing robot-

assisted radical prostatectomy (NS-RARP) utilizing three-dimensional printing and hydroge. BJU Int. 2020;

6. Li P, Jiang S, Yu Y, Yang J, Yang Z. Biomaterial characteristics and application of silicone rubber and PVA hydrogels mimicked in organ groups for prostate brachytherapy. J Mech Behav Biomed Mater. 2015;

7. Farshad M, Barbezat M, Flüeler P, Schmidlin F, Graber P, Niederer P. Material characterization of the pig kidney in relation with the biomechanical analysis of renal trauma. J Biomech. 1999;

8. Melnyk R, et al. Mechanical and functional validation of a perfused, robot-assisted partial nephrectomy simulation platform using a combination of 3D printing and hydrogel casting. World J Urol. 2019;

9. Veneziano D, Poniatowski LH, Reihsen TE, Sweet RM. Preliminary evaluation of the SimPORTAL major vessel injury (MVI) repair model. Surg Endosc. 2016;30(4):1405–12.

10. Villegas L, Schneider BE, Callery MP, Jones DB. Laparoscopic skills training. Surg Endosc. 2003;17(12):1879–88.

11. Gilbody J, Prasthofer AW, Ho K, Costa ML. The use and effectiveness of cadaveric workshops in higher surgical training: a systematic review. Ann Roy College Surgeons Engl. 2011;

12. Ross HM, Simmang CL, Fleshman JW, Marcello PW. Adoption of laparoscopic colectomy: results and implications of ASCRS hands-on course participation. Surg Innov. 2008;

13. Carey JN, Minneti M, Leland HA, Demetriades D, Talving P. Perfused fresh cadavers: method for application to surgical simulation. Am J Surg. 2015;210(1):179–87.

14. Minneti M, Baker CJ, Sullivan ME. The development of a novel perfused cadaver model with dynamic vital sign regulation and real-world scenarios to teach surgical skills and error management. J Surg Educ. 2018;

15. Faure JP, Breque C, Danion J, Delpech PO, Oriot D, Richer JP. SIM Life: a new surgical simulation device using a human perfused cadaver. Surg Radiol Anat. 2017;

16. Stone J, Melnyk R, Wu G, Rashid H, Joseph JV, Ghazi A. V4-01 Patient specific rehearsal using 3d printing for complex partial nephrectomy cases. J Urol. 2017;197(4):e375.

Chapter 15
Creating Standards for 3D Soft-Tissue Modelling

Emre Huri, Osman Tunç, Young Lae Moon, and Dae Ok Kim

15.1   Introduction

Medical images from hospitals consist of a two-dimensional (2D) dataset and provide human body information as a slice, but the human body has three-dimensional (3D) morphology. If we should simulate this 3D morphology, we might be able to obtain more information about the body as well as contribute in the clinical environment to both treatment and surgical outcomes. Our objective is to generate 3D medical data from 2D images. We know that two dimensional images are radiological data that clinicians encounter every day in daily clinical practice. 3D modeling requires good knowledge of human anatomy, good technology knowledge and ability to use appropriate software. Determining the clinical purpose of 3D modeling, clarification of the expectations is essential in determining the software type to be used. Although doctors expend a great deal of time and effort in this process, the resultant 3D data are different in each institute. The standardization trials, therefore, provide standard, easy, and accurate 3D data for clinical fields and even for industrial markets. IEEE Standards documents are developed within the IEEE Societies and the Standards Coordinating Committees of the IEEE Standards Association

E. Huri (✉)
Department of Urology, Hacettepe University, Ankara, Turkey
e-mail: emrehuri@hacettepe.edu.tr

O. Tunç
Btech Innovation Company, METU Technopolis, Ankara, Turkey
e-mail: osman.tunc@btech.com.tr

Y. L. Moon
YM Orthopedic Hospital, Gwangju, South Korea

D. O. Kim
Medical Biochemistry Lab and Researching Bio 3D Printing, Chosun University, Gwangju, Republic of Korea

© Springer Nature Switzerland AG 2021
E. Huri, D. Veneziano (eds.), *Anatomy for Urologic Surgeons in the Digital Era*,
https://doi.org/10.1007/978-3-030-59479-4_15

(IEEE-SA) Standards Board. IEEE develops its standards through a consensus development process, approved by the American National Standards Institute, which brings together volunteers representing varied viewpoints and interests to achieve the final product. This chapter will provide general information about the standardization work we do within IEEE-SA, does not cover standards.

15.2 Scope

The standardization trials reduce the 3D printing output variability of soft and hard tissue in medical images and defines a defined model data file format standard for consistent 3D printing. Standardization involves acquiring model data with physical density and size characteristics through medical tomography image calibration and developing digital file format data using image segmentation technology. In the soft and hard tissue cases, image processing and segmentation are required, however there is no standardization for intensity range because it is taken by various devices and protocols such as MRI or CT, or injection protocol. However, it is known that providing radiological images in thin slices (1–5 mm) allows segmentation to be performed more accurately in 3D modeling. Otherwise, the excessive cross-section slices will lead to a lack of details in the 3D visualization of organ.

In medical imaging and modeling procedures for soft tissue 3D printing will include the following features:

– Pre-processing for image enhancement.
– Segmentation in medical image for soft tissue 3D printing.
– Post-processing for false positive reduction.

15.3 Overview of Medical Imaging and Modeling Procedures for Soft Tissue 3D Printing

The application of computational methods to medical images (CT, MRI, and so on) has made it possible to create three-dimensional (3D) targeted anatomical models. In addition, additive manufacturing, or 3D printing as it is commonly known, is a process used together to create 3D patient-specific objects.

15.4 Methods

(a) *Image Isotropic Conversion*

If we have few slices of patient's images, when we reconstruct back to 3D, there will be a lot of "empty space" in between the image. Isotropic conversion is adding

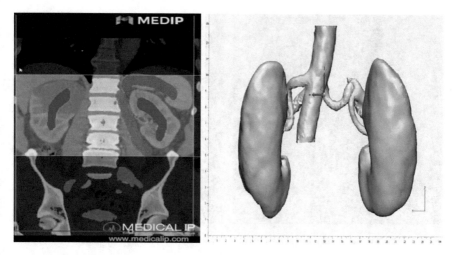

Fig. 15.1 Reconstruction of 3D medical data generated by isotropic conversion (segmentation of kidney—3D visualization)

more slice in between so that we can get more images and we can have more smooth visualization (by sampling and calculation from data points of each two images) (Fig. 15.1).

(b) *Image Enhancement*

In medical imaging tomography, the noise is inevitable due to different imaging principles. Therefore, it is necessary to remove these noises before segmentation to ensure a good quality segmentation result. Gaussian Low Pass Filter uses a normal distribution function to remove noise from the image, while the Laplacian of Gaussian Filter is a filtering method that highlights the edges of the images. By doing so, you can either remove the noise in the medical image or pre-processing the techniques that emphasize certain areas to increase the quality of the final segmentation result.

(c) *Image Segmentation*

Image segmentation is the process of partitioning a digital image into multiple segments. The goal of medical image segmentation is to simplify and/or change the representation of an image into something that is more meaningful and easier to analyze (Figs. 15.2 and 15.3).

(d) *False Positive Reduction*

Extraction results inevitably include false positives (FP). Removal of these FP is necessary, which may require different methods depending on the extraction algorithm. For instance, in the graphic to be shown the red area on the left is the FP area of the extraction of the bronch, and the results are effectively removed by various tests. The importance of the FP removal process can be found in this example.

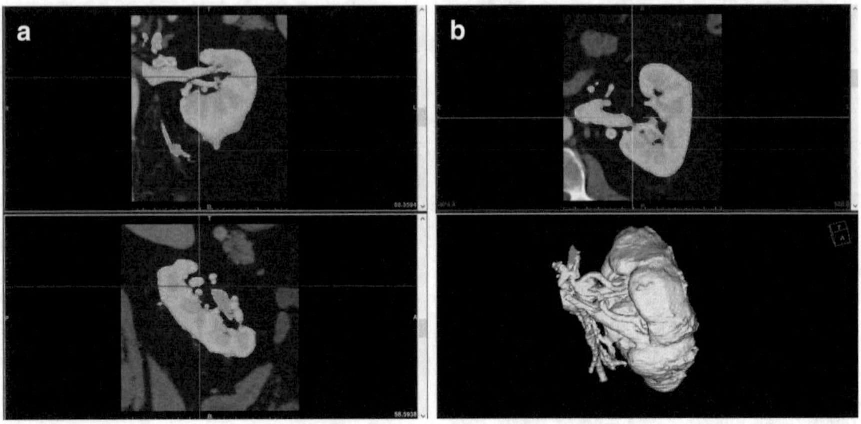

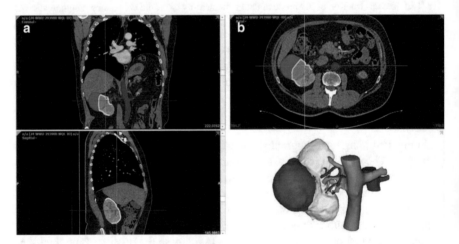

Fig. 15.2 Soft tissue segmentation (**a**) CT image (**b**) kidney region of CT image

Fig. 15.3 Soft tissue segmentation (**a**) 3D visualization (**b**) segmented vessel region of CT image

15.5 MedTRain3DModsim and Standardization Experience

The MedTRain3DModsim Erasmus + European Union Project, which started on October 2016 and completed on October 2018, was led by Hacettepe University in Ankara, Turkey, and partner organizations Chosun University, South Korea; Charles University, Czech Republic; and Rome 3 University, Italy and Hellenic Urological Association, Greece. The full name of the project was 'Novel Educational Materials in Medical Training with 3D Modeling Application and Simulation Modalities (Virtual Reality and Augmented Reality)', which was the first project funded by the Turkish National Agency. The aim of the project was to extract and reconstruct 3D realistic anatomical models from computer tomography (CT) (Digital Imaging and Communications in Medicine, DICOM) images with various software packages and print or simulate them in 3D for educational purposes. The project focused on models of solid organs and the urinary system, including the prostate, kidney, ureter, and liver.

One of the intellectual outcomes (IO) was "*Standardization of 3D Medical Models*", the description of IO was evaluation of several model's characteristics for standardization. The summary of applied methodology was to evaluate and create standardization on different specifications of the models including visualize 3D volume image, accuracy for augmented reality target recognition (the affected part—marker), accuracy for target recognition (the affected part—marker) tracking, real-time rendering speed for target recognition (the affected part—marker) and 3D objects, matching level for target recognition (the affected part—marker) and 3D objects and real-time 3D rendering speed for VR simulation etc. However, the group worked collaboratively with IEEE-EMBS Standard Association 3D Based Medical Application Working Group to maintain standards of virtual and 3D printed medical models.

15.6 Stepwise 3D Modeling Technique for 3D Medical Printed Urological Organ Models

All 3D anatomical modeling studies are realized by transferring MRI and CT scans to Mimics® software via DICOM files. Radiological images are monitored in the axial, coronal and sagittal projections. HU (Hounsfield Unite) values were assigned to 2D radiological images for masking. The segmentation is performed by checking the anatomical boundaries of various structures. Different MRI sequences are used for segmentation of different structures. All MRI and CT scans are superposed to make them a unique structure. After then, a design module "3-matic" is used for detailed modeling. STL files are then transferred to the 3D printer.

15.6.1 Preparation of Urological Models

Alternative medical training tools are needed as adjuncts to those currently used. The primary drivers to develop new sources of training are limitations in traditional training methods, complexity of procedures, the rise of new procedures, and variance in human anatomy due to age and pathologies. In MedTRain3DModsim Project, we aimed extraction and reconstruction of 3D realistic anatomical models from CT/DICOM images with variable software packages and printing them three dimensionally for educational purposes.

15.6.2 *Benefits*

- Identify the international standards of 3D medical modeling and applications for solid organ models as a first time in the world (IEEE-SA 3D Based Medical Application WG Collaboration)
- Decrease the cost with using virtual based 3D printed and edited models for surgical implementation and simulation, learning anatomy in medical fields specifically on urology and general surgery, no more expensive machines and simulators
- Using technology and printed materials for better understanding 3D surgical anatomy
- Creating 3D printed medical models for dry lab training (in laparoscopic/endoscopic/robotic surgeries)
- EBU (European Board of Urology) Curriculum for residency training will be used for creation useful 3D printed surgical and organ models in urological section
- Virtual training curriculum on medical models will be one of the target at the end of the Project
- Once digital definitions (STL files) are secured, the specimen can be reproduced in any quantity.
- A unique pathology can be imaged and then shared amongst multiple institutions. For biomodels, several studies also report the advantage of enlarging the specimen to increase visibility for hard-to-see structures.
- For simulation, a key advantage of 3D printing, versus in vivo training, is the ability to complete entire procedures in a no-risk environment.
- Without simulators, residents develop procedural skill in a step-wise fashion; obtaining competence in one step before advancing to the next step, at a later date on a different patient. 3D printed simulators do not suffer from these limitations, and therefore may accelerate resident training.
- 3D printed simulators affords trainees the ability to repetitively perform and perhaps master the basic maneuvers that are the cornerstone of the procedure.
- Do not forget that Simulators are an adjunct to in vivo training. Training solely on a simulator cannot ensure competence in the procedure and does not obviate the need for in vivo training or proctored cases

15.6.3 *Methodology*

Reconstruction of computer based 3D anatomical models from standardized DICOM images, firstly there will be used software packages such as MIMICS® and Medical IP® for extracting adequate anatomical info to the model. Additional software will be used for volume rendering, texturing processes to create realistic human models. These models will be shown as virtual reality view. These virtual models will be converted for producing real 3D printed educational materials, processing the printed organ/system models will also be performed to mimics the surgical models in appropriate manner. 3D printing is the vehicle for production of anatomical replicas for two intents. One: study and visualization (static biomodels) and, two: simulation of medical procedures (physical simulators). In the project, we both use "static biomodels" and "physical simulators" for training purposes. For static biomodels, 3D printed training tools are compared to 2D radiographic imaging (computed tomography [CT]), 3D digital models, palatinate models and cadaveric specimens. For physical simulators, the comparisons are drawn against cadaveric dissection, virtual reality simulators and in vivo training during surgical procedures. We prefer to make comparisons with 2D CT and cadaveric models during the training activities.

15.6.4   Workflow

The processes began with CT or magnetic resonance imaging (MRI) data, from patients or cadavers, that generated Digital Imaging and Communications in Medicine (DICOM) files. These were then imported into software programs where the anatomy was segmented to create the desired anatomic structures. Where needed, this data was further modified and repaired. Next, polygonal mesh (STL) files were generated for 3D printing. These data can be used for virtual reality model or printed model. Following 3D printing, the anatomical replicas were used as-is, coated, painted or dyed. For the physical simulators, we will use 3D printed replicas combined with other materials to imitate tissue, such as silicone, hydrogel etc. For urinary system replicas, all 3D printed models including lumen will be adaptable to endoscopic urologic devices. In this project, we used two types of 3D printed models; the first one, using 3D printing to create molds that are then used to cast anatomic structures in materials that better simulate human tissue, the second one is 3D printed anatomic replicas without using mold, directly one to one similar to STL file. The cast materials include silicone, polyurethane, hydrogel, gelatin/ agar mixture and high-acyl gum. The post-processes models after production were shown in Fig. 15.4.

15.7   Kidney (Basic)

Kidney 3D planning and modeling studies were achieved with Mimics® (Fig. 15.5). DICOM files of CT scans were imported into Mimics. Radiological images were visualized on axial, coronal and sagittal planes. Masking process was assume using HU (The gray values of CT images are expressed according to the Hounsfield) values on 2D radiological images. Segmentation of the structures was done by following the anatomical boundaries. Surface rendering was used to produce 3D models of different anatomical structures. Then, a design module 3-matic was used for detailed modeling. Then, the STL files were exported to 3D printer.

Radiological Data Requirements: Contrast CT Scan, Slice Thickness: 0.5–1.5 mm

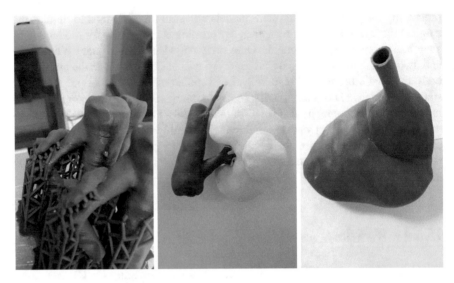

Fig. 15.4 Post-process after production

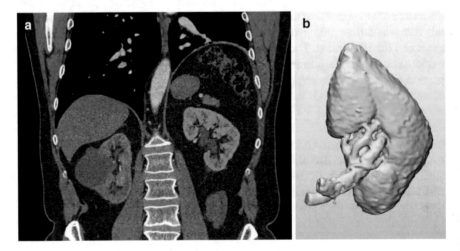

Fig. 15.5 CT image (**a**) segmentation of kidney—3D visualization (**b**)

15.8 Kidney (with Renal Tumor)

In this study: First, the DICOM files of contrast CT scan were imported to Mimics software followed by the segmentation of 3D models of the kidney, tumor, vessel by the software (Fig. 15.6). The model created in Mimics was exported to the design module of 3-matic for modeling.

Radiological Data Requirements: Contrast CT Scan, Slice Thickness: 0.5–1.5 mm

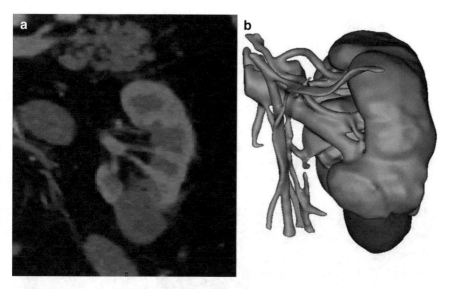

Fig. 15.6 CT image (**a**) segmentation of kidney and with tumor—3D visualization (**b**)

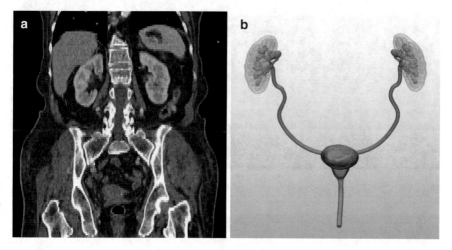

Fig. 15.7 CT image (**a**) segmentation of kidney and ureter—3D visualization (**b**)

15.9   Ureter

CT images were analyzed retrospectively and modeled with 3D printing where the DICOM files on axial, coronal, and sagittal plan were converted to STL files (segmentation images) by Mimics®. The lumen and wall were created with data processing via manual smoothing and hollow command in 3-matic (Fig. 15.7).

Radiological Data Requirements: Contrast CT Scan, Slice Thickness: 0.5–1.5 mm

15.10   **Bladder** (Fig. 15.8)

Radiological Data Requirements: Contrast CT Scan, Slice Thickness: 0.5–1.5 mm

15.11   **Prostate**

Prostate 3D anatomical modeling studies (Fig. 15.9) were realized with Mimics. DICOM files of mp-MRI were imported into Mimics.

Radiological Data Requirements: Contrast mp-MR

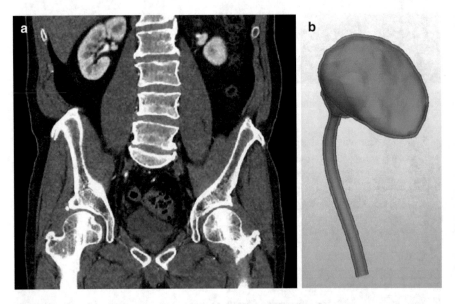

Fig. 15.8 CT image (**a**) segmentation of bladder—3D visualization (**b**)

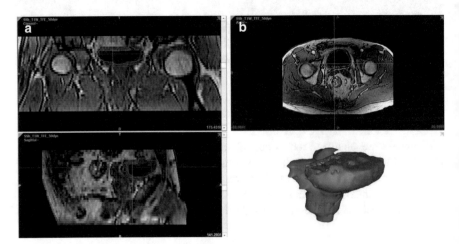

Fig. 15.9 MRI image (**a**) segmentation of prostate and bladder—3D visualization (**b**)

15.12   Sacrum (Fig. 15.10)

Radiological Data Requirements: CT Scan, Slice Thickness: 0.5–1.5 mm
The variables of models in terms of image process, modeling process, production and post-process are shown in Fig. 15.11.

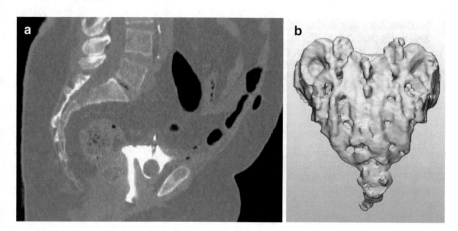

Fig. 15.10   CT image (**a**) segmentation of sacrum bone—3D visualization (**b**)

MODELS VARIABLES	KIDNEY	URETER	BLADDER	PROSTATE+URETHRA	PELVICB BONE	SACRUM	SILICON KIDNEY	VESSEL
Image Process Variable								
Pixel size	0.5 mm	0.5 mm	0.5 mm	0.5 mm	0.5 mm	0.5 mm	N/A	0.5 mm
Slice thickness	1 mm	1 mm	1 mm	1 mm	1 mm	1 mm	N/A	1 mm
Modeling Process Variables								
Modeling Time	⁻8 hour	⁻3 hour	⁻4 hour	⁻3 hour	⁻5 hour	⁻4 hour	⁻12 hour	⁻3 hour
Anatomic suitability	±1 mm	±1 mm	±1 mm	±1 mm	±1 mm	±1 mm	±1 mm	±1 mm
Production and Post Process Variables								
Production Technology	SLA	SLA	SLA	SLA	FDM	FDM	Tersine MÜhendislik	SLA
Production resolution	0.025	0.025	0.1	0.1	0.2	0.2		0.1
Production Period	⁻16 hour	⁻8 hour	⁻10 hour	⁻9 hour	⁻32 hour	⁻18 hour	⁻36 hour	⁻10 hour
Post process Period	⁻3 hour	⁻2 hour	⁻1 hour	⁻2 hour	⁻2 hour	⁻2 hour	⁻5 hour	⁻2 hour
Material Type (soft/hard)	Resin/Hard	Resin/Hard	Resin/Hard	Resin/Hard	PLA/Hard	Resin/Hard	silicon/soft	Resin/Hard

Fig. 15.11   Variables of models

Suggested Reading

1. 3333.2.1-2015 – IEEE Recommended Practice for Three-Dimensional (3D) Medical Modeling. 2015.
2. Moon YL. 3D medical application. http://www.youtube.com/user/ylm2103.
3. Lim CW, Seon JM, Moon YL. Orthopaedic 3D printing and simulation. Ann Joint. 2018;3:66.
4. Goo HW, Park SJ, Yoo SJ. Advanced medical use of three-dimensional imaging in congenital heart disease: augmented reality mixed reality virtual reality and three-dimensional printing. Korean J Radiol. 2020;21(2):133–45.
5. Tatar I, Huri E, Selcuk I, Moon YL, Paoluzzi A, Skolarikos A. Review of the effect of 3D medical printing and virtual reality on urology training with 'MedTRain3DModsim' Erasmus + European Union Project. Turk J Med Sci. 2019;49(5):1257–70.

Part IV
Understanding Anatomy and Translating It to Everyday Surgery

Chapter 16
Exploration of Pelvic Anatomy: Cadaveric Dissection Atlas

Ilker Selcuk and Emre Huri

16.1 Retroperitoneum

The retroperitoneum is the space which is under the peritoneum. The peritoneum is a serous membrane that covers the anterior and posterior abdominal walls from the level of diaphragm superiorly to the level of pelvic floor inferiorly [1]. The retroperitoneal space is the potential area located between the parietal peritoneum anteriorly and the transversalis fascia posteriorly. The retroperitoneal anatomic structures; adrenal gland, kidney, ascending colon, descending colon, rectum, ureter, abdominal aorta and its branches, inferior vena cava and its tributaries, superior hypogastric plexus and pelvic autonomic nerves, could be accessed by cutting the anterior peritoneal covering. This peritoneal membrane is called parietal peritoneum and the extensions of parietal peritoneum covering the visceral structures is called visceral peritoneum.

The essential anatomical structures of pelvic retroperitoneum are explained here in the manner of surgical anatomy.

16.1.1 Pelvic Avascular Spaces

These spaces are named according to the anatomical location of pertinent organs and they provide the surgical maneuvers to be completed safely. A combination of sharp and blunt dissection is performed to adequately develop these spaces which

I. Selcuk (✉)
Department of Gynecologic Oncology, University of Health Sciences, Ankara City Hospital Maternity Hospital, Ankara, Turkey

E. Huri
Department of Urology, Hacettepe University, Ankara, Turkey

© Springer Nature Switzerland AG 2021
E. Huri, D. Veneziano (eds.), *Anatomy for Urologic Surgeons in the Digital Era*,
https://doi.org/10.1007/978-3-030-59479-4_16

are located under the parietal peritoneal covering. Pelvic avascular spaces maintain a safe surgical zone for most of the pelvic procedures regarding uterus, rectum or bladder and pelvic sidewall. During pelvic lymphadenectomy, the surgeon should open the pararectal and paravesical space. Moreover, during the radical hysterectomy, the vesicovaginal and rectovaginal space should also be opened to achieve the parametrial and paracolpial resection.

Pelvic avascular spaces:
- Prevesical (Retropubic) space
- Paravesical space
- Pararectal space
- Presacral (Retrorectal) space
- Vesicovaginal space
- Rectovaginal space

16.1.1.1 Prevesical (Retropubic) Space

It is posterior to the pubic bone and anterior to the bladder. Prevesical space is also called retropubic space or space of Retzius. Grasping the median umbilical ligament (Urachus) with downward traction and cutting it from the level of the junction part of the parietal peritoneum and anterior abdominal wall opens a cleavage to the space of Retzius. Blunt dissection towards the symphysis pubis is preferred to develop the prevesical space entirely. During anterior or total exenteration procedures, urogynecologic procedures (Burch's colposuspension) or radical cystectomy, this step is extremely important. Dorsal clitoral neurovascular bundle is found at the midline of this space, and additionally, retropubic space is rich in venous vessel structures [2].

Borders of the prevesical space (Figs. 16.1 and 16.2):

- Anterior: Pubic symphysis
- Posterior: Bladder
- Superior: Parietal peritoneum
- Lateral: Arcus tendineus fascia pelvis

16.1.1.2 Paravesical Space

Paravesical space is adjacent to the bladder, laterally, at the posterior surface of the pubic bone. It is also at the lateral part of the paravaginal and prevesical space. Paravesical space is divided into two parts by the obliterated umbilical artery, the lateral part unites with the obturator space (fossa).

Borders of the paravesical space (Figs. 16.3, 16.4, and 16.5):

- Medial: Bladder, vagina, space of Retzius, superior vesical artery
- Lateral: Obturator fossa, obturator internus muscle, external iliac vessels

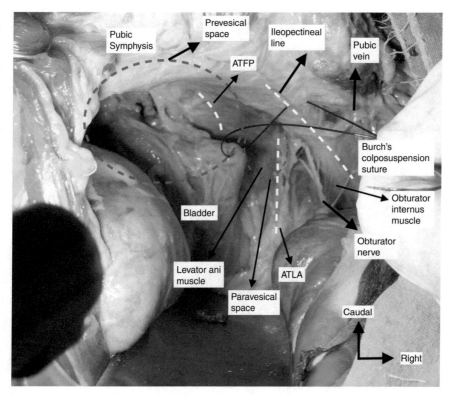

Fig. 16.1 Borders of the prevesical space (Abbreviations: *ATFP* Arcus tendineus fascia pelvis, *ATLA* Arcus tendineus levator ani)

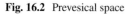

Fig. 16.2 Prevesical space

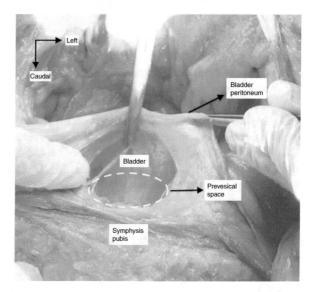

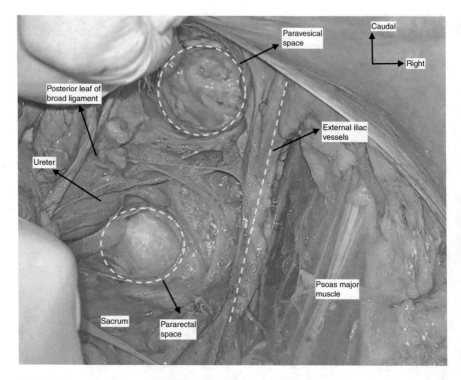

Fig. 16.3 Paravesical space, right pelvic sidewall

- Posterior: Uterine artery, cardinal ligament, lateral parametrium
- Anterior: Pubic bone, superior pubic ramus
- Inferior: Levator ani muscle

Clinical tip

After identification of the entry point of the round ligament to the inguinal canal which is superior to the inguinal ligament, 2–3 cm inferomedial to that point, the paravesical space could easily be developed bluntly after cutting the covering tissue of parietal peritoneum. During pelvic lymphadenectomy, the lateral part of paravesical space is important to dissect the obturator lymph nodes and this approach could provide the visualization of the pubic vein or artery called corona mortis [3]. Corona mortis is based mainly on the venous anastomotic vessels between the inferior epigastric vessels and obturator vessels [4]. During the radical hysterectomy, the medial part of the paravesical space (medial to obliterated umbilical artery) is used to dissect the parametrium.

Obturator fossa

Obturator fossa is lateral to the paravesical space and contains obturator lymph nodes, nerve, artery, and vein. Separation of external iliac artery and vein from the adjacent psoas major muscle also provides exposure to the obturator fossa from the lateral part.

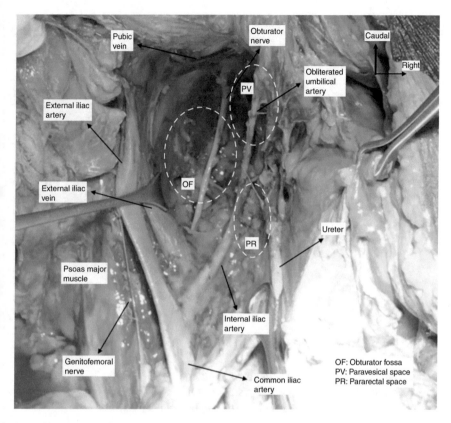

Fig. 16.4 Obturator fossa, left pelvic sidewall

Borders of the obturator fossa (Fig. 16.4):

- Medial: Obliterated umbilical artery
- Lateral: Obturator internus muscle
- Superior: External iliac vessels
- Inferior: Obturator internus muscle, intersection with the levator ani muscle
- Anterior: Obturator membrane
- Posterior: Origin of the internal iliac vessels

16.1.1.3 Pararectal Space

Pararectal space is lateral to the rectum and it should be developed in the same manner with the angle of the sacral bone. The ureter divides the pararectal space into two parts; the medial part is named Okabayashi's space and the lateral part is named Latzko's space.

Fig. 16.5 Pararectal space, right pelvic sidewall

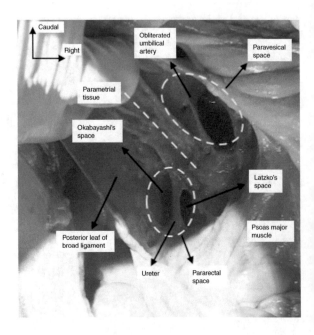

Borders of the pararectal space (Figs. 16.3–16.5):

- Medial: Rectum, uterosacral ligament, ureter
- Lateral: Internal iliac artery, the posterior division
- Anterior: Uterine artery, cardinal ligament, lateral parametrium
- Posterior: Sacrum

Clinical tip

After entering the retroperitoneum, the posterior leaf of the broad ligament is pulled towards the sacrum and firstly the pelvic ureter is identified under the infundibulo-pelvic ligament. The ureter divides the pararectal space into two compartments and the medial part is between the ureter and rectum that consists of the end part of the hypogastric nerve deeply and the hypogastric nerve continues as the inferior hypogastric plexus within the bundles of pelvic splanchnic nerves (Detailed knowledge in pelvic autonomic nerves) [5]. This space (Okabayashi's) is considerably important during the nerve-sparing radical hysterectomy [6]. During pelvic lymphadenectomy while dissecting the interiliac nodes or during ligation of internal iliac artery for postpartum bleeding or pelvic hemorrhage developing the pararectal space will medialize the ureter and provide a clear and safe margin [7].

16.1.1.4 Presacral (Retrorectal) Space

Presacral space is also called retrorectal space. It is a potential retroperitoneal area anterior to the presacral fascia and posterior parietal peritoneum covers it. During posterior or total exenteration procedures or low anterior resection, presacral space provides a surgical field. Presacral space contains the hypogastric nerve at the lateral edges bilaterally and the superior hypogastric plexus is found at the superior part of this space anterior to the aortic bifurcation and left common iliac vein [8].

Borders of the presacral space (Figs. 16.6 and 16.7):

- Anterior: Distal portion of the mesentery of sigmoid colon, rectum and the posterior parietal peritoneum covering it
- Posterior: Promontorium and sacrum, presacral fascia
- Inferior: Levator ani and coccygeus muscle
- Superior: Posterior parietal peritoneum
- Lateral: Ureter and internal iliac vessels, hypogastric nerve

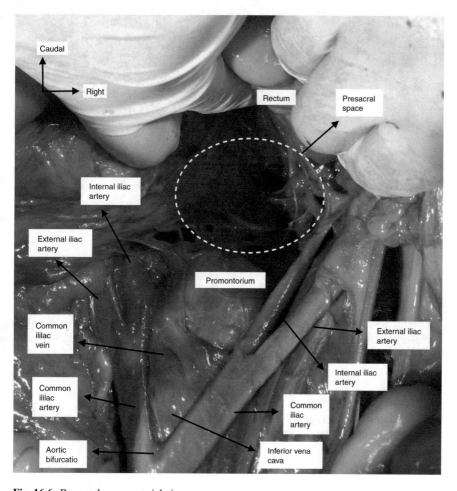

Fig. 16.6 Presacral space, cranial view

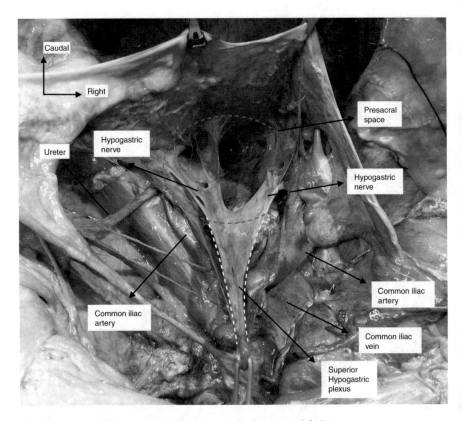

Fig. 16.7 Presacral space and superior hypogastric plexus, cranial view

16.1.1.5 Vesicovaginal Space

This space is developed by cutting the vesicouterine peritoneal reflection and retracting the bladder caudally. Vesicovaginal space is dissected with sharp and blunt maneuvers from the midline, excessive lateral dissection will injure the vesical veins that are lying on the bladder pillars. Vesicovaginal space is important to achieve a total hysterectomy and the caudal dissection level of the bladder defines the radicality and excision margin of the vagina [9].

Borders of the vesicovaginal space (Fig. 16.8):

- Anterior: Bladder, Trigone
- Posterior: Anterior vaginal wall, distal portion of uterine cervix
- Lateral: Bladder pillars, pubocervical ligament
- Inferior: Urogenital diaphragm

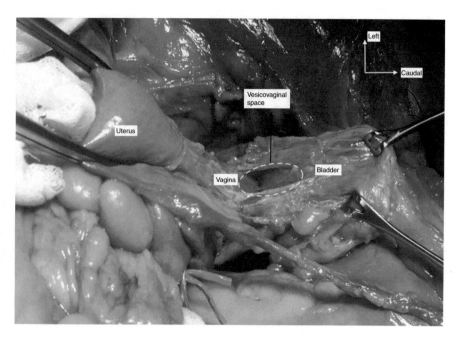

Fig. 16.8 Vesicovaginal space

16.1.1.6   Rectovaginal Space

Cutting the rectouterine peritoneal fold (Pouch of Douglas) between the uterosacral ligaments will maintain access to the rectovaginal space. Dissection should be performed towards the vagina and caudally, otherwise perirectal fatty tissue might be injured and it receives the arterial supply from the branches of the middle rectal artery.

Clinical tip
Endometriosis, ovarian tumors, and an abscess will enclose this field, in that situation pararectal space is developed, the ureter is lateralized from the uterosacral ligament and dissection is carried out from lateral to medial over the uterosacral ligaments. Additionally, in the case of a cervical mass, both the vesicovaginal and rectovaginal spaces should be developed with the paravesical space.

Borders of the rectovaginal space (Fig. 16.9):

- Anterior: Posterior vaginal wall
- Posterior: Anterior wall of the rectum and perirectal fatty tissue
- Lateral: Uterosacral ligament, rectal pillars

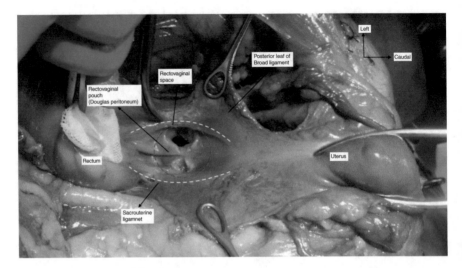

Fig. 16.9 Rectovaginal space

16.1.2 Pelvic Ureter

Pelvic ureter crosses over the common iliac artery from lateral to medial at the level of the pelvic brim and runs attached to the deep part of the posterior leaf of the broad ligament. It lies on the medial side of the internal iliac artery, lateral to the uterosacral ligament and enters the medial portion of cardinal ligament just under the isthmic part of the uterus. At this level, the uterine artery crosses over the ureter and ureter passes through the ureteric tunnel within the parametrium just before entering the Trigone at the anterolateral part of the upper vagina. At the level of ureteric tunnel, the ureter is surrounded by the veins of the bladder. The ureter enters the posterolateral part of the Trigone and takes a 1.5 cm course in the bladder wall [10].

Since the ureter does not have a specific vessel for vascular supply, it receives arterial branches from the common iliac, internal iliac, uterine, superior gluteal, vaginal, middle rectal, inferior and superior vesical arteries (Fig. 16.10).

Clinical tip
The mid-part of the ureter (between the pelvic brim and lower third) is less vascularized than the other parts. During radical hysterectomy procedure, especially while dissecting the vesicouterine ligament, this step has an increased risk of injury to the lower third, distal part of the ureter. During dissection of the ureter, care must be taken to preserve the adventitia and the fatty tissue covering the ureter which is clinically called mesoureter [11, 12].

Potential three sites of ureter injury during pelvic surgical procedures (Fig. 16.11):

- During infundibulopelvic (IP) ligament ligation where the ureter passes postero-inferior to it (site I)
- During uterine artery ligation where the ureter is below the uterine artery nearby the uterine isthmus (site II)
- At the anterolateral part of the upper vagina especially during radical hysterectomy (site III)

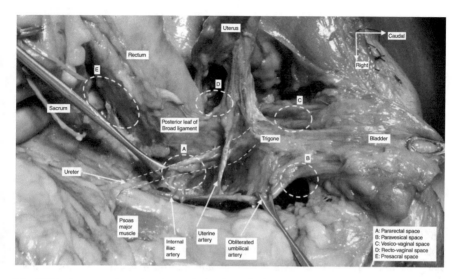

Fig. 16.10   Pelvic ureter, right pelvic sidewall

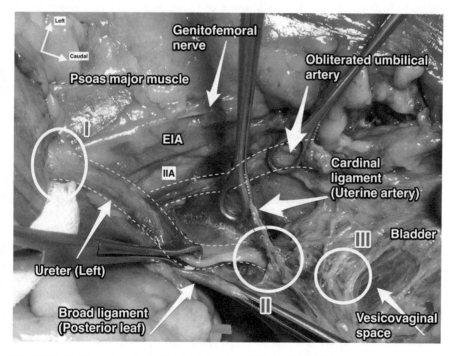

Fig. 16.11   Pelvic ureter, sites of injury, left pelvic sidewall (Abbreviations: *EIA* external iliac artery, *IIA* internal iliac artery)

Clinical tip

During dissection of the anterior parametrium for radical hysterectomy, the ureter is unroofed from the ureteric tunnel and the bladder pillars (clinically termed vesicouterine ligament), this dissection may cause bleeding which arises from the veins of the bladder [13]. This hemorrhage is frequently stopped with minimal pressure, thermal energy must be used cautiously to prevent any thermal injury to the ureter.

16.1.3   Pelvic Autonomic Nerves

Presynaptic sympathetic fibers which pass through the paravertebral ganglions (lateral to the aorta) without making a synapse and reach to the prevertebral ganglions (anterior to the aorta) are called lumbar splanchnic nerves (T5-L2/L3). Lumbar splanchnic nerves synapse at the prevertebral ganglions; celiac ganglion, aorticorenal ganglion, superior mesenteric ganglion, and inferior mesenteric ganglion; after that, postsynaptic nerve fibers run to the abdominopelvic viscera through the periarterial plexuses (celiac plexus, superior hypogastric plexus, and inferior hypogastric plexus) which are formed by the condensation of sympathetic and parasympathetic nerve fibers. Superior mesenteric plexus, intermesenteric plexus and inferior mesenteric plexus are secondary extensions of celiac plexus, besides intermesenteric plexus primarily lies anterior to the abdominal aorta and gives fibers to join the superior hypogastric plexus [14, 15]. The superior hypogastric plexus which transmits postsynaptic sympathetic nerve fibers lies within the aortic bifurcation, anterior to the left common iliac vein and superior to the presacral space. The superior hypogastric plexus runs in front of the Promontorium, and is divided into right and left hypogastric nerves; those lie at the lateral part of presacral space bilaterally, medial to the internal iliac artery and posterolateral to the rectum (Fig. 16.7) [16].

Presynaptic parasympathetic nerve fibers arise from S2 to S4 and run together with those spinal nerves. After they leave the spinal nerves, they are called pelvic splanchnic nerves which run deep to the parametrium under the deep uterine vein and join obliquely to the extensions of the hypogastric nerve to form the inferior hypogastric plexus which lies under the ureter and parallel to the uterosacral ligament, on the lateral surface of rectum, and base of vagina and bladder bilaterally (Fig. 16.12). The inferior hypogastric plexus contains postsynaptic sympathetic, presynaptic and postsynaptic parasympathetic fibers, and general visceral afferent fibers. Pelvic splanchnic nerves synapse at the ganglions located near the target organ and afterwards, they give the postsynaptic nerve fibers. Postsynaptic nerve fibers are located at the secondary plexuses which are the extensions of the inferior hypogastric plexus, found on the lateral side of the rectum, uterine cervix and bladder bilaterally; called middle rectal plexus, uterovaginal plexus and vesical plexus, respectively [17].

General visceral afferent fibers; the pain, and stretching sense from bladder, rectum and uterus go within the pelvic splanchnic nerves. Pelvic splanchnic nerves

Fig. 16.12 Inferior hypogastric plexus and pelvic splanchnic nerves, right pelvic sidewall (Abbreviations: *IHP* inferior hypogastric plexus, *PSN* pelvic splanchnic nerves, *IIA* internal iliac artery, *EIA* external iliac artery, *EIV* external iliac vein)

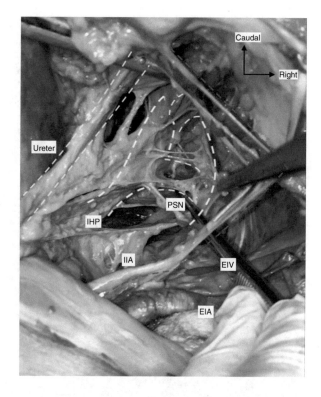

also maintain the motor impulse for the smooth muscle of hindgut and bladder. Lumbar splanchnic sympathetic nerves contribute to the formation of both superior and inferior hypogastric plexus, they maintain the innervation of the bladder neck.

16.1.4   Pelvic Vasculature

16.1.4.1   Common Iliac Artery and Vein

The aorta is divided into right and left common iliac artery at the level of L4-L5 vertebra called aortic bifurcation and the common iliac arteries lie on the anterolateral side of the lumbar body. Anterior to the sacroiliac joint the common iliac artery is divided into the external and internal iliac artery (Fig. 16.6).

Clinical tip

The common iliac veins join to form the inferior vena cava at a lower level than the aortic bifurcation and the left common iliac vein lies posterior to the left common iliac artery, anterior to the Promontorium. During dissection of presacral lymph nodes or medial common iliac nodes, the left common iliac vein will be injured. The left common iliac vein is also important during the sacrocolpopexy procedures [18].

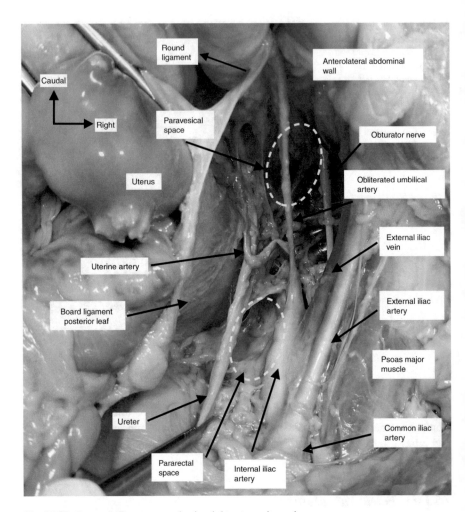

Fig. 16.13 External iliac artery and vein, right retroperitoneal space

16.1.4.2 External Iliac Artery and Vein

The external iliac artery is the direct extension of the common iliac artery that is named the femoral artery after passing below the inguinal ligament. After entering the retroperitoneum, firstly the external iliac vessels are noticed on the medial side of the psoas major muscle [19]. The external iliac vein lies medially to the artery on the posteroinferior surface, and the branches and tributaries of the external iliac artery and vein are located at the anterior surface of the vessels (Fig. 16.13).

Inferior epigastric artery

The inferior epigastric artery originates from the distal part of the external iliac artery posterior to the inguinal ligament (Fig. 16.14). It is accompanied with the inferior epigastric vein. Together they shape the lateral umbilical fold. The inferior

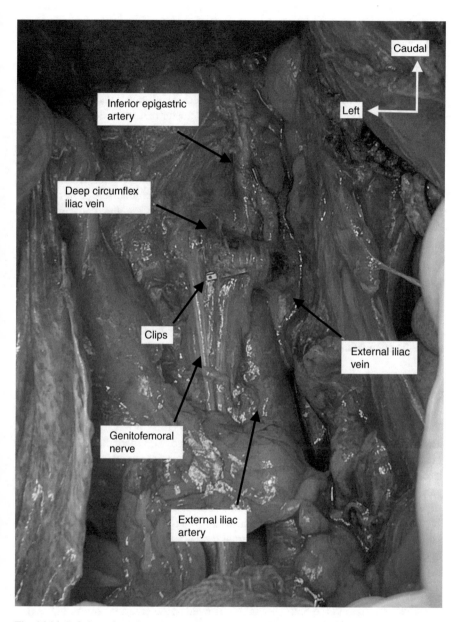

Fig. 16.14 Inferior epigastric artery and deep circumflex iliac vein, left pelvic sidewall

epigastric artery runs in the subperitoneal tissue, then ascends obliquely upward at the medial margin of the deep inguinal ring, and it is the deep artery of the anterior abdominal wall. This lateral umbilical fold is anatomically close to the round ligament [2]. The inferior epigastric vein accompanies the arterial counterpart. Corona mortis is a connection between the external iliac or inferior epigastric vessels and the obturator vessels. Corona mortis is mainly shaped by the pubic vein and rarely it is structured by an arterial anastomosis (Fig. 14.4).

Deep circumflex iliac artery

The deep circumflex iliac artery originates proximal to the inferior epigastric artery and runs towards the lateral part of the deep anterior abdominal wall. Deep circumflex iliac artery courses laterally and vertically posterior to the inguinal ligament, then turns medially at the level of the iliac crest. It has anastomoses with the ascending branch of the lateral circumflex femoral artery. During its course, it gives a branch at the level of the anterior superior iliac spine, which lies between the internal oblique muscle and transversus abdominis muscle, that has anastomoses with the lumbar and inferior epigastric vessels. Deep circumflex iliac vein joins the external iliac vein after crossing over the external iliac artery, it is noticed proximal to the inferior epigastric artery (Fig. 16.14).

Clinical tip

The distal border of pelvic lymphadenectomy is the deep circumflex iliac vein. Dissection of lymph nodes distal to this part increases the risk of lymphorrhea. Clip ligation of the lymph channels is suggested to prevent lymphocele formation [20]. While dissecting the obturator lymph nodes, care should be taken not to injure the pubic vein which lies posterior to the superior pubic ramus. Corona mortis is mostly a venous connection rather than an arterial anastomosis.

16.1.4.3   Internal Iliac Artery and Vein

The internal iliac artery is the most variably branching artery. The internal iliac artery passes down into the pelvis inferomedially and is divided into the anterior and posterior division. The anterior division continues with the obliterated umbilical artery to the anterior abdominal wall within the medial umbilical fold. The proximal part of the umbilical artery gives the branch of the superior vesical artery that lies superolateral to the bladder and forms the medial border of the paravesical space. The ureter is medial to the internal iliac artery and the internal iliac vein lies on the posterolateral surface between the internal iliac artery and medial part of the psoas major muscle. The internal iliac vein has a lot of collateral tributaries which are especially lying below the obturator nerve (Fig. 16.15) [21].

- The anterior trunk of the internal iliac artery: Anterior trunk gives branches to the pelvic viscera and the branches are distributed at the anterior portion of the pelvic brim. Umbilical artery, uterine, superior vesical, inferior vesical, vaginal, obturator, middle rectal, internal pudendal and inferior gluteal artery are the branches of the anterior trunk (Figs. 16.16 and 16.17).
- The posterior trunk of the internal iliac artery: Posterior trunk is at the inferomedial portion of the pelvic brim. The iliolumbar artery, lateral sacral artery and superior gluteal artery are the branches of the posterior division. They have anastomoses with other arteries; iliolumbar-forth/fifth lumbar artery, lateral sacral-median sacral artery and superior gluteal-inferior gluteal/internal pudendal artery (Fig. 16.18).

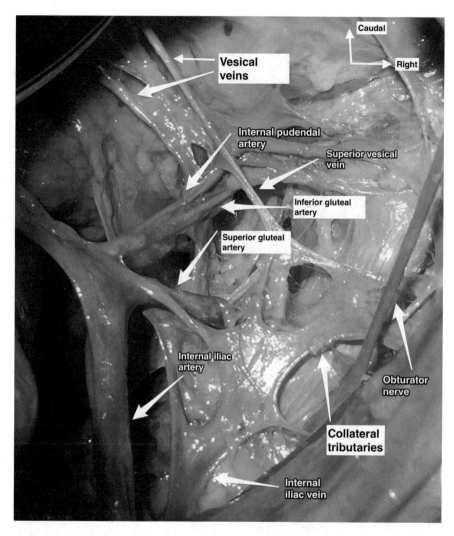

Fig. 16.15 Collateral tributaries of the internal iliac vein, right pelvic sidewall

Obturator artery and vein

The obturator artery is the lateral branch originating from the anterior division of the internal iliac artery, which lies below the obturator nerve ahead to the obturator canal.

Obturator vein drains into the internal iliac vein and lies mostly below the obturator artery (Fig. 16.19).

Clinical tip

Aberrant obturator artery may be seen up to 20–30% in the population and originates from the external iliac artery or inferior epigastric artery. Aberrant obturator artery crosses the external iliac vessels and runs ahead to the obturator canal inferomedially.

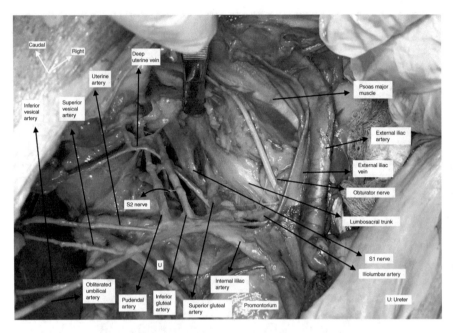

Fig. 16.16 Internal iliac artery and branches, right pelvic sidewall

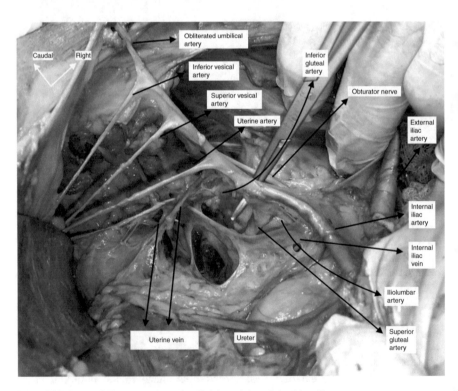

Fig. 16.17 Internal iliac artery, anterior division, right pelvic sidewall

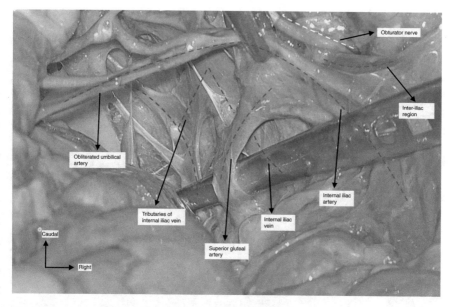

Fig. 16.18 Internal iliac artery, posterior division, right pelvic sidewall

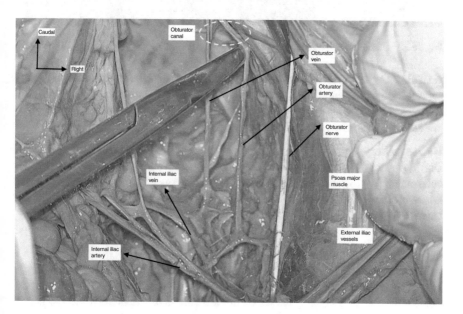

Fig. 16.19 Obturator vessels, right pelvic sidewall

Obliterated umbilical artery

The obliterated umbilical artery is the end branch of the internal iliac artery, diverging from the anterior division and becomes the medial umbilical ligament at the anterior abdominal wall. It divides the paravesical space into two parts and the superior vesical artery diverges from the proximal part of the umbilical artery. Superior

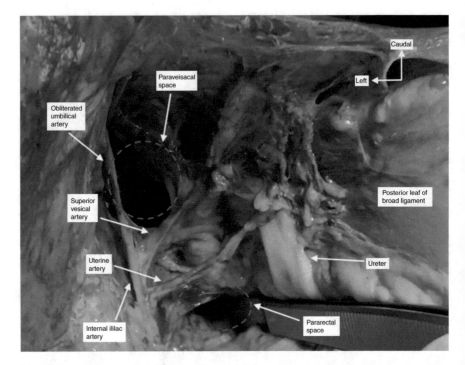

Fig. 16.20 Uterine artery, left pelvic sidewall

vesical artery supplies the upper part of the bladder and the inferior vesical artery supplies the base. Ligation of the superior vesical artery during pelvic surgery/radical hysterectomy does not alter the bladder functions. Upward traction of the obliterated umbilical artery reveals the uterine artery.

Uterine artery
Uterine artery diverges from the anterior division of the internal iliac artery and lies anteromedially towards the isthmic part of the uterus and uterine cervix. Uterine artery crosses over the ureter. The uterine artery lies within the cardinal ligament between the anterior and posterior layers of the broad ligament (Fig. 16.20).

Clinical tip: How to identify the uterine artery?
After developing the paravesical space, dissection of the obliterated umbilical artery in a cephalad manner will facilitate the identification of the uterine artery or after developing the pararectal space following the course of the ureter from the pelvic brim to the point where it crosses under the uterine artery is another option.

Internal pudendal artery
The internal pudendal artery lies anterior to the piriformis muscle, passes through the greater sciatic foramen and enters the ischio-anal fossa through the lesser sciatic foramen. The dorsal artery of the clitoris is the branch of the internal pudendal artery (Fig. 16.16).

Inferior gluteal artery

The inferior gluteal artery passes between the S1 and S2 (sacral) nerves and leaves the pelvis through the greater sciatic foramen (Fig. 16.16).

References

1. Selcuk I, Ersak B, Tatar I, Gungor T, Huri E. Basic clinical retroperitoneal anatomy for pelvic surgeons. Turk J Obstet Gynecol. 2018;15(4):259–69.
2. Loukas M, Benninger B, Tubbs RS. Gray's clinical photographic dissector of the human body. 1st ed. Saunders; 2012.
3. Selcuk I, Uzuner B, Boduc E, Baykus Y, Akar B, Gungor T. Pelvic lymphadenectomy; step-by-step surgical education video. J Turk Ger Gynecol Assoc. 2019;
4. Selcuk I, Tatar I, Firat A, Gungor T, Huri E. Is corona mortis a historical myth? A perspective from gynecological oncologist. J Turk Ger Gynecol Assoc. 2018;
5. Selcuk I, Tatar I, Huri E, Gungor T. Anatomical and functional basis of pelvic autonomic nerves with regard to radical hysterectomy. JCOG. 2018;28(4):163–9.
6. Fujii S. Anatomic identification of nerve-sparing radical hysterectomy: a step-by-step procedure. Gynecol Oncol. 2008;111(2 Suppl):S33–41.
7. Selcuk I, Uzuner B, Boduc E, Baykus Y, Akar B, Gungor T. Step-by-step ligation of the internal iliac artery. J Turk Ger Gynecol Assoc. 2019;20(2):123–8.
8. Karram M, Baggish M. Atlas of pelvic anatomy and gynecologic surgery. 4th ed. Elsevier; 2016.
9. Morrow PC. Surgical anatomy. In: Morrow PC, editor. Morrow's gynecologic cancer surgery. 2nd ed. South Coast Medical Publishing; 2012.
10. Sargon M. Anatomi Akıl Notları. 2. baskı ed. Ankara: Güneş Tıp Kitabevleri; 2017.
11. Jackson LA, Ramirez DMO, Carrick KS, Pedersen R, Spirtos A, Corton MM. Gross and histologic anatomy of the pelvic ureter: clinical applications to pelvic surgery. Obstet Gynecol. 2019;133(5):896–904.
12. Nakamura M, Tanaka K, Hayashi S, Morisada T, Iwata T, Imanishi N, et al. Local anatomy around terminal ureter related to the anterior leaf of the vesicouterine ligament in radical hysterectomy. Eur J Obstet Gynecol Reprod Biol. 2019;235:66–70.
13. Fujii S, Takakura K, Matsumura N, Higuchi T, Yura S, Mandai M, et al. Precise anatomy of the vesico-uterine ligament for radical hysterectomy. Gynecol Oncol. 2007;104(1):186–91.
14. Standring S. Gray's anatomy: the anatomical basis of clinical practice. 41st ed. Elsevier; 2016.
15. Agur AMR, Dalley AF. Grant's Atlas of Anatomy. 12th ed. Philadelphia: Wolters Kluwer/Lippincott Williams and Wilkins; 2009.
16. Clemente CD. Clemente's anatomy dissector. 3rd ed. Lippincott Williams & Wilkins (LWW); 2010.
17. Ripperda CM, Jackson LA, Phelan JN, Carrick KS, Corton MM. Anatomic relationships of the pelvic autonomic nervous system in female cadavers: clinical applications to pelvic surgery. Am J Obstet Gynecol. 2017;216(4):388e1–e7.
18. Snell RS. Clinical anatomy by regions. 9th ed. Lippincott Williams & Wilkins (LWW); 2011.
19. Tekelioğlu T, Tuncer HA, Sahin EA, Selcuk I. Pelvisin Vasküler Anatomisi. In: Ayhan A, Celik H, Dursun P, editors. Jinekolog Onkolog Bakış Açısıyla; Postpartum Kanama. Ankara: Güneş Tıp Kitabevleri; 2017.
20. Lv S, Wang Q, Zhao W, Han L, Wang Q, Batchu N, et al. A review of the postoperative lymphatic leakage. Oncotarget. 2017;8(40):69062–75.
21. Selcuk I, Yassa M, Tatar I, Huri E. Anatomic structure of the internal iliac artery and its educative dissection for peripartum and pelvic hemorrhage. Turk J Obstet Gynecol. 2018;15(2):126–9.

Chapter 17
Pelvic District: Approaches to Prostatic Diseases

Paolo Dell'Oglio, Silvia Secco, Christian Wagner, Dogukan Sokmen, Volkan Tugcu, and Antonio Galfano

17.1 Introduction

The trans-perineal radical prostatectomy (RP) was the first approach described by Young in 1905 and implemented into the clinical practice [1]. Subsequently, Millin in 1948 proposed the retropubic RP [2] that was associated with a significant blood loss. Only when Walsh [3] in the early 1980s improved the anatomical understanding of the pelvic structures, the perineal approach became less attractive and the retropubic one took the lead.

Robot-assisted radical prostatectomy (RARP) was introduced in 2000 with the aim of overcoming the morbidity related to the open RP [4, 5] and now has become the operation of choice for both localized and locally advanced prostate cancer [6, 7]. Since the introduction of RARP several variations on the original description of this operation have been reported, such as the posterior Retzius-sparing RARP (RS-RARP) [8] and the perineal RARP (R-RPP) [9, 10] (Fig. 17.1).

In this chapter we describe the key steps of RARP and the anatomical landmarks that can be found during three different approaches (anterior vs. posterior vs. perineal). Increased anatomical understanding of the same anatomical structures from a different point of view, will guide surgeons to safely complete a full RARP procedure regardless of the approach used.

P. Dell'Oglio · S. Secco · A. Galfano (✉)
Department of Urology, ASST Grande Ospedale Metropolitano Niguarda, Milan, Italy

C. Wagner
Department of Urology, St. Antonius-Hospital Gronau GmbH, Gronau, Germany

D. Sokmen · V. Tugcu
Department of Urology, Istanbul Bakirkoy Dr. Sadi Konuk Training and Research Hospital, University of Health Sciences, Istanbul, Turkey

© Springer Nature Switzerland AG 2021
E. Huri, D. Veneziano (eds.), *Anatomy for Urologic Surgeons in the Digital Era*,
https://doi.org/10.1007/978-3-030-59479-4_17

Fig. 17.1 Different
approaches for robot-
assisted radical
prostatectomy

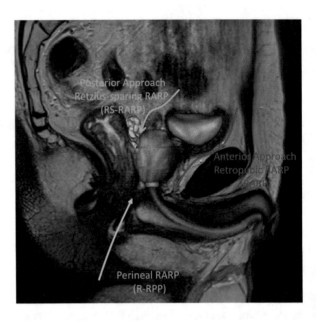

17.1.1   Standard Retropubic RARP (Anterior Approach)

This approach is for sure the most common one, passing through the same anatomical field as open RP. Several techniques were described [11–14]. Here we will focus on the most crucial steps according to the related anatomical issues.

After secure placement of the patient in a steep Trendelenburg (30–35°) and the transperitoneal port placement under direct vision (Fig. 17.2), the medial umbilical ligaments are identified and the peritoneum is opened laterally following them down to the level of the vas deferens. The bladder detachment allows optimal exposure and is most favourable when an extended lymph node dissection (LND) is planned. In case an extraperitoneal approach is chosen, the Retzius space is developed with a dedicated dilatation balloon and the port are placed.

To clearly identify the bladder neck and proceed with its dissection in a safe manner, some key steps are required. We strongly recommend performing these **steps before bladder neck incision,** especially for naïve surgeons. First, the fat over the prostatic ligament, the anterior surface of the prostate and the bladder neck is removed scarifying the dorsal vein of the penis (Fig. 17.3a). Second, the endopelvic fascia is incised with cold scissors, starting close to the prostate base and pushing medially the prostate (Fig. 17.3b). The muscle fibres of the levator ani muscle should be swept off the prostate fascia laterally, and the round shape of the prostate can be followed until reaching the urethral region, avoiding vascular damage that will stain the surgical field (Fig. 17.3c–d). All these aforementioned steps allow for optimal identification of prostate margins, dorsal vascular complex-DVC (Santorini Plexus) that is directly attached to the prostate and, eventually, accessory pudendal arteries that need to be preserved to increase functional outcomes. The anatomical

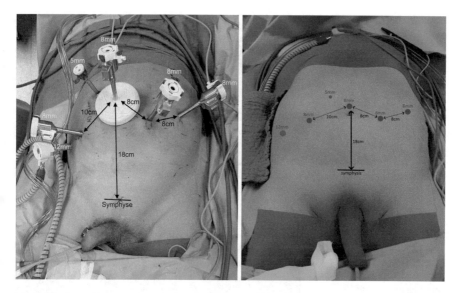

Fig. 17.2 Steps of standard retropubic robot-assisted radical prostatectomy (anterior approach). Port placement

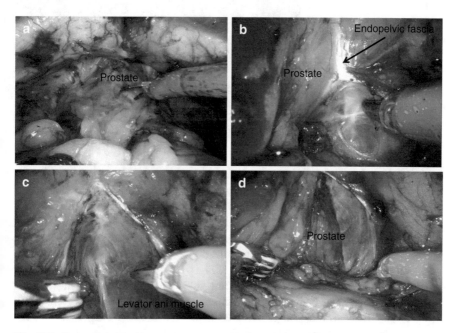

Fig. 17.3 Steps of standard retropubic robot-assisted radical prostatectomy (anterior approach). Removal of the fat over pubo-prostatic ligaments, anterior prostate and bladder neck (**a**); incision of the endopelvic fascia (**b–d**)

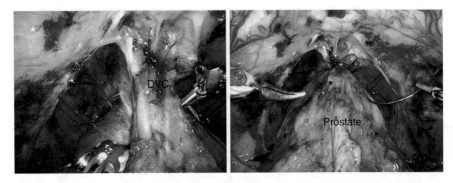

Fig. 17.4 Steps of standard retropubic robot-assisted radical prostatectomy (anterior approach). Ligation of the dorsal vascular complex (DVC) [before bladder neck dissection]

Fig. 17.5 Steps of standard retropubic robot-assisted radical prostatectomy (anterior approach). Bladder neck dissection (ventral approach)

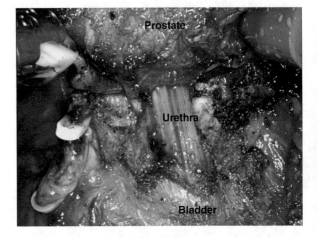

landmarks of the urethra, prostate apex and DVC can be visualized laterally by gently pushing the prostatic apex medially. A better understanding of the anatomical planes of the apex, can be obtained with the ligation of the DVC. The suture is placed right underneath the DVC in a small notch that marks the borderline between urethra and DVC, as shown in Fig. 17.4. The ligation of the DVC might also be performed after bladder neck and lateral lobe dissection or after its complete dissection (selective DVC ligation) [15, 16] (Fig. 17.11c).

The **bladder neck** is approached starting from its ventral surface. Intermittent traction on the catheter balloon and assessment of tissue resistance pressing medially with robotic instruments at the level of the junction between the prostate and the bladder might help to identify the bladder neck. The dissection is started in the midline, maintaining the bladder stretch with careful continuous traction in the cephalad direction. The longitudinal fibres of the bladder neck can be easily distinguished from the circular fibres of the detrusor muscle (Fig. 17.5). After transecting

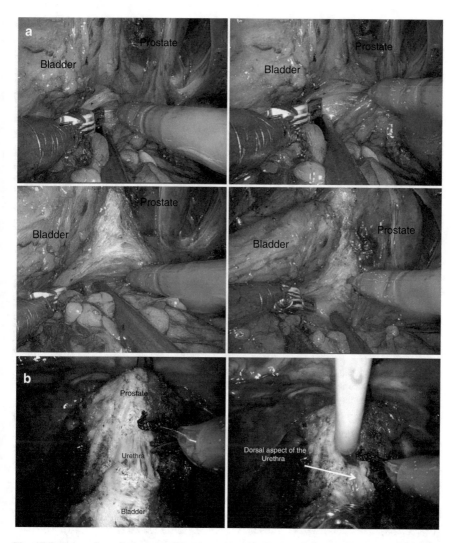

Fig. 17.6 Steps of standard retropubic robot-assisted radical prostatectomy (anterior approach). (**a, b**) Bladder neck dissection (dorso-lateral approach)

the ventral bladder neck, the urethra is visualized and opened. The dorsal dissection of the urethra and bladder neck is carried out, carefully watching out for the ureteric orifices (when feasible) and median lobes. Some surgeons [14] prefer to start the dissection of the bladder neck through a dorso-lateral approach and thereafter continuing the incision ventrally in the midline (Fig. 17.6).

To reach the plane of the vas deferens and **seminal vesicles**, the prostate is lifted up and the vesico-prostatic fibres are transected. In the midline the vas deferens come into view, and dissection is carried out down until the tip of the seminal

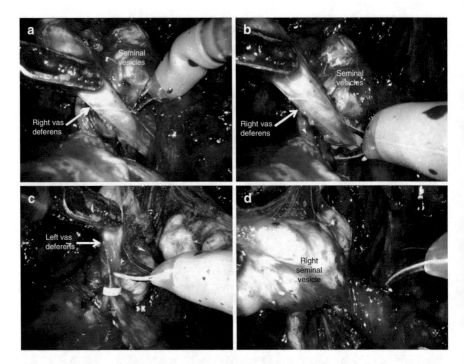

Fig. 17.7 Steps of standard retropubic robot-assisted radical prostatectomy (anterior approach). Dissection of vas deferens (**a–c**) and seminal vesicles (**d**)

vesicles (Fig. 17.7a). Herein the vas deferens are cut (Fig. 17.7b–c). Dissection of the seminal vesicles is then performed, lifting first the vas deferens and then the seminal vesicles and gently pushing off the tissue of surrounding seminal vesicles fascia (then forming the Denonvillier's fascia) with accurate pint-point coagulation/ clipping of the seminal vesicle arteries (Fig. 17.7d).

In case a **nerve-sparing** procedure is planned, key is how the dorsal prostate dissection is performed. Both seminal vesicles are lifted up in a symmetrical way (Fig. 17.8a). The Denonvillier's fascia is grasped and incised (Fig. 17.8b). The capsule of the prostate must be identified, and Denonvillier's fascia should be spared and pushed off the prostate dorsally down to the apex of the prostate (bloodless plane) (Fig. 17.8c, d). To facilitate the nerve sparing, the dorsal dissection should be carried out laterally, following the curvature of the prostate capsule. The nerve sparing can be completed pushing laterally the bundle in an antegrade direction (Fig. 17.9) or using a retrograde approach (Fig. 17.10) or a combination of both. The retrograde approach requires a lateral dissection of the neurovascular bundle, which can sometimes be more challenging because the veins in the prostatic fascias have to be transected and might stain the surgical field. In case extrafascial approach is chosen, the Denonvillier's fascia is dissected free and left on the posterior surface

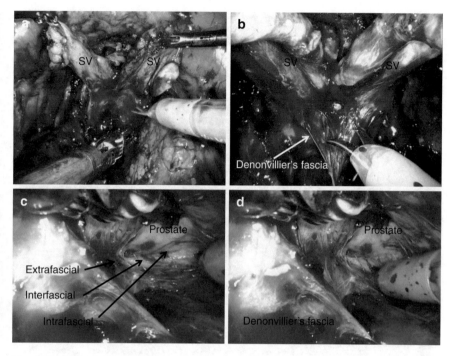

Fig. 17.8 Steps of standard retropubic robot-assisted radical prostatectomy (anterior approach). Seminal vesicles lifted up in a symmetrical way (butterfly) (**a**); Denonvillier's fascia incision (**b**); dissection of the posterior space between the prostate and the rectum (**b–d**)

of the prostate. Thereafter, the prostatic pedicles are clipped and dissected. The prostate is free from the lateral attachments.

The ultimate step of the prostatic dissection is the **apical dissection**. During this step keys are the constant cranial traction on the prostate and the rotation of the prostate to improve the visualization of the dissection area of the apex. After the DVC is transected (Fig. 17.11a, b), a loss of resistance indicates that only the urethral stump is attached to the prostate, containing the sphincter muscle. The prostate is gently released from the urethral stump and the urethra is transected (Fig. 17.12) following the anatomical shape of the gland and preserving the maximal length.

A posterior reconstruction approximating the Denonvillier's fascia with rhabdosphincter muscle with a running suture might be performed before vesico-urethral anastomosis (the so called "Rocco's stitch") (Fig. 17.13a). It increases the haemostasis and minimizes the traction on the anastomosis. The modified Van Velthoven **anastomosis** (Fig. 17.13b) is then carried out, using a barbed suture with two needles, starting from 6 to 12 o'clock anticlockwise on the right side and from 6 to 12 o'clock clockwise on the left side. A transurethral catheter or suprapubic catheter can be placed. Placing a drain is optional.

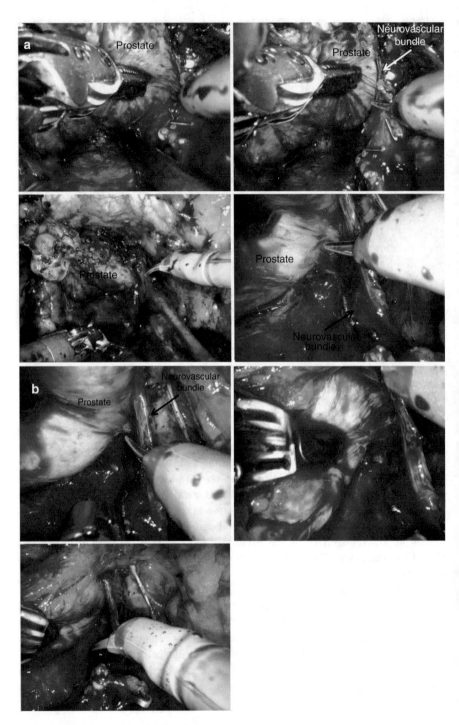

Fig. 17.9 Steps of standard retropubic robot-assisted radical prostatectomy (anterior approach). (**a, b**) Nerve sparing (antegrade approach)

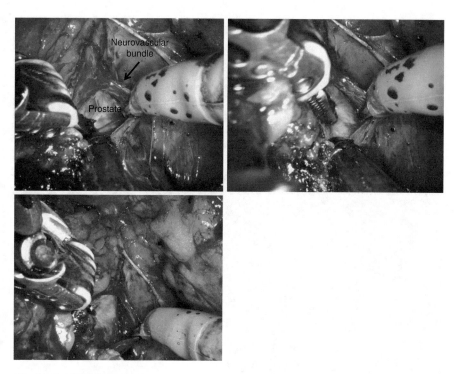

Fig. 17.10 Steps of standard retropubic robot-assisted radical prostatectomy (anterior approach). Nerve sparing (retrograde approach)

17.1.2   Retzius-Sparing RARP (Posterior Approach)

In this approach we have to deal with several anatomical issues.

Patient placement is in line with the anterior approach. Figure 17.14 depicts port placement.

We suggest to position the grasper on the second arm and to use a 30° lens, placed downwards during the initial steps and upwards after the dissection of the seminal vesicles.

The procedure starts accessing the rectovesical pouch. In order to expand the surgical field as much as possible and to reduce the risk of damage of the bowel, release of the adhesions of the sigma might be necessary. Moreover, in some patients (i.e. obese or with small pelvis) where the lower part of the sigma is not straight, it could be useful to place a stitch with a straight needle (we call it "Pansadoro stitch" from an original idea of prof. Vito Pansadoro) coming from the upper 5 mm assistant trocar to make tension on the epiploic appendices and straighten the rectum (Fig. 17.15). When the rectovesical pouch is free, a peritoneotomy at the anterior surface of the Douglas space is performed and the vas deferens are identified and transected always bearing in mind that the distal ureter is behind. The **seminal vesicles** are carefully dissected until the prostatic base is identified. To further increase

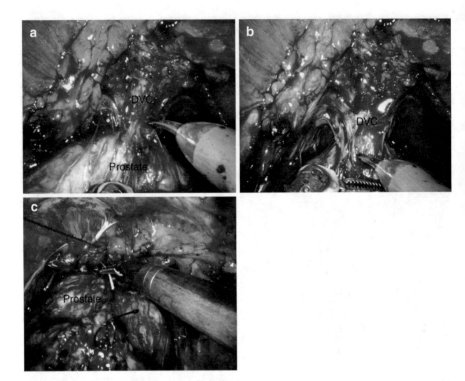

Fig. 17.11 Steps of standard retropubic robot-assisted radical prostatectomy (anterior approach). Dissection (**a, b**) and (**c**) ligation of the dorsal vascular complex (DVC) [selective DVC ligation]

the surgical field, we strongly recommend placing two transabdominal suprapubic stitches that lift and support the bladder and retract the seminal vesicles (Fig. 17.16).

Thereafter, with a 30° upwards scope, the **nerve-sparing** level has to be chosen according to the oncological safety and functional needs. In the case of RS-RARP, this step is performed after the seminal vesicles isolation with an antegrade or retrograde approach. We recommend incising the Denonvillier's fascia starting from an extrafascial plan and approximating to the prostatic capsule in order to reach an inter- or intrafascial plane according to the oncological situation (Fig. 17.17). The easiest place to find the desired plane is in the midline of the Denonvillier's fascia, where less vessels are present and the plane is clearer. Once isolated the posterior aspect of the prostate down to the apex, we usually dissect the prostatic pedicles and push laterally the bundles downwards in an antegrade direction (Fig. 17.18). Going to the apex along the midline and coming back to the bundles allows to isolate better the prostatic pedicle.

In case of an extracapsular disease, the extrafascial approach is always feasible also with the RS-RARP [17]. Similarly to the anterior approach, the Denonvillier's fascia is dissected and left on the posterior surface of the prostate. After dissection of the prostatic pedicles, laterally to the prostate, a dissection with clips is carried out until the levator ani muscle is identified (Fig. 17.19). Thereafter the prostate is free from the lateral attachments.

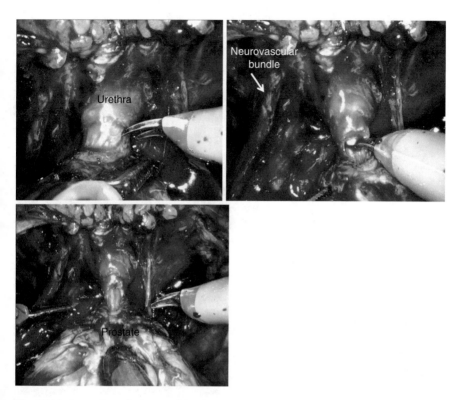

Fig. 17.12 Steps of standard retropubic robot-assisted radical prostatectomy (anterior approach). Incision of the urethra

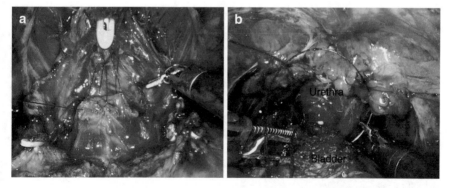

Fig. 17.13 Steps of standard retropubic robot-assisted radical prostatectomy (anterior approach). Posterior reconstruction (**a**) and vesico-urethral anastomosis (**b**)

Fig. 17.14 Steps of
Retzius-sparing robot-
assisted radical
prostatectomy (posterior
approach). Port placement

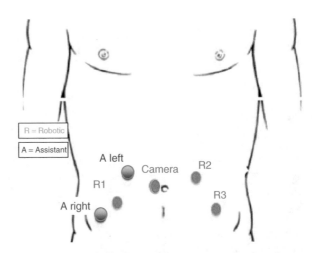

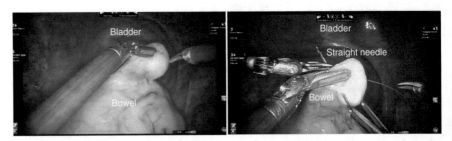

Fig. 17.15 Steps of Retzius-sparing robot-assisted radical prostatectomy (posterior approach). Pansadoro stitch

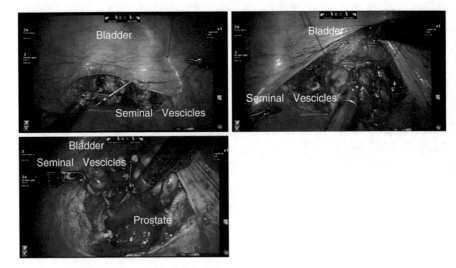

Fig. 17.16 Steps of Retzius-sparing robot-assisted radical prostatectomy (posterior approach). Transabdominal suprapubic stitches

Fig. 17.17 Steps of Retzius-sparing robot-assisted radical prostatectomy (posterior approach). Denonvillier's fascia incision and dissection of the posterior space between the prostate and the rectum

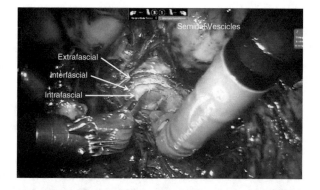

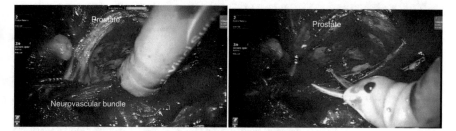

Fig. 17.18 Steps of Retzius-sparing robot-assisted radical prostatectomy (posterior approach). Nerve sparing (antegrade approach)

Fig. 17.19 Steps of Retzius-sparing robot-assisted radical prostatectomy (posterior approach). Extrafascial approach

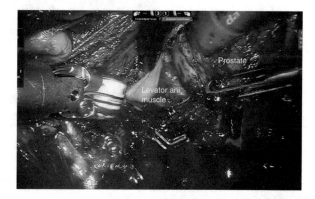

Once isolated the posterior and lateral surfaces of the prostate, the exposition of the **bladder neck** is obtained retracting the seminal vesicles downwards with the grasper. During RS-RARP, the bladder neck is approached starting from its dorsal surface. From this point of view, we find a first layer represented by the vesicoprostatic muscle. Under this layer the circular muscle fibres of the bladder are encountered. These can be bluntly dissected and separated from the prostate. We suggest using few pint-point coagulations only to stop bleedings and to continue with the dissection, following the fibres laterally as far as possible before opening the bladder neck (Fig. 17.20). Two tips can be very useful at this point: first, we carefully surround the anterior surface of the bladder neck with the bipolar Maryland forceps. This manoeuvre improves the space and the visibility of this structure that otherwise would be hidden. Second, we put two quickly absorbable sutures (Vycril rapide 3-0) at 6 and 12 o' clock in the bladder neck, in order to fix the mucosa and to easily recognize both starting and ending points of the anastomosis (Fig. 17.21). This is very practical especially in case of small bladder neck. Moreover, it helps keeping the bladder neck closed during the dissection and avoids urine spillage against the camera.

The **apex** is usually the last part of the prostate to be isolated. The posterior aspect of the apex was already isolated during the development of the posterior surface of the prostate. The anterior part of the apex is prepared in a standard fashion, with two main differences: (1) whenever oncologically safe, the Santorini

Fig. 17.20 Steps of Retzius-sparing robot-assisted radical prostatectomy (posterior approach). Bladder neck dissection

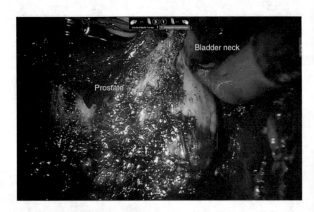

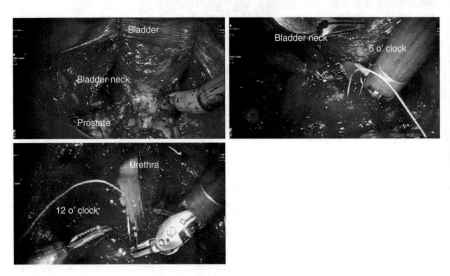

Fig. 17.21 Steps of Retzius-sparing robot-assisted radical prostatectomy (posterior approach). Placement of two short stitches at 6 and 12 o'clock of the bladder neck

plexus is spared; in fact, once sectioned the anterior part of the bladder neck, the followed surgical plane passes between the DVC and the anterior surface of the prostate; (2) the bladder is not in the lower back part of the screen but it is in the upper anterior part of it. Having the 30° scope upwards allows to have a good vision also in these circumstances (Fig. 17.22). Some Authors perform the apical incision before the isolation of the bladder neck. In our opinion this can be done, but it increases the difficulty of the surgery. A delicate preparation of the apex is generally recommended to avoid a breakage which might increase difficulties in the positive surgical margins (PSMs) interpretation.

Finally, the **vesico-urethral anastomosis** can be performed in different ways. After several trials and attempts, nowadays we recommend to perform a standard van Velthoven modified anastomosis, starting from 12 o' clock [18]. Specifically, we generally use two separate barbed sutures of 15 cm (V-loc 3-0) that helps avoiding the presence of the wire in the middle of the surgical field in a small surgical field. We are used to start from the left anterior quarter, then we do the anterior and posterior right quarter, and finally we close it with the posterior left quarter (Fig. 17.23). At the end of the anastomosis, we usually remove the trans-urethral catheter and we position a suprapubic tube, that is inserted under direct

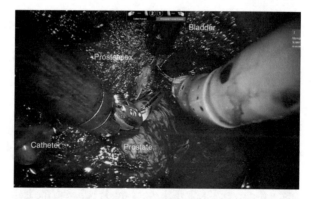

Fig. 17.22 Steps of Retzius-sparing robot-assisted radical prostatectomy (posterior approach). Dissection of the anterior surface of the prostate from the Santorini plexus

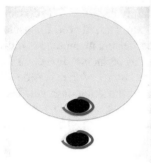

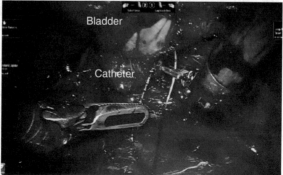

Fig. 17.23 Steps of Retzius-sparing robot-assisted radical prostatectomy (posterior approach). Vesico-urethral anastomosis

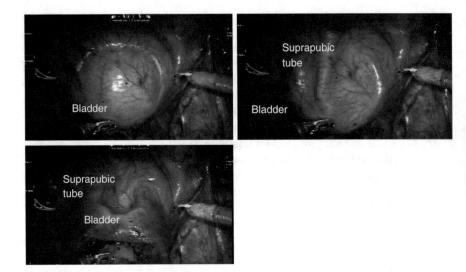

Fig. 17.24 Steps of Retzius-sparing robot-assisted radical prostatectomy (posterior approach). Suprapubic tube placement

vision with the intent of improving comfort and avoiding inadvertent traction on the anastomosis (Fig. 17.24) [19].

17.1.3 Perineal RARP (R-RPP)

After secure placement of the patient in a lithotomy position with a 15° Trendelenburg, a sterile glove is placed in the rectum, and the edges of the glove are sewn to the perineal skin.

An **open surgical step** is required to prepare the perineum for the robotic docking: a 6-cm semilunar incision is made between the ischial tuberosities (Fig. 17.25). The subcutaneous tissue is dissected and the central tendon of the perineum is incised. Bilateral ischio-rectal fossas are bluntly and sharply dissected. The dissection is held from the inferior side to the apex of the prostate. The puborectal muscle groups are incised across. When the dissection limit reaches the membranous urethra and when it is visible at the top of the prostate, the perineum dissection is ended. The subcutaneous tissue that is placed below the limits of the incision is deeply dissected on the superficial perineal fascia to insert the single-port gel. The tissue that hangs down from the top of the perineal incision is suspended by using a suture passing below the skin under the scrotum. This suture is fixed on the skin with clips to improve the optical appearance of robotic dissections. The position of the robotic and assistant trocars is shown in Fig. 17.26.

The robotic steps start with the development of the posterior prostatic space to expose the levator ani muscle. The Denonvillier's fascia is identified and incised followed by the dorsal prostate dissection along the length of the prostate. The **nerve-sparing** level is decided at this time, and it is performed in a retrograde

Fig. 17.25 Steps of perineal robot-assisted radical prostatectomy. Perineal incision

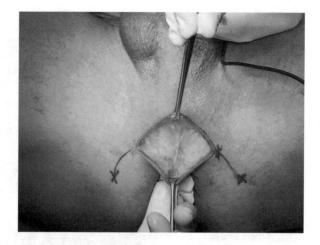

Fig. 17.26 Steps of perineal robot-assisted radical prostatectomy. Robotic docking

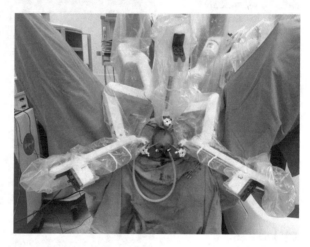

direction (Fig. 17.27). Thus, the posterior and lateral surfaces are the first parts of the prostate to be isolated (Fig. 17.28). Once the posterior plane is delineated, the Denonvillier's fascia is opened closely to the cranial part of the posterior surface of the prostate to identify the **seminal vesicles**, that are isolated. At this point, the membranous urethra is dissected and cut, prosecuting with a retrograde dissection of the anterior surface of the **apical and anterolateral surface of the prostate,** leaving the DVC intact, as in the Retzius-sparing approach. The prostatic lateral pedicles are clipped and dissected. After the lateral dissection of the two-side prostate is completed, the last part of the prostate to be managed is the **bladder neck.** Once identified, it is cut with monopolar scissors, starting from the anterior side and prosecuting backwards. The urethral catheter is retracted after the anterior incision. If there is a median lobe, it is hung up with the help of a stay suture for an easier dissection. After the bladder neck dissection is carried out, the robot is undocked and the specimen is retrieved. The robotic system is re-docked to perform the **vesico-urethral anastomosis.** Two thorn-sutures are used in a running fashion (Fig. 17.29).

Fig. 17.27 Steps of perineal robot-assisted radical prostatectomy. Apical dissection

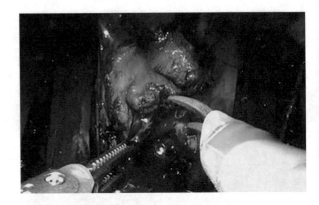

Fig. 17.28 Steps of perineal robot-assisted radical prostatectomy. Lateral prostate lobe dissection

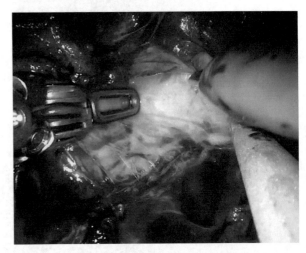

Fig. 17.29 Steps of perineal robot-assisted radical prostatectomy. Vesico-urethral anastomosis

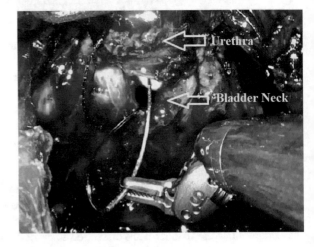

Fig. 17.30 Steps of perineal robot-assisted radical prostatectomy. Jackson-Pratt drain placement

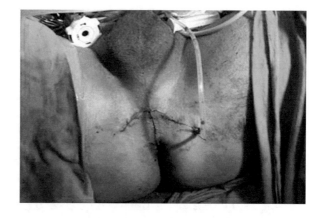

The first suture is placed on the anterior bladder neck at 12 o'clock from outside to inside proceeding in a clockwise fashion until 6 o'clock. Similarly, the second suture is used in a counterclockwise direction to complete the anastomosis. When anastomosis is completed, a 22-Ch urethral catheter is positioned and a proof of water-tightness is performed. The robot is undocked and a drainage catheter is left. The layers are closed according to their anatomy (Fig. 17.30).

17.2 Discussion

The **retropubic RARP** is still the most commonly used approach by robotic surgeons dealing with RARP. General consensus is reached that this is less challenging compared to other approaches especially in non-expert hands. As a matter of fact, all anatomical structures involved appears in their "familiar way" and, generally, robotic arms have more space of movement which is key in narrow pelvis, obese patients and big prostate. Moreover, if performed with a transperitoneal approach, it allows also for an optimal exposure of the lymphatic regions that need to be harvested in case an extended LND is planned (i.e. the external iliac, the obturator fossa and the internal iliac lymph nodes). Differently from the other available RARP approaches, bladder detachment is mandatory to reach the Retzius space and some of the anterior structures involved in continence preservation (such as puboprostatic ligaments, endopelvic fascia and DVC) are not preserved. This upheaval of the normal anatomy do translate in better exposure (i.e. better understanding of all the landmarks of the prostate), but at the same time might translate in worse functional outcomes [20]. Indeed, despite evidences suggest excellent functional outcomes in those patients treated with standard approach (rate of erectile function-EF- and urinary continence-UC-recovery in high volume centres and in the best-case scenario is approximately 40% and >90%, respectively) [6, 7, 21], there is still a margin of improvement.

In 2010 a **RS-RARP** approach was described for the first time. Its purpose is to improve functional outcomes recovery [8]. The rationale of this technique stems on the preservation of all crucial anterior anatomical structures advocated to play a role in the maintenance of potency and continence, passing through the Douglas space. This allows high immediate (up to 92%) and long-term (up to 96%) UC recovery [18]. A recent systematic review and meta-analysis [20] provided evidence that the RS-RARP is associated with faster and better long-term UC recovery relative to the standard RARP, without increasing the risk of complications. Conversely, according to the last randomized controlled trial published by Menon et al. [22], no statistical significant difference was observed for EF recovery between the two approaches at 1-year follow-up (69.2 vs. 86.5% for anterior and posterior approach, respectively). However, this new approach is not devoid of limitations. First, it is reasonable to question whether the narrow surgical field of the RS-RARP translates into higher rate of PSMs. This is particularly true when we are approaching the anterior surface of the prostate where the room for the robotic arms movement is decimate. Indeed, recent evidence suggests a higher rate of PSMs especially in case of tumours that are located or have invaded the anterior fibromuscular stroma [20]. These findings might be biased by the fact that all available studies included in this last systematic review relied on surgeons with an extensive expertise for standard RARP and an initial expertise for RS-RARP. The largest available studies that compare standard RARP vs. RS-RARP performed by a single surgeon with extensive experience in both approaches [17] observed that the rate of PSMs did not differ between the two techniques. Despite these promising findings and the increasing adoption of this technique by several international centres [23], other experts are still reluctant to perform the RS-RARP. They argue that there can be an intrinsic *higher risk* of PSMs in surgeons not familiar with the technique due to narrower/deeper space and less exposure compared to the standard approach [24]. Second, approaching the bladder neck from its dorsal surface, does not allow visualization of the ureteral orifices. This represents one of the major drawbacks of the RS-RARP. Despite no adverse outcomes are reported in terms of damage of the ureteral orifices, future techniques should be discovered to allow ureteral orifices identification and safer vesico-urethral anastomosis. Third, since the bladder neck is open, the third robotic arm needs to be used to close the bladder and avoid urine spillage against the camera. In case of big prostate, the apical dissection might be trickier without the use of the third arm. However, recent data confirmed the feasibility of the posterior approach also in larger prostate with similar oncological and functional outcomes [25]. Fourth, the small and limited space related to this RP procedure might increase the difficulties in obese patients. However, no data is available on the feasibility of RS-RARP in this setting. The increase application of the Da Vinci Single port (SP) robotic system will allow better access and manoeuvrability, limiting instrument clashing and facilitating all RS-RARP surgical steps, especially in patients with larger prostate and higher body mass index [26].

In 2014 the feasibility of **R-RPP** was described in three male cadavers [9]. Thereafter, several authors confirmed the feasibility and safety of this approach in the human setting [10, 27–29]. From an anatomic standpoint of view, it is a reasonable approach considering only the location of the prostate. It provides a straight access to the prostate in contrast to the retropubic and RS-RARP. This access avoids accidental visceral damage or major vessels injury during intraperitoneal approach and represents the more appropriate anatomical way to do RP in those patients with previous abdominal or pelvic surgeries. Additionally, there is no need of steep Trendelenburg like in the other two approaches; since this fact, it potentially reduces the risk of rhabdomyolysis and facial edema [30]. Moreover, as the posterior approach the bladder is not mobilized, the endopelvic fascia, the puboprostatic ligaments and the DVC are not opened and accessory pudendal arteries are avoided. This should result in shorter operative time, less blood loss and excellent functional outcomes. In the largest series of patients who underwent R-RPP (n = 95) [29] the immediate and 1-year UC recovery were 41 and 91%, respectively. EF recovery at 1 year was 77%. Excellent and comparable oncological outcomes to standard RARP were also reported [28]. Other anatomical advantages of this approach are represented by the location of the proximal bladder neck in the surgical field that, being straight to the robotic camera, allows the visualization of the ureteral orifice during the vesico-urethral anastomosis. Another advantage of the R-RPP approach is that eliminates the need for pneumoperitoneum. Therefore, it might represent the future gold standard for obese patients considering the higher incidence of case abortion secondary to the excessive airway and pneumoperitoneal pressure reported in this subset of patients [31]. Moreover, the absence of abdominal insufflation might translate into shorter return to bowel function and less postoperative discomfort; on the contrary, perineal pain and sitting down could be more problematic in R-RPP. Specific studies should be carried out on this topic. One of the major disadvantages of the R-RPP is the deep and narrow surgical field that ends in limited vision. This is partially compensated by the advantages of robotic surgery and by the increasing adoption of the Da Vinci SP platform to perform R-RPP that allows to work in narrow and deeper space reducing robotic arms conflict relative to SI system [32]. Accurate selection of the patient is mandatory. Indeed, it is a well-established procedure for patients with organ-confined PCa. Conversely, studies are needed to demonstrate the oncological safety of this approach in case of advanced disease. Last but not least, R-RPP in large prostate might be challenging considering the fact that surgical field is already narrow. Indeed, only few cases described the feasibility and safety of R-RPP in patients with large prostate.

17.3 Conclusions

In this chapter we presented an overview of the anatomical landmarks that can be found during different approaches for RARP, from standard to perineal approach, passing through the RS-RARP. We highlighted advantages and pitfalls of the different approaches, showing how different ways can lead to similar oncological and functional outcomes. Future randomized studies are needed to identify what is the best-tailored approach according to patients characteristics.

References

1. Young HH. The early diagnosis and radical cure of carcinoma of the prostate. Being a study of 40 cases and presentation of a radical operation which was carried out in four cases. 1905. J Urol. 2002;167:939–46; discussion 47.
2. Millin T. Retropubic prostatectomy. J Urol. 1948;59:267–80.
3. Walsh PC, Lepor H, Eggleston JC. Radical prostatectomy with preservation of sexual function: anatomical and pathological considerations. Prostate. 1983;4:473–85.
4. Abbou CC, Hoznek A, Salomon L, Olsson LE, Lobontiu A, Saint F, et al. Laparoscopic radical prostatectomy with a remote controlled robot. J Urol. 2001;165:1964–6.
5. Menon M, Shrivastava A, Tewari A, Sarle R, Hemal A, Peabody JO, et al. Laparoscopic and robot assisted radical prostatectomy: establishment of a structured program and preliminary analysis of outcomes. J Urol. 2002;168:945–9.
6. Dell'Oglio P, Mottrie A, Mazzone E. Robot-assisted radical prostatectomy vs. open radical prostatectomy: latest evidences on perioperative, functional and oncological outcomes. Curr Opin Urol. 2020;30:73–8.
7. Costello AJ. Considering the role of radical prostatectomy in 21st century prostate cancer care. Nat Rev Urol. 2020;17(3):177–88.
8. Galfano A, Ascione A, Grimaldi S, Petralia G, Strada E, Bocciardi AM. A new anatomic approach for robot-assisted laparoscopic prostatectomy: a feasibility study for completely intrafascial surgery. Eur Urol. 2010;58:457–61.
9. Laydner H, Akca O, Autorino R, Eyraud R, Zargar H, Brandao LF, et al. Perineal robot-assisted laparoscopic radical prostatectomy: feasibility study in the cadaver model. J Endourol. 2014;28:1479–86.
10. Kaouk JH, Akca O, Zargar H, Caputo P, Ramirez D, Andrade H, et al. Descriptive technique and initial results for robotic radical perineal prostatectomy. Urology. 2016;94:129–38.
11. Guillonneau B, Vallancien G. Laparoscopic radical prostatectomy: the Montsouris technique. J Urol. 2000;163:1643–9.
12. Menon M, Tewari A, Peabody J, Team VIP. Vattikuti Institute prostatectomy: technique. J Urol. 2003;169:2289–92.
13. Rocco B, Coelho RF, Albo G, Patel VR. [Robot-assisted laparoscopic prostatectomy: surgical technique]. Minerva urologica e nefrologica = Ital J Urol Nephrol. 2010;62:295–304.
14. Ficarra V, Gan M, Borghesi M, Zattoni F, Mottrie A. Posterior muscolofascial reconstruction incorporated into urethrovescical anastomosis during robot-assisted radical prostatectomy. J Endourol. 2012;26:1542–5.
15. Bianchi L, Turri FM, Larcher A, De Groote R, De Bruyne P, De Coninck V, et al. A novel approach for apical dissection during robot-assisted radical prostatectomy: the "collar" technique. Eur Urol Focus. 2018;4:677–85.
16. Antonelli A, Palumbo C, Veccia A, Fisogni S, Zamboni S, Furlan M, et al. Standard vs delayed ligature of the dorsal vascular complex during robot-assisted radical prostatectomy: results from a randomized controlled trial. J Robot Surg. 2019;13:253–60.
17. Lee J, Kim HY, Goh HJ, Heo JE, Almujalhem A, Alqahtani AA, et al. Retzius sparing robot-assisted radical prostatectomy conveys early regain of continence over conventional robot-assisted radical prostatectomy: a propensity score matched analysis of 1,863 patients. J Urol. 2020;203:137–44.
18. Galfano A, Di Trapani D, Sozzi F, Strada E, Petralia G, Bramerio M, et al. Beyond the learning curve of the Retzius-sparing approach for robot-assisted laparoscopic radical prostatectomy: oncologic and functional results of the first 200 patients with >/= 1 year of follow-up. Eur Urol. 2013;64:974–80.
19. Galfano A, Secco S, Panarello D, Barbieri M, Di Trapani D, Petralia G, et al. Pain and discomfort after Retzius-sparing robot-assisted radical prostatectomy: a comparative study between suprapubic cystostomy and urethral catheter as urinary drainage. Minerva urologica e nefrologica = Ital J Urol Nephrol. 2019;71:381–5.

20. Checcucci E, Veccia A, Fiori C, Amparore D, Manfredi M, Di Dio M, et al. Retzius-sparing robot-assisted radical prostatectomy vs the standard approach: a systematic review and analysis of comparative outcomes. BJU Int. 2020;125:8–16.
21. Coughlin GD, Yaxley JW, Chambers SK, Occhipinti S, Samaratunga H, Zajdlewicz L, et al. Robot-assisted laparoscopic prostatectomy versus open radical retropubic prostatectomy: 24-month outcomes from a randomised controlled study. Lancet Oncol. 2018;19:1051–60.
22. Menon M, Dalela D, Jamil M, Diaz M, Tallman C, Abdollah F, et al. Functional recovery, oncologic outcomes and postoperative complications after robot-assisted radical prostatectomy: an evidence-based analysis comparing the Retzius sparing and standard approaches. J Urol. 2018;199:1210–7.
23. Galfano A, Secco S, Bocciardi AM, Mottrie A. Retzius-sparing robot-assisted laparoscopic radical prostatectomy: an international survey on surgical details and worldwide diffusion. Eur Urol Focus. 2020;6(5):1021–3.
24. Stonier T, Simson N, Davis J, Challacombe B. Retzius-sparing robot-assisted radical prostatectomy (RS-RARP) vs standard RARP: it's time for critical appraisal. BJU Int. 2019;123:5–7.
25. Galfano A, Panarello D, Secco S, Di Trapani D, Barbieri M, Napoli G, et al. Does prostate volume have an impact on the functional and oncological results of Retzius-sparing robot-assisted radical prostatectomy? Minerva urologica e nefrologica = Ital J Urol Nephrol. 2018;70:408–13.
26. Agarwal DK, Sharma V, Toussi A, Viers BR, Tollefson MK, Gettman MT, et al. Initial experience with da Vinci single-port robot-assisted radical prostatectomies. Eur Urol. 2020;77:373–9.
27. Tugcu V, Akca O, Simsek A, Yigitbasi I, Sahin S, Tasci AI. Robot-assisted radical perineal prostatectomy: first experience of 15 cases. Turk J Urol. 2017;43:476–83.
28. Tugcu V, Akca O, Simsek A, Yigitbasi I, Sahin S, Yenice MG, et al. Robotic-assisted perineal versus transperitoneal radical prostatectomy: A matched-pair analysis. Turk J Urol. 2019;45:265–72.
29. Eksi M, Colakoglu Y, Tugcu V, Sahin S, Simsek A, Evren I, et al. Robot assisted radical perineal prostatectomy; review of 95 cases. BJU Int. 2020;27.
30. Hsu RL, Kaye AD, Urman RD. Anesthetic challenges in robotic-assisted urologic surgery. Rev Urol. 2013;15:178–84.
31. Wiltz AL, Shikanov S, Eggener SE, Katz MH, Thong AE, Steinberg GD, et al. Robotic radical prostatectomy in overweight and obese patients: oncological and validated-functional outcomes. Urology. 2009;73:316–22.
32. Garisto J, Bertolo R, Wilson CA, Kaouk J. The evolution and resurgence of perineal prostatectomy in the robotic surgical era. World J Urol. 2020;38(4):821–8.

Chapter 18
Retroperitoneal District: Approaches to Renal Diseases

Giuseppe Simone, Gabriele Tuderti, Giovanni E. Cacciamani, Aldo Brassetti, Nima Nassiri, and Inderbir Gill

18.1   Anatomic Overview of Retroperitoneum

The retroperitoneum is the posterior compartment of the abdomen defined anteriorly by parietal peritoneum and posteriorly by transversalis fascia and the lumbar spine. The cephalic border of the retroperitoneum is the diaphragm and it extends into the pelvis. There are three zones (central, flank, and pelvic). The retroperitoneal space contains the kidneys, adrenal glands, the pancreas, spinal nerve roots, the abdominal aorta, the inferior vena cava, parts 2–4 of the duodenum, the ascending and descending colon, the rectum, retroperitoneal lymph nodes. Retroperitoneal lymph nodes are classified by their relationship to the great vessels and their branches. Above the bifurcation of the aorta, lymph nodes are either para-aortic, inter-aorto-caval, paracaval, retro-aortic or retro-caval. Below the bifurcation of the aorta, there are pre-sacral, common iliac, external iliac, internal iliac, obturator, hypogastric, and pre-sciatic lymph nodes. The lymph node of Cloquet (Rosenmüller) is the lowest of the external iliac lymph nodes.

Gabriele Tuderti and Giovanni Cacciamani contributed equally.

G. Simone (✉) · G. Tuderti · A. Brassetti
Department of Urology, "Regina Elena" National Cancer Institute, Rome, Italy

G. E. Cacciamani · N. Nassiri · I. Gill
Institute of Urology, University of Southern California, Los Angeles, CA, USA
e-mail: nima.nassiri@med.usc.edu

18.2   Localised Renal Tumours: Management and Treatment

Renal diseases candidate for surgical resolution are mostly represented by neoplasms. Accordingly, surgical treatment has to be planned in order to achieve the best outcomes for the patients.

Partial nephrectomy (PN) is the surgical option to be taken into account whenever a renal tumor is considered resectable, offering comparable oncological outcomes to radical nephrectomy (RN) [1, 2], with improved outcomes in terms of renal function preservation [3].

Nowadays, indications for PN are essentially based on tumor size and tumor position; however, their cut-off might depend on surgeon expertise. Regardless, we consider absolute contraindications to PN evidence of urinary tract infiltration at preoperative imaging or gross haematuria.

In the era of widespread diffusion of minimally-invasive techniques, most of PN or RN surgeries are performed through a laparoscopic or robotic approach, as open approach is addressed only when the surgeon considers the case is going to perform not feasible with a minimally-invasive approach.

RN surgery may be safely performed through pure laparoscopy, with a three-trocars access, while robotic can be required in more challenging clinical scenarios, such as locally advanced tumors, or in patients with renal vein or inferior vena cava (IVC) tumor thrombus arising from a renal tumor.

As concerns minimally-invasive approach adoption for PN, robotic surgery plays a leading role, while pure laparoscopy may be addressed only to small and exophytic renal masses, easier to be managed.

In this contest, another important issue to consider is the management of renal hilum.

Apart from the standard main artery clamping, during the last decade several subtypes of approaches have been developed, with the common purpose to reduce at minimum the ischemia time during the tumor resection, and consequently reducing the risk of post-operative renal function deterioration [4, 5]. We support the off-clamp technique, in which the renal hilum is not isolated at all, but the surgeon focuses directly to the tumor area and perform the tumor resection [6]. However, we recommend this approach only to experienced surgeons.

18.3   Transperitoneal Approach for Minimally Invasive Radical Nephrectomy and Partial Nephrectomy

18.3.1   Robotic Trans-peritoneal Right Partial Nephrectomy

In the trans-peritoneal approach of robotic PN, trocars placement depends from which robotic platform is available (Si, Xi, etc.). However, in most of cases, a 5-trocar access is usually performed. The camera port is placed on the para-rectal

Fig. 18.1 Ports configuration for robotic transperitoneal partial nephrectomy

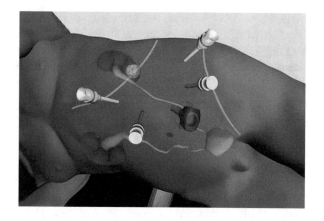

line, at the level of the umbilicus, through an open access and Hasson trocar placement; once pneumoperitoneum is achieved, the two robotic arms ports are placed 2 cm below the rib margin and 2 cm medially to the anterior-superior iliac spine, respectively, in order to create a perfect triangulation with the camera. Two 12 mm assistant ports are placed between the robotic ports and the camera port for each side, in order to create a U-shaped configuration (Fig. 18.1).

Instruments used by the console surgeon are: a curved monopolar scissors, a prograsp forceps, a needle holder.

Instruments used by the assistant surgeon are: a blunt tip grasper, a sealing device (we usually adopt 10 mm Ligasure Atlas™), one or two suction devices (very useful in the enucleation phase, as one is used for irrigation, in order to maintain a clean dissection plane, and the other one is used for suction), Hem-o-lok clips with Hem-o-lok clip applier. Pneumoperitoneum is maintained at 12 mmHg, and raised at 20 mmHg during the enucleation phase.

When approaching the right kidney, the first step is to gently medialize the ascending colon and the duodenum (Kocher maneuver). If it is necessary to isolate the upper pole, a liver retractor might be necessary to lift the right lobe of the liver anteriorly and provide adequate exposure. Once exposed the kidney surrounded by its perirenal fat, through off-clamp technique we directly incise the Gerota's capsule in the area where the tumor is located, until we reach the renal parenchyma. At this point we identify the mass, and, after margins scoring, the resection is accomplished and the specimen put in an endocatch bag. The surgical field is maintained clean by the assistant which adopts two suction devices, one for irrigation and one for suction. Finally, renorrhaphy is performed through a running suture, with a sliding clip-technique. If the surgeon planned to do an on-clamp procedure, the first step is to identify psoas muscle. Once the psoas muscle is clearly identified, the ureter and the gonadal vein have to be detected, and then the dissection proceeds cephalad toward the renal hilum. Once isolated the renal artery, the Gerota's capsule is incised and the renal tumor is identified. Once performed margins scoring, a bulldog clamp is applied to the renal artery and the dissection is performed, being aware of the ischemia time. After tumor enucleation, the specimen is put in an endocatch bag, renorrhaphy is completed, bulldog clamp is removed and blood flow is restored. Finally, when haemostasis control is achieved, Gerota's capsule is closed with a running suture and hem-o-lok clips. A drain is recommended to be left, and trocars are gently removed, being aware of any bleeding from the ports' access.

18.3.2 Videolaparoscopic Trans-peritoneal Right Radical Nephrectomy

As concerns trans-peritoneal pure laparoscopic right RN, a four-trocar access is performed: two 12 mm ports, one for camera and one for the surgeon, and two 5 mm ports, one for the surgeon and one for assistant. The camera port is placed on the para-rectal line, at the level of the umbilicus, through an open access and Hasson trocar placement; once pneumoperitoneum in achieved, the two surgeon ports are placed on the mid-clavicular line, on the right side and on the left side of the camera (the distance depends from the dimension of the patient's abdomen); the assistant port is placed on the anterior axillary line, in line with the camera port. Instruments used by the surgeon are: a sealing device (we usually adopt 10 mm Ligasure Atlas™), a blunt tip grasper, a suction device, a right-angled dissector, a monopolar scissors, titanium clips with clip applier, Endo-GIA stapler. The assistant surgeon uses alternatively or a suction device or a blunt tip grasper. Pneumoperitoneum is maintained at 12 mmHg.

As for the on-clamp PN procedure, the first step is to identify psoas muscle. Once the psoas muscle is clearly identified, the ureter and the gonadal vein have to be detected and then the dissection proceeds cephalad toward the renal hilum. Once the renal artery and the renal vein are carefully prepared, through adoption of the right-angled dissector, suction device and sealing device, the artery is clipped (two clips at the proximal side) and transected. The vein is usually sealed and transected through Stapler, being aware of any thinner accessory vessels which might be accidentally injured. Once completed the nephrectomy, the specimen is secured in an endocatch bag. A drain is left in the renal fossa and trocars are gently removed, being aware of any bleeding from the ports' access. The specimen is removed through a little axial incision medial to the right anterior-superior iliac spine.

18.3.3 Robotic Trans-peritoneal Left Partial Nephrectomy

Trocar positioning and instruments adopted are already described in the Robotic trans-peritoneal Right PN section.

When approaching the left kidney, the descending colon is firstly medialized. As previously highlighted, if an off-clamp approach is planned, Gerota's capsule is directly incised in order to achieve the tumor and perform the resection. On the contrary, if an on-clamp approach is considered, the psoas muscle plan is identified, and, after identified the ureter and the gonadal vein, the dissection proceeds cephalad towards the renal hilum. If an isolation of the upper pole is necessary, the lienorenal attachments are released, allowing the spleen and the tail of the pancreas to reject medially, thus providing optimal exposure to the renal hilum as well. Once isolated the renal artery, the Gerota's capsule is incised and the renal tumor is identified. Once performed margins scoring, a bulldog clamp is applied to the renal artery and the dissection is performed, being aware of the ischemia time. After tumor enucleation, the specimen is put in an endocatch bag, renorrhaphy is completed, bulldog clamp is removed and blood flow is restored. Finally, when haemostasis control is achieved, Gerota's capsule is closed with a running suture and hem-o-lok clips. A drain is recommended to be left, and trocars are gently removed, being aware of any bleeding from the ports' access.

18.3.4 Videolaparoscopic Trans-peritoneal Left Radical Nephrectomy

Trocar positioning and instruments adopted are already described in the Videolaparoscopic trans-peritoneal Right RN section.

Key surgical steps are the same of the on-clamp robotic left PN technique. Once the renal artery and the renal vein are carefully prepared, through adoption of the right-angled dissector, suction device and sealing device, the artery is clipped (two clips at the proximal side) and transected. The vein is usually sealed and transected through Stapler, being aware of any thinner accessory vessels which might be accidentally injured. Once completed the nephrectomy, the specimen is secured in an endocatch bag. A drain is left in the renal fossa and trocars are removed, being aware of any bleeding from the ports' access. The specimen is removed through a little axial incision medial to the left anterior-superior iliac spine.

18.4 Retroperitoneal Approach for Minimally Invasive RN and PN

The retroperitoneal approach for RN or PN is ideally suited for the patient with a hostile abdomen, either from intrinsic intraabdominal disease or from extensive prior abdominal surgery, and the patient with a posterior or posteromedial renal mass that is difficult to expose through an intraabdominal approach. This approach avoids bowel mobilization, intraabdominal adhesions, and the need to flip the kidney. Below are the general steps to performing a robotic retroperitoneal nephrectomy, with pearls highlighted.

Under general anesthesia, the patient is placed in steep flank position, approaching 90°, with the side of the renal mass uppermost. The bed is fully flexed to create space between the ribs and the iliac crest. The primary camera port is placed in the mid-axillary line between the 12th rib and the iliac crest. Access is obtained to the retroperitoneum using a small open incision. A balloon dilator system is used to open approximately 800–1500 mL of retroperitoneal space. If an inadvertent peritoneotomy is made, billowing of the peritoneum encroaches upon the operating space. This can be troubleshooted by either closing the peritoneotomy laparoscopically if small or opening the peritoneum widely. A self-retaining balloon port is then placed after this space has been created. The posterior robotic port, which is the left working arm for right sided cases and the right working arm for left sided cases, is placed between the erector spinae muscle and the lowest rib behind the posterior axillary line. The anterior robotic port, which is the right working arm for right sided cases and the left working arm for left sided cases is placed along the anterior axillary line at the level of the umbilicus. The fourth robotic arm is the most anterior robotic port and is placed at the lateral edge of the ipsilateral rectus muscle. Finally, the assistant port is placed just medial to the anterior superior iliac spine, between the camera port and the anterior robotic arm. An air seal port is recommended for use as the assistant port. A wide separation of ports is recommended to prevent clashing of the robotic arms. The peritoneal reflection is teased off of the anterior musculature prior to placement of secondary ports. A horizontally oriented psoas muscle is the most important landmark. Initially, we incise Gerota's fascia parallel to the psoas muscle. We then identify all renal vasculature and circumferentially mobilize them. We then mobilize the kidney to identify the tumor. For masses amenable to partial nephrectomy, we then perform intraoperative ultrasonography with the help of an ultrasound technician, and mark the lines of resection on the surface of the kidney using monopolar electrocautery. We then clamped the renal artery first with two Scanlan bulldogs to ensure appropriate cessation of arterial inflow. Venous structures may or may not be clamped depending on hilar anatomy. The tumor is then excised in usual fashion without electrocautery using robotic scissors. After the tumor is excised, we reconstruct the partial nephrectomy bed using 2-0 V-Loc suture for the inner medullary layer. A horizontal mattress cortical approximation using 2-0 Vicryl sutures ensues. At this point, we check our closure for residual bleeding and achieve perfect hemostasis with additional interrupted Vicryl sutures as needed. We then unclamp the renal arteries and again confirm perfect hemostasis. Total warm ischemia time is minimized as much as possible. Percentage excised and percentage of kidney saved is recorded. In cases of radical nephrectomy, a single 60 mm vascular load endo-GIA is fired across the hilum when both arterial and venous structures are taken in unison. Alternatively, these may be ligated separately, with arterial ligation preceding venous. A Blake drain is left behind the kidney in all partial nephrectomies and in radical nephrectomies on a case by case basis. The specimen is removed intact and sent it to pathology. At this point, we close all fascial incisions greater than 8 mm followed by closure of superficial layers of the skin. All smaller incisions are closed in two layers.

18.5   Locally Advanced Renal Tumours with Inferior Vena Cava Thrombus

18.5.1   Basis of Robotic Management of Renal Tumours with Venous Thrombosis

Around 10% of patients with Renal Cell Carcinoma have venous tumour thrombosis which can involve the renal vein, the inferior vena cava (IVC) or the right atrium in very rare advanced cases, representing a significant adverse prognostic factor. Accordingly, aggressive surgical resection is widely accepted as the default management option for patients with venous tumour thrombus. However, uncertainties remain over the best approach for surgical treatment of these patients.

Surgical management of patients with (IVC) tumor thrombus arising from a renal tumor requires IVC thrombectomy, RN and ipsilateral retroperitoneal lymphadenectomy (RPLND), and surgical procedure may be different, according to thrombus level (Table 18.1). If performed through an open approach, this complex major surgical operation requires a large muscle-cutting abdominal or thoracoabdominal incision to achieve the necessary surgical access for vascular control and thrombectomy.

In the last decade, initial experiences for robotic management of level 0 (renal vein) and level I–II thrombi were reported. Robot-assisted surgery for level III caval thrombi was first reported in 2015, and standardised in 2017, corroborated by 1-year outcomes [7]. Spurred by these initial publications, additional centers have recently reported early experiences attesting to the increasing interest within the field for robot-assisted caval thrombectomy surgery. Although the literature is relatively poor, we believe that the robotic approach might reliably duplicate open surgery, and thus allow more teams to embark safely on robot-assisted caval thrombectomy surgery. Our step-by-step standardized anatomic-based robotic approach is primarily focused towards minimizing the chances of intraoperative tumor thromboembolism and major hemorrhage, the two major complications of IVC thrombectomy surgery.

As preoperative work-up, patients undergo cross-sectional abdominal imaging (CT and MRI). Preoperative trans-esophageal ecocardiography is also essential to potentially identify the cranial extremity in the case of level III IVC thrombus. Angioembolization of the tumor-bearing kidney is performed in the majority of cases.

Table 18.1 Classification of tumor thrombus level according to the Mayo staging system

Level 0	Thrombus extending to the renal vein
Level I	Thrombus extending into the IVC to no more than 2 cm above the renal vein
Level II	Thrombus extending into the IVC to more than 2 cm above the renal vein but not to the hepatic vein
Level III	Thrombus extending into the IVC to above the hepatic vein but not to the diaphragm
Level IV	Thrombus extending into the supradiaphragmatic IVC or right atrium

18.5.2 Robotic Instrumentation

The four-arm Si or Xi da Vinci Surgical System (Intuitive Surgical Inc, Sunnyvale, CA, USA) with a six- to seven-port approach are used, including two assistant ports. Bariatric-length robotic ports might be useful to reduce external robotic arms clashing. Apart from the standard robotic instruments adopted for robotic renal surgery, a double-fenestrated grasper is used to pass posterior to the IVC, to establish a Rummel tourniquet control of the retrohepatic/intrahepatic IVC.

The patient is placed in a 75° lateral decubitus position, with the table fully flexed. For both right- or left-sided tumors, the patient is initially secured right side up to facilitate IVC exposure and control. For right-sided tumors, the procedure proceeds directly to a right RN following IVC thrombectomy; for left-sided tumors, the patient is repositioned left side up and the robot's redocked following IVC thrombectomy.

Port configuration is similar to the one for robotic PN, except for the two robotic trocars which are placed more medially, as the surgery target is IVC and renal hilum. Moreover, a fourth arm robotic trocar is positioned medially to the left robotic port.

18.5.3 Inferior Vena Cava Control (for Right- or Left-Sided Tumors)

The primary concept we support in this surgical scenario is the "IVC-first, kidney-last" approach, in a minimal IVC touch manner, to reduce chances of tumor embolism and major bleeding. The right colon and duodenum are reflected medially to expose the IVC. Retroperitoneal dissection begins infrarenally in the midline, to expose the inter-aortocaval region.

Dissection of the infrarenal IVC involves control of all encountered lumbar veins and the gonadal vein, which are closed with Hem-o-lok clips (Teleflex, Wayne, PA, USA) and cut, or sealed and transected with 10 mm Ligasure device. The infrarenal IVC is encircled with a double-loop tourniquet (Rummel), using a vessel loop passed through a half-inch piece of rubber drain tube and secured in place with a Hem-o-lok clip. Dissection is carried cephalad within the inter-aortocaval region. The left renal vein is mobilized and encircled with a Rummel tourniquet.

For proximal IVC control, careful interaortocaval dissection is performed towards the liver.

For level III thrombi, the relevant number of short hepatic veins is controlled with robotic Hem-o-lok clips and/or 10 mm Ligasure. Releasing the short hepatic veins is essential to retract the caudate lobe; this maneuver exposes an additional 3–4 cm of the IVC, allowing high intrahepatic access to the retro-hepatic IVC. Furthermore, in order to maximize exposure of retro-hepatic IVC, triangular ligament is transected, and the liver partially rotated medially. The right main adrenal vein is controlled with Hem-o-lok clips or 10 mm Ligasure, and the right lateral border of the suprarenal IVC is dissected. Retrocaval dissection of the intrahepatic IVC is performed. A double-fenestrated grasper is used to encircle the IVC with a Rummel tourniquet in this high retrohepatic location. The right renal hilum is dissected and the right renal vein is exposed.

18.5.4 Management of the Upper Boundary of IVC Thrombus

When dealing with level III IVC thrombus, a meticulous knowledge of the thrombus cranial edge level is crucial, because if the thrombus is located below major hepatic veins it might be sufficient to put the proximal tourniquet just above the thrombus head; in this case an intraoperative ultrasound probe might easily identify thrombus limits. A further tool to control the cranial edge of the tumor thrombus is represented by the use of indocyanine green (ICG) guidance.

Under ICG guidance, IVC blood flow can be checked in order to better define the thrombus limits and to identify the area of absence of blood flow, due to the neoplastic thrombus which occupies part of the caval lumen (Fig. 18.2).

On the contrary, at the level of the proximal tourniquet, the intravenous injection of ICG shows a normal blood flow (Fig. 18.3).

After confirming the proper control of cranial IVC thrombus edge, the previously applied tourniquet can be cinched down.

After thrombus excision, IVC suture, and touriquet's removal, near infrared fluorescence may be used to inspect IVC lumen and to confirm proper restoration of IVC flow.

On the other hand, if the thrombus edge involves major hepatic veins hostium, thus the suprarenal tourniquet should be placed above. In this scenario, Pringle maneuver (clamping of porta hepatis, containing portal vein, common hepatic artery and common bile duct) is usually performed in open surgery, to prevent massive blood loss if the IVC is clamped above the major hepatic veins.

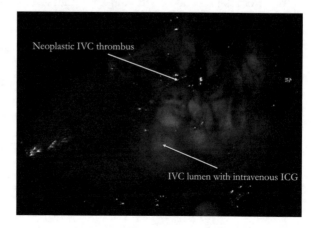

Fig. 18.2 Checking of IVC thrombus limits through intraoperative ICG guidance

Fig. 18.3 Evidence of
normal blood flow at the
level of the proximal IVC
tourniquet through
intraoperative ICG
guidance

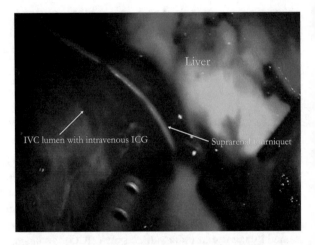

Fig. 18.4 Cavotomy and
thrombus removal

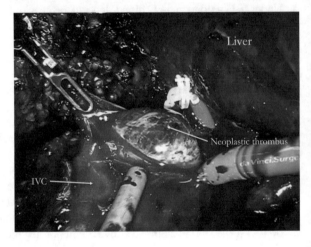

If performing robotic IVC thrombectomy, all these surgical maneuvers might be
very challenging and complex. Accordingly, one strategy to manage the cranial
margin of the thrombus is to use an occluding balloon Fogarty catheter to control
the upper boundary of the IVC thrombus, under transesofageal ultrasound
guidance [8].

The 9 French Fogarty catheter is inserted in the IVC, and placed safe all above
the thrombus.

The balloon is inflated, and the catheter is attracted distally to completely occlude
the IVC.

After Fogarty catheter is inserted in the IVC, Trans esophageal ultrasound imaging is mandatory to highlight the cranial part of the thrombus, to identify major
hepatic veins, and to recognize the right atrium. Moreover, transesophageal ultrasound is used to ensure the proper placement of the catheter tip on the cranial edge
of the thrombus before inflating the balloon.

Once inflated and distally attracted, cavotomy is performed and the thrombus is progressively mobilized (Fig. 18.4).

18.5.5 Right-Sided Robotic Caval Thrombectomy

All Rummel tourniquets have to be in the appropriate position, with a sufficient margin around the thrombus. This is achieved with visual confirmation (appropriate narrowing of the cava on cinching the Rummel tourniquet) and/or a drop-in ultrasound probe.

The right renal artery is clipped and transected in the interaortocaval region. Anesthesiologist is alerted that caval blood flow will be temporarily halted.

The initial maneuver is to cinch the distal (infrarenal) IVC tourniquet. Once assured that the patient is able to tolerate caval cross-clamping, the left renal vein and proximal IVC Rummel tourniquets are cinched sequentially, thus excluding the thrombus-bearing caval segment. The thrombus-bearing right renal vein is transected with an Endo GIA stapler (vascular load; Covidien). The excluded caval segment is now rotated and circumferentially inspected 360° to reconfirm visually that all feeding lumbar veins have been secured. An appropriately performed cavotomy is created toward the right edge of the IVC, adjacent to the right renal vein ostium; the cavotomy should be well planned so that subsequent caval reconstruction does not overly narrow its lumen.

The thrombus is carefully dissected free from the IVC lumen without local spillage. The right renal vein ostium, along with its staple line, and any infiltrated or densely adherent IVC wall are excised en-bloc with the thrombus; the tumor thrombus specimen is immediately placed in a 10-mm Endocatch bag, precluding local seeding. The IVC lumen is copiously irrigated and flushed with heparinized solution.

Caval reconstruction is performed with a 3-0 or 4-0 prolene suture with a single-layer running stitch. Tourniquets are released sequentially (left renal vein, suprarenal IVC, infrarenal IVC) and caval flow restored. Right RN and ipsilateral RPLND are then completed in the standard fashion.

18.5.6 Left-Sided Robotic Caval Thrombectomy

The following maneuvers are different for left-sided tumors. Temporary cessation of blood flow to the right kidney is necessary to properly exclude the caval segment for controlled thrombectomy. The right renal artery and vein are controlled with individual bulldog clamps, prior to cinching the infra- and suprarenal IVC tourniquets. The thrombus-bearing left renal vein is transected with an Endo GIA stapler (left-sided tumors routinely undergo preoperative angioinfarction). After caval thrombectomy and reconstruction, caval flow is restored and the right kidney revascularized. The patient is repositioned left side up for left RN and ipsilateral RPLND.

References

1. Ljungberg B, Albiges L, Abu-Ghanem Y, et al. European Association of Urology guidelines on renal cell carcinoma: the 2019 update. Eur Urol. 2019;75:799–810.
2. Van Poppel H, Da Pozzo L, Albrecht W, et al. A prospective, randomised EORTC intergroup phase 3 study comparing the oncologic outcome of elective nephron-sparing surgery and radical nephrectomy for low-stage renal cell carcinoma. Eur Urol. 2011;59:543–52.
3. Scosyrev E, Messing EM, Sylvester R, et al. Renal function after nephron-sparing surgery versus radical nephrectomy: results from EORTC randomized trial 30904. Eur Urol. 2014;65:372–7.
4. Simone G, Capitanio U, Tuderti G, et al. On-clamp versus off-clamp partial nephrectomy: Propensity score-matched comparison of long-term functional outcomes. Int J Urol. 2019;26:985–91.
5. Simone G, Gill IS, Mottrie A, et al. Indications, techniques, outcomes, and limitations for minimally ischemic and off-clamp partial nephrectomy: a systematic review of the literature. Eur Urol. 2015;68:632–40.
6. Simone G, Misuraca L, Tuderti G, et al. Purely off-clamp robotic partial nephrectomy: Preliminary 3-year oncological and functional outcomes. Int J Urol. 2018;25:606–14.
7. Chopra S, Simone G, Metcalfe C, et al. Robot-assisted level II-III inferior vena cava tumor thrombectomy: step-by-step technique and 1-year outcomes. Eur Urol. 2017;72:267–74.
8. Kundavaram C, Abreu AL, Chopra S, et al. Advances in robotic vena cava tumor thrombectomy: intracaval balloon occlusion, patch grafting, and vena cavoscopy. Eur Urol. 2016;70:884–90.

Chapter 19
Radical Cystectomy: Abdominal District and Neobladder Configurations

Andrea Minervini, Andrea Mari, Gianni Vittori, Marco Carini, and Walter Artibani

19.1 Introduction

Radical cystectomy (RC) with extended lymphadenectomy and urinary diversion is currently the most commonly used treatment in patients with muscle-invasive invasive bladder cancer (MIBC) and with high-grade non-MIBC non-responding to endovesical immunological therapy [1, 2]. Although, in renal and prostate cancer surgery, minimally invasive approaches increased exponentially at the beginning of last century [3, 4], their use in RC was delayed due to the high oncological concerns due to the high risk of recurrence after this treatment [5]. Historically, in 1992 the first radical cystectomy with laparoscopic technique was reported in literature, however the technical difficulties have limited its spread and adoption [6]. In the years to follow, the increasing adoption of robotic system in urologic centers together to the higher ability of surgeons in minimally invasive surgery led to the introduction of the Robot-Assisted Radical Cystectomy (RARC) which replicates the surgical principles of the open radical cystectomy (ORC) [7]. Recent randomized clinical trials confirmed the oncologic safety of RARC and its non-inferiority compared to ORC in terms of perioperative outcomes and recurrence-free survival [8, 9].

Indeed, the robotic system provides unequalled highly magnified three-dimensional stereoscopic and detailed view of all the anatomical structures. It is essential for minimally invasive, either laparoscopic or robot-assisted, surgery a good knowledge about the different anatomical structures of the anterior abdominal wall.

A. Minervini (✉) · A. Mari · G. Vittori · M. Carini
Department of Urology, University of Florence, Florence, Italy

Unit of Oncologic Minimally-Invasive Urology and Andrology, Careggi Hospital, Florence, Italy

W. Artibani
Department of Urology, Azienda Ospedaliera Universitaria Integrata (A.O.U.I.), Verona, Italy

© Springer Nature Switzerland AG 2021
E. Huri, D. Veneziano (eds.), *Anatomy for Urologic Surgeons in the Digital Era*,
https://doi.org/10.1007/978-3-030-59479-4_19

19.2 Anatomical Landmarks of the Anterior Abdominal Wall

After trocar positioning, when the camera is inserted into the male pelvis, it is required special orientation and confidence with several anatomical landmarks.

Five tissue folds stand out on the inner anterior abdominal wall, subdividing it in different portions. In the middle wall, the median umbilical ligament, a fibrous cord running through the transversalis fascia and the peritoneum, formed as the allantois stalk during fetal development that lasts through life (urachus), form the median umbilical fold, connecting the apex of the urinary bladder and the navel. On both sides of the median umbilical fold are appreciable the medial umbilical folds, that accommodating the remnants of the fetal umbilical arteries, set the limit of two depressions, the supra-vesical fossae. Medial umbilical ligaments play a crucial role during cystectomy; they help the surgeon to identify the upper vesical pedicle, including the superior vesical artery. A representation of these anatomic landmarks in robotic surgery are depicted in Fig. 19.1. The lateral umbilical folds are formed from both inferior epigastric arteries. Hernia classification is based on the different location of the hernial sac, in reference to the lateral umbilical fold. Direct inguinal hernias arise from a weakness on the wall of the medial inguinal fossa. Lateral inguinal fossa is a s shallow concave stretch of peritoneum, placed laterally the deep inguinal ring, entry to the inguinal canal. In case of indirect inguinal hernia, the components of the spermatic cord could accompany the hernial sac through the inguinal canal. Below the inguinal ligament, made of external abdominal oblique aponeurosis and connecting the anterior superior iliac spine to the pubic tubercle, a

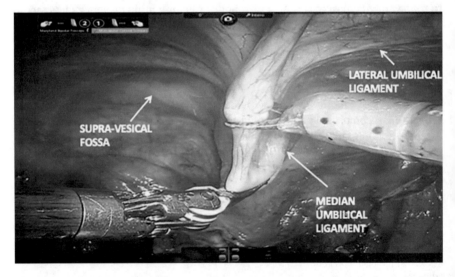

Fig. 19.1 The median umbilical ligament, a fibrous cord running through the transversalis fascia and the peritoneum. It connects the apex of the urinary bladder and the navel. On both sides of the median umbilical fold are appreciable the medial umbilical folds that set the limit of the supra-vesical fossae

fibromuscular structure, the iliopectineal arch, subdivides this space in two sectors: the muscular lacuna laterally, which contains the iliopsoas muscle and the femoral nerve, and the vascular lacuna medially, with the external iliac vessels. The lacunar ligament, which connects the inguinal ligament, arises medially to the external iliac vein and is the caudal extent landmark during lymphadenectomy for bladder or prostate cancer [10, 11].

19.3   Topographical Anatomy of the Female Pelvis

An overview on the pelvis shows the female pelvic bone, characterized by the sacral promontory and the two wide iliac wings; in this region are located organs of the peritoneal and subperitoneal pelvic cavity, such as the urinary bladder, ureters, uterus, vagina, ovaries, oviducts, and the rectum. The upper half of the urinary bladder, the uterus, the adnexa, and the anterior wall of the rectum are partially covered by the parietal peritoneum. The uterus is placed between the urinary bladder and the rectum, developing the rectouterine excavation (Douglas' fold) and the vesicouterine excavation. These anatomic landmarks in robotic surgery are depicted in Fig. 19.2. Different pairs of ligaments help to maintain the position of the uterus

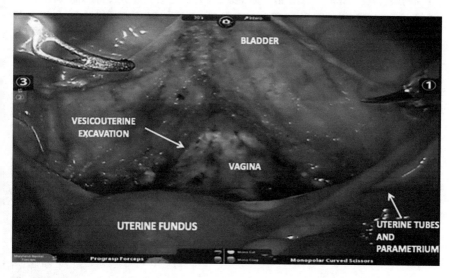

Fig. 19.2 The uterus is located within the pelvic region immediately behind and almost overlying the bladder, and in front of the sigmoid colon. The fundus is the uppermost rounded portion of the uterus and is the most evident portion in robotic surgery with a transperitoneal approach. The *rectouterine excavation* (Douglas' fold) and the *vesicouterine excavation* are the spaces between the uterus and the bladder anteriorly and between the uterus and the rectum posteriorly. The uterine tubes are connected to the uterus superiorly. This part of the tubes is called *isthmus* as it is the narrowest segment. The round ligaments of the uterus originate at the uterine horns in the parametrium and exits the pelvis via the deep inguinal ring. The parametrium stands in front of the cervix and extends laterally between the layers of the broad ligaments. It connects the uterus to other tissues in the pelvis

within the pelvis: the cardinal ligaments (transverse cervical ligaments), containing the uterine arteries, the uterine venous plexus, and the parts of the distal third of the ureters, connect the cervix to the lateral pelvic wall; the broad ligament of the uterus, a double-layer fold of peritoneum that attaches the lateral portions of the uterus to the lateral pelvic sidewalls; the suspensory ligaments, which contain the ovarian vessels and connect the ovaries to the lateral wall of the pelvis; the ovarian ligaments, that connect the ovaries to the uterus; the round ligaments, a connection between the deep inguinal ring and the uterine horns; the rectouterine folds that form the recto-uterine excavation; the endopelvic fascia, that with its parietal and the visceral layers covers the borders of the subperitoneal space (cavum retzii) and forms the superior layer of the fascia of the pelvic diaphragm. Pubovesical ligaments thus contribute to stability of urinary bladder, by anchoring it to the symphysis pubis and with lateral connections to the superior layer of the fascia of the pelvic diaphragm [10, 12–14].

19.4   Topographical Anatomy of the Male Pelvis

Male pelvis has a typical heart shape and bones are typically smaller and narrower compared to female gender. In the pelvis are located the urinary bladder, the ureters, the prostate, the seminal vesicles, the deferent ducts, and the rectum. The rectovesical excavation represents the caudal pouch of the abdominal cavity and it is located between the urinary bladder and the rectum. The rectovesical fold mark the borders of the excavation laterally, including the inferior hypogastric plexus. The deferent ducts along their path raise a peritoneal fold, forming the paravesical fossa. Similarly, to female pelvis, the pelvic fascia consists of two layers: a parietal layer, that covers the lateral wall of the pelvis, and the endopelvic fascia, which is the visceral layer overlaying the pelvic organs. On the lateral surfaces of the prostate, the endopelvic fascia continues with the prostate visceral fascia, which is multilayered and contains collagen, smooth muscle and fat. The prostate visceral fascia contains a lateral sheath which covers the lateral glandular prostate and a posterior thickened sheath, also known eponymically as Denonvilliers' fascia. This corresponds to the recto-vaginal fascia in the female and it is detached from the rectal fascia propria by a prerectal cleavage plane. Distally, the fascia becomes thickener just distal to the prostate-urethral junction and has direct continuity with the midline raphe ending in the perineal body or central tendon of the perineum. These anatomic landmarks in robotic surgery are depicted in Figs. 19.3 and 19.4.

19.5   Anatomy of the Urinary Bladder

The urinary bladder is a muscular-membranous organ, standing preperitoneally behind the symphysis. The peritoneum covers parts of the ventral and dorsal wall. The bladder can be divided into the corpus, constituted by two lateral walls, a dorsal wall and a ventral wall, the bladder neck and the trigone.

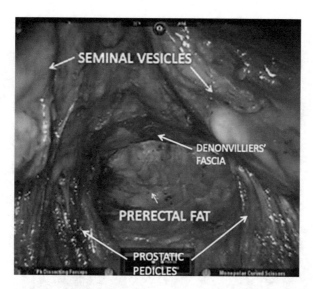

Fig. 19.3 The seminal vesicles are positioned below the urinary bladder and lateral to the vas deferens. The seminal vesicles are an important landmark during the development of the rectovesical excavation in robotic surgery while performing a transperitoneal approach. They are located dorsolaterally to the urinary bladder and posteriorly to the prostate. On the lateral surfaces of the prostate, the endopelvic fascia continues with the prostate visceral fascia which is multilayered and contains collagen, smooth muscle and fat. The prostatic pedicles provide the main arterial supply of the gland and provides branches to both the inferior bladder and the ejaculatory system. The inferior branches distribute as a plexus in the prostatic apex and anastomoses with the superior branches

The trigone constitutes the base of the bladder and it is limited by the internal urethral orifice, continuing into the bladder neck, and the orifices of the ureters. The ureters enter obliquely into the bladder wall and their inner smooth muscle layers form with the inner fibers of the contralateral ureter the superficial trigone.

The bladder is adjacent to the small intestine and sigmoid colon. In men, the bladder neck contacts the prostate. In women, the bladder trigone and bladder neck stand cranially to the vagina, while the uterus is located posterior to the bladder.

The shape, size and topographical position of the bladder is variable, depending on its filling state. In the supine position, the empty bladder is totally contained in the minor pelvis, lying at about the level of the symphysis pubis. As soon as the bladder is refilled, it rises over the pelvis, while always maintaining extraperitoneal domicile. In females, the bladder lies directly upon the pelvic diaphragm; in males, instead the bladder neck and the pelvic diaphragm are separated by the interposed prostate gland [15].

The urinary bladder wall is structured into several layers: the mucosa and the submucosa, the detrusor muscle (constituted by inner longitudinal, middle circular and outer longitudinal fibers), and adipose and connective tissues surrounding the bladder. The urinary bladder generally receives bilaterally the superior and the inferior vesical arteries, which sometimes are constituted by a pedicle of different

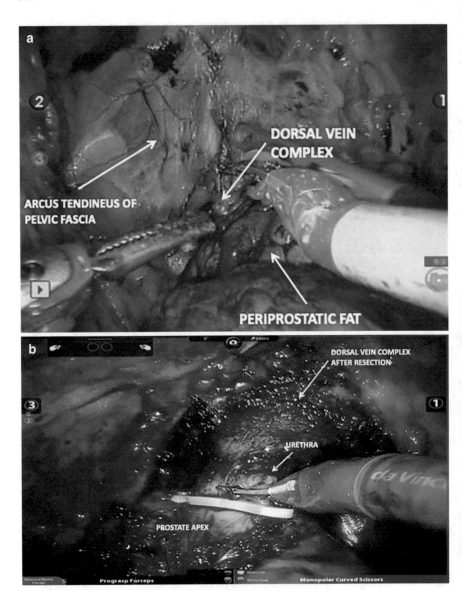

Fig. 19.4 The anterior surface of the prostate is narrow and convex from side to side. It stands posteriorly to the pubic symphysis, from which it is separated the dorsal vein complex. The prostate is anteriorly connected to the pubic bone on either side by the puboprostatic ligaments. The parietal pelvic fascia includes the endopelvic fascia which lies on the anterior surface of the prostate, the lateral parietal fascia which covers the levator ani laterally, and the tendinous arch of the pelvic fascia. During robotic surgery, once the Retzium space is developed, the endopelvic fascia is isolated and the puboprostatic ligaments stand anteriorly to the prostate apex and the dorsal venous complex. A proper control and division of the dorsal venous complex allows the procedure to be performed with minimal blood loss and provides excellent exposure of the prostatic apex and urethra (**a**). After performing a careful dissection of the apex of the prostate and of the urethra, a large Hemo-o-lok clip is positioned to ensure a hermetic seal and to prevent urine spillage (**b**)

vessels. The superior vesical arteries descend in the medial umbilical ligament from the internal iliac artery. The inferior vesical arteries arise from a common branch of the middle rectal artery and reach also the prostate through prostatic branches. Several venous plexuses, extensively communicating with prostatic venous plexuses in males and the vaginal venous plexuses in females, provide the drainage of the blood on both sides of the base of the bladder.

The urinary bladder is bilaterally innervated together with the adjacent organs by the inferior hypogastric plexus (pelvic plexus) through parasympathetic and sympathetic nerve fibers. The inferior hypogastric plexus arises at the crossing of the ureter and the common iliac artery on both sides from fibers of the superior hypogastric plexus, and fibers of the sacral and pelvic splanchnic nerves. From the inferior hypogastric plexus, numerous branches are distributed to the viscera of the pelvis (middle rectal plexus, vesical plexus, prostatic plexus, and uterovaginal plexus) accompanying the branches of the internal iliac artery. The pudendal nerve is part of the somatic nervous system and innervates the striated parts of the external urethral sphincter among others. After distribution of the lumbosacral plexus, the pudendal nerve leaves the pelvis by surrounding the ischial spine and proceeds through the pudendal canal (Alcock's canal) at the bottom of the inferior pubic bone.

19.6   Urinary Derivation: Innovative Approaches

Over the years, several urinary derivations have been developed. Urinary diversions can be defined as heterotopic or orthotopic, continent or incontinent, direct or connected through different segments of the digestive tract. In orthotopic neobladder, continence is dependent on the activity of the striated external sphincter, and voiding is performed by increasing the abdominal pressure obtained by a manoeuvre of valsalva (abdominal press) and with contemporaneous relaxation of the pelvic floor muscles. The ileum is preferred for intracorporeal bladder reconstruction due to its easy accessibility and higher functional and metabolic results compared to other segments. Furthermore, its digestive anastomosis has the lowest fistulas rate formation allowing the highest compliance with low contraction pressures [16] Indeed, whichever is the surgical approach, the final choice of the digestive segment is often dictated by the possibility of the segment to come into contact with the urethra. However, if the anastomosis is under tension, a mesenteric plasty can be made. Other precautions are also very important: the selection and isolation technique of the intestinal segment should carefully respect the digestive vascularization. Vessels are easily identified when the mesentery is lifted avoiding the standard transillumination test performed in open surgery. The required length is usually measured taking care of the regular measure of robotic instruments. According to Studer technique, the mesenteric incision at the distal extremity of the segment should be wide, while the proximal extremity should be little but efficient. Ileo-ileal anastomosis is one of the most delicate steps of this surgical procedure, since intestinal anastomotic leakage is responsible for the highest morbidity and mortality in the postoperative period. The mesenteric edge must be cleared, to allow a good application of the sutures on the serous without any fat interposition. The anastomosis confection begins on this side, and it is important not to include the mucosa for a good matching of the two interfaces. The mesentery is closed preferably after the continuity is restored, to avoid tearing during mobilization of the plasty. The opening is performed with monopolar scissors on the antimesenteric edge of the intestine. The realization of the different configurations will be facilitated by placing some suture wires as landmark and the construction of a frame using a few separate stitches. In this phase it is mandatory to sacrifice any tissue of doubtful vitality.

Closure of the new reservoir is long and is therefore made by over-sewing braided absorbable sutures: the creation of a sealed, but not ischemic suture is of paramount importance. As suturing can be tedious and longer with a robotic approach compared to open surgery, staple suturing has been proposed, although it has been associated with stone development inside the intestinal derivation. Therefore, two solution are possible: the use of absorbable staples or the realization of an everted suture. Even though new stapling devices are now available, allowing absorbable continent sutures, the hand-sewn reservoir functions appear to be still more favourable compared to that of stapled ones, discouraging the absorbable staples use [17].

The uretero-intestinal anastomosis is an important phase of urinary diversion development. Stenosis of uretero-intestinal anastomosis still remains the most common late complication of the orthotopic neobladder reconstruction. The ideal technique of ureteral reimplantation should be simple and might aim to preserve the ureteral vascularization, ensuring a free flow of urine from kidneys to the reservoir and preventing its flowing back up the ureters in the direction of the kidneys. Several techniques of ureteral reimplantation have been described and all of them requiring ureteral stenting in the postoperative course. In robotic surgery, real-time indocyanine green angiography using the Firefly technology (Intuitive Surgical, Sunnyvale, CA, USA) may help to preserve ureteral blood supply and prevent ureteral stenosis [18].

In the last decade, the RARC has been increasingly used as a viable alternative to open surgery for the treatment of muscle-invasive or high-grade non-MIBC unresponsive to endovesical immunological therapy. In some centers, despite a robotic approach is used for the demolitive phase, an extracorporeal urinary derivation (ECUD) is performed. However, intracorporeal urinary derivation (ICUD) has become popular since the procedure was first described by Beecken et al., in 2003, adopting Hautmann W-shaped reconfiguration, with an operative time of 8.5 h [19]. Moreover, ICUD has recently increased its spread due to the improvement and simplification of surgical technique, that along with the development of modified reconfigurations, has led to some benefits, including less intra-operative blood loss, expedited return of bowel function, less operative time and shorter hospital stay with faster resumption of daily activities [20, 21]. A recent report from the International Robotic Cystectomy Consortium has indicated also that the ICUD, due to the avoiding of wound incision, the lower postoperative pain and the decreased bowel exposure, is feasible and it is associated with a lower risk of complications compared with ECUD [22]. Nevertheless, the RARC with totally

intracorporeal neobladder remains a technically challenging and complex procedure and a high experience by the surgeon should be required. Among the most
innovative approaches of robot-assisted neobladder reconfiguration, undoubtedly
deserve to be mentioned two intracorporeal neobladder (ICNB) techniques: the
Vescica Ileale Padovana (V.I.P) and the FloRIN (Florence Robotic Intracorporeal
Neobladder).

19.7   Padua Neobladder Configuration

The Vescica Ileale Padovana (VIP) was first described in 1989 as a technique for
total bladder replacement [23]. It represents the second most commonly performed
neobladder technique in Italy [24] and it has gained popularity also in Europe and
Northern America due to its simplicity, technical advantages, and functional outcomes. Reproducing open surgical technique principles, in 2018 Cacciamani et al.
has described their initial experience of robot-assisted VIP (RA-VIP) [25]. Also
Simone et al. previously discussed the use of robotic approach to perform VIP [26].
In the first paper, Cacciamani et al. describe a surgical technique that basically replicates the open procedure, however staplers are avoided, and only reabsorbable
sutures were used. Furthermore, in this technique, a shorter ileal segment (40 vs.
55–65 cm) is used reducing the absorption surface and leading to a smaller post-
voiding residual [25].

   For this neobladder configuration, the following ileal segments are used: 8 cm
for the right plate, 10 cm for the neck configuration, 8 cm for the left plate and
16 cm folded in a "U" configuration to create an 8-cm dome (Fig. 19.5). A 40 cm
ileal segment, thus, is isolated 10–15 cm upstream the ileocecal valve; in order to
reach the membranous urethra, the distal handle (16 cm) is lowered in shape of
U. The ileal-urethral anastomosis is performed in a similar way to Camey 2 technique: a cut is made at the most sloped part of the neobladder neck, at the top of the
U-shaped handle; the urethroileal anastomosis is performed with two end-knotted
2-0 Monocryl Visi-Black running sutures. The difference is that the ileal orifice of
the urethral anastomosis is very close to the posterior mesentery insertion. The
intestine is opened along its entire length on the antimesenteric edge. The ureters are
then replaced on each arm of this first handle and the ureteroileal anastomosis is
performed according to the modified split-nipple technique with 4-0 Monocryl
(Ethicon, Somerville, NJ, USA) interrupted sutures. The most caudal part of this
first handle is tubularized forward and backwards, 4–5 cm long. The proximal handle is folded inward, approximating two 8-cm segments, resembling an inverted
U. The neobladder is thus shaped as a triangle with 8-cm sides and the vertex at the
inverted U-shaped neobladder neck. The inner borders are then sutured to each
other by a 3.0 absorbable running suture, configurating, with the subsequent folding, the neobladder dome. The superior part is subsequently sewed to the inferior
handle. Finally, the new Padua ileal neobladder is anchored on both sides to psoas
muscles with single absorbable stitches.

Fig. 19.5 The Vescica
Ileale Padovana (VIP)
neobladder

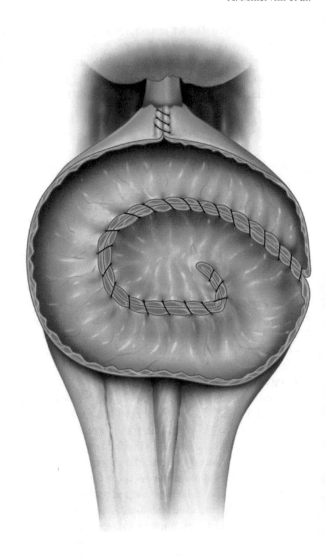

19.8 Florence Robotic Intracorporeal Neobladder (FloRIN)

The Florence Robotic Intracorporeal Neobladder (FloRIN) is a new reconfiguration strategy, described and performed since 2017 [27]. The FloRIN reconfiguration has been proposed to create a neobladder with a similar shape to the natural bladder with a fast and simple intracorporeal technique to perform during robotic surgery. The FloRIN reconfiguration includes the following main surgical steps: isolation of 50 cm of ileum; bowel anastomosis; urethro-ileal anastomosis and creation of an asymmetrical 'U'-shape (30 cm distally and 20 cm proximally to anastomosis),

Fig. 19.6 The Florence
robotic intracorporeal
neobladder (FloRIN)

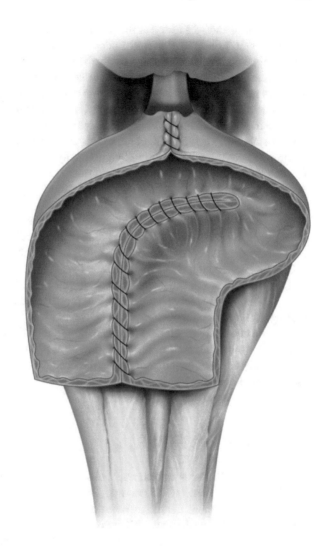

ileum detubularization; posterior wall reconfiguration as an 'L'; bladder neck reconstruction; anterior folding of the posterior plate to reach the 12 o'clock position; uretero-enteral 'orthotopic' bilateral functional and oncological outcomes and to reduce operative time (Fig. 19.6).

In detail, a single landmark stich is placed 20 cm away from the ileocecal valve. Then, a 50 cm distal ileal segment is isolated, and a second landmark stitch is positioned in the point of least traction, indicating where the future neobladder neck-urethral anastomosis will take place. An asymmetric U-shape ileum is isolated: this is 25 and 20 cm long distally and proximally from the point of urethral anastomosis, respectively.

The ileum is then dissected at the points marked in advance with the endo-GIA 60 mm Echelon FlexTM Powered Endopath® Stapler (ethicon endo surgery), and the intestinal continuity is restored by realizing a latero-lateral anastomosis.

The urethral-ileal anastomosis is performed using a double armed 3-0 Stratafix suture. In men, to avoid the caudal retraction of the urethra-sphincter complex and to reconstruct the posterior fibers of the raphe, a posterior reconstruction is performed between the recto-urethral muscle, Denonvillers fascia and perimesenter-free tract of the distal loop. The neobladder neck is reconstructed from the anterior part of the urethral-ileal anastomosis suturing longitudinally a 2–5 cm section in cranial sense. The detubularization of the selected ileal tract is then performed and the posterior plane is reconfigured as an "L" to widen the posterior plate of the neobladder. The posterior plate is folded anteriorly, roughly 5 cm right from the proximal edge of the posterior closure with the purpose to create two symmetrical segments. The length of the neobladder neck is decided depending on the possibility of the posterior plate, once overturned, to reach the neobladder neck at 12 o'clock position.

The FloRIN configuration is technically feasible with acceptable time efficiency [28]. Even in this case, satisfactory results have been achieved, showing in the first cases studied good reservoir capacity, low pressure with no reflux, and complete voiding [29]. However, further prospective clinical studies with larger patient cohorts are necessary to validate this innovative surgical technique. This configuration seems to be safe also in terms of mid-term postoperative complications and oncological and functional outcomes [30]. Indeed, further studies and external validation should be important to confirm these results.

19.9   Studer Neobladder

The Studer neobladder is an orthotopic diversion configurated through the isolation of a distal ileal segment 54–56 cm long, 25 cm proximal to the ileocecal valve. The isolated ileum segment ileum is rotated of 120° on its mesenteric axis to allow to connect the proximal segment with the right paracolic gutter (Fig. 19.7).

The distal end of the ileal segment, 40–44 cm long, is opened along its antimesenteric border whereas the proximal 15 cm maintain their tubularization, so called "afferent limb". The opened segment is then folded into itself, to assume a U-shape. In the afferent tubular ileal segment, the ureters are then separately anastomosed, in an end-to-side fashion, according to Nesbit technique, at around 12–14 cm upward the pouch. This segment constitutes an anti-reflux system, whose principle is based on the abdominal pressure exerted during micturition by the valsalva maneuver. The two posterior edges of the open handle are sutured one to the other. Then the bottom of the U is folded on its limbs, using one stitch passed in U, giving a spherical reservoir. The lower half of the anterior wall is closed; the closure of the top half can also be started. The area of the neo pouch still open is modulated in order to define the declivous point of the pocket. It is preferably placed close to the meso, outside of the suture lines, more than 2–3 cm from the crossing of the intestinal segments. A small incision is made in this area to configurate the neobladder neck-urethral anastomosis.

Fig. 19.7 The Studer
neobladder

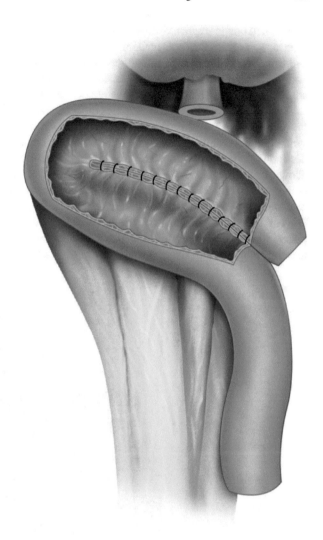

19.10   Hautmann W Neobladder

After bowel examination, a 60-cm segment of the terminal ileum is isolated; the most dependable part of the ileal tract should be long enough to reach the pelvis at the top of the symphysis pubis at skin level, to ensure the configuration of a tension-free neobladder neck-urethral anastomosis. Transillumination of the mesentery is performed to identify the arterial arcades supplying the isolated segment. The bowel is divided 20–25 cm proximal to the Bauhin's valve in the avascular window of Treves and upstream in a suitable avascular plane between the superior mesenteric arcades. Continuity of the bowel is then restored by end-to-end anastomosis. After the isolated bowel segment is thoroughly cleaned and rinsed with saline or an iodine solution, an antimesenteric incision of the ileum is carried out, sparing only the 2–3 cm short chimneys on both sides of the 'W' and the future site of the ileo-urethral anastomosis. Four ileum branches are then arranged in the shape of a 'W' with 2–3 cm-long chimneys on each side of the 'W', thanks to five to six traction sutures (Fig. 19.8). Once the W acquires the desired shape, the ileal plate is configurated by sewing together the cut edges of the antimesenteric borders, using 2-0 synthetic absorbable suture on a straight needle, creating the posterior wall. The declinous point of the pouch is therefore located, using surgeon's index finger, allowing the confection of urethral-neobladder anastomosis. Once it is realized, the ureters are spatulated and stented with 7 or 8 F catheters, before configuring their anastomosis with the W-shaped ileum tract, according to Le Duc technique [31]. To prevent the splints dislocation, an absorbable suture (4-0 polyglycolic acid) is placed through the ureter and bladder wall 1 cm away from the anastomosis; the ureteral stents are the passed through the anterior neobladder wall [32].

Fig. 19.8 The Hautmann W neobladder

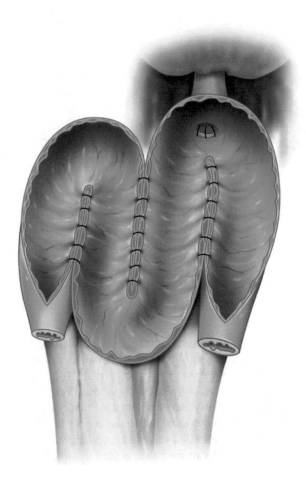

Technical modifications have been made later. The author proposed a urethral anastomosis without an anti-reflux system in the internal arms of the W. In case of a short ureter, it is possible not to open the handle at both ends, performing a direct anastomosis with the spatulated ureter. Moreover, according to some authors, the ileal segment used for reconstructing an Hautmann type neobladder could be shorter (40 cm) than the usual 60–70 cm, to avoid various metabolic dysfunctions and to reduce urinary retention rate.

19.11   Ves.pa Neobladder

Starting from the extensive experience with VIP (Vescica Ileale Padovana) [23], Ves.pa neobladder (from the Latin Vesica Patavina) has been proposed as a novel surgical technique for a totally intracorporeal robot-assisted orthotopic pouch, in order to simplify neobladder configuration with exclusively intracorporeal suturing and reducing operative times, while respecting the essential principles of ideal urinary diversion.

A 45-cm ileum segment is tubularized, leaving a 5 cm distal segment closed. A hole is created 15 cm from the distal edge and a urethral anastomosis is confected over a Foley catheter. A posterior plate is then created with a 2-needle, 3/0, double-running barbed suture: the first part sutures the external margin of the proximal edge to the internal margin at 15 cm; the second part of the running suture goes in the opposite direction, linking the internal margin in a retrograde fashion (from the 15 cm point to the 5 cm point) with the external margin (from 40 to 30 cm). Once the posterior plate is complete, the edges of the anterior and posterior plates are aligned for suturing by cross-folding and the anterior wall of the neobladder is closed with a running 2-0 suture. The right ureter is spatulated and anastomosed to the afferent limb with Bricker's technique or, if dilated, according to Wallace. The left ureter is anastomosed directly on the anterior wall of the neobladder [33].

19.12   Y Pouch

The Y pouch, also known as a Tanta pouch, was first described by the Egyptian group in 1988 [34]. The Y pouch was reconstructed using 40 cm of terminal ileum, which consists of the central detubularized segments arranged in a U shape and two limbs for ureteroileal anastomosis [35].

For creation of the Y pouch neobladder, after completion of the radical cysto-prostatectomy and lymphadenectomy, both ligated ureters are left in their respective side, and there is no need to transpose either ureter below the sigmoid mesocolon [35]. An estimated 40-cm segment of terminal ileum, 25 cm away from the ileocecal valve is identified as the bowel segment is measured by visual estimation, as well as relation to pelvic anatomy. The ileal segment is then brought down to the pelvis, to ensure adequate mesenteric length, allowing for a tension-free urethra-ileal anastomosis. The 40-cm segment is arranged and detubularized on the antimeseneric edge in a U-shaped configuration that is made out of two central segments of 14 cm each and two limbs of 6 cm each [35]. A stitch in placed as landmark in the most distal portion of the U-shaped loop, where the urethroileal anastomosis is performed. The posterior plat is then made with 3/0 V-Loc running suture, starting from the distal part of the U, joining the medial edges of the detubularized segments. After bowel continuity is restored, by performing end-to-end or anatomical side-to-side anastomosis using an Endo-GIA stapler, the anterior plate is closed and the ureters are anastomosed to the dorsal aspect of the two limbs with 4/0 Vicryl sutures, adopting the Nesbit technique.

References

1. Babjuk M, Bohle A, Burger M, et al. EAU guidelines on non-muscle-invasive urothelial carcinoma of the bladder: update 2016. Eur Urol. 2017;71:447–61.
2. Alfred Witjes J, Lebret T, Comperat EM, et al. Updated 2016 EAU guidelines on muscle-invasive and metastatic bladder cancer. Eur Urol. 2017;71:462–75.
3. Schiavina R, Mari A, Antonelli A, et al. A snapshot of nephron-sparing surgery in Italy: a prospective, multicenter report on clinical and perioperative outcomes (the RECORd 1 project). Eur J Surg Oncol. 2015;41:346–52.
4. Ficarra V, Novara G, Ahlering TE, et al. Systematic review and meta-analysis of studies reporting potency rates after robot-assisted radical prostatectomy. Eur Urol. 2012;62:418–30.
5. Mari A, Campi R, Tellini R, et al. Patterns and predictors of recurrence after open radical cystectomy for bladder cancer: a comprehensive review of the literature. World J Urol. 2018;36:157–70.
6. Sanchez de Badajoz E, Gallego Perales JL, Reche Rosado A, Gutierrez de la Cruz JM, Jimenez Garrido A. Radical cystectomy and laparoscopic ileal conduit. Arch Esp Urol. 1993;46:621–4.
7. Wilson TG, Guru K, Rosen RC, et al. Best practices in robot-assisted radical cystectomy and urinary reconstruction: recommendations of the Pasadena Consensus Panel. Eur Urol. 2015;67:363–75.
8. Bochner BH, Dalbagni G, Marzouk KH, Sjoberg DD, Lee J, Donat SM, Coleman JA, Vickers A, Herr HW, Laudone VP. Randomized trial comparing open radical cystectomy and robot-assisted laparoscopic radical cystectomy: oncologic outcomes. Eur Urol. 2018;74:465–71.
9. Parekh DJ, Reis IM, Castle EP, et al. Robot-assisted radical cystectomy versus open radical cystectomy in patients with bladder cancer (RAZOR): an open-label, randomised, phase 3, non-inferiority trial. Lancet (London, England). 2018;391:2525–36
10. Wein AJ. Campbell-Walsh urology, 11th ed (4 Volumes Set). 2015. p. 4168.
11. Kahle W, Platzer W, Fritsch H, Kühnel W, Frotscher M. Color atlas of human anatomy. New York: Thieme; 2015.
12. Otcenasek M, Baca V, Krofta L, Feyereisl J. Endopelvic fascia in women: Shape and relation to parietal pelvic structures. Obstet Gynecol. 2008;111:622–30.
13. Fritsch H, Lienemann A, Brenner E, Ludwikowski B. Clinical anatomy of the pelvic floor. Adv Anat Embryol Cell Biol. 2004; https://doi.org/10.1007/978-3-642-18548-9.
14. Smith RP, Roger P, Netter FH, Frank H, Smith RP, Roger P. Netter's obstetrics and gynecology. Philadelphia, PA: Saunders/Elsevier; 2008.
15. Hodges CV. Surgical anatomy of the urinary bladder and pelvic ureter. Surg Clin North Am. 1964;44:1327–33.

16. Hohenfellner M, Burger R, Schad H, Heimisch W, Riedmiller H, Lampel A, Thuroff JW, Hohenfellner R. Reservoir characteristics of Mainz pouch studied in animal model. Osmolality of filling solution and effect of oxybutynin. Urology. 1993;42:741–6.
17. Montie JE, Pontes JE, Powell IJ. A comparison of the W-stapled ileal reservoir with hand-sewn reservoirs for orthotopic bladder replacement. Urology. 1996;47:476–81.
18. Shen JK, Jamnagerwalla J, Yuh BE, et al. Real-time indocyanine green angiography with the SPY fluorescence imaging platform decreases benign ureteroenteric strictures in urinary diversions performed during radical cystectomy. Ther Adv Urol. 2019;11. https://doi.org/10.1177/1756287219839631
19. Beecken W-D, Wolfram M, Engl T, Bentas W, Probst M, Blaheta R, Oertl A, Jonas D, Binder J. Robotic-assisted laparoscopic radical cystectomy and intra-abdominal formation of an orthotopic ileal neobladder. Eur Urol. 2003;44:337–9.
20. Haber GP, Campbell SC, Colombo JR, Fergany AF, Aron M, Kaouk J, Gill IS. Perioperative outcomes with laparoscopic radical cystectomy: "pure laparoscopic" and "open-assisted laparoscopic" approaches. Urology. 2007;70:910–5.
21. Richards KA, Kader K, Pettus JA, Smith JJ, Hemal AK. Does initial learning curve compromise outcomes for robot-assisted radical cystectomy? A critical evaluation of the first 60 cases while establishing a robotics program. J Endourol. 2011;25:1553–8.
22. Ahmed K, Khan SA, Hayn MH, et al. Analysis of intracorporeal compared with extracorporeal urinary diversion after robot-assisted radical cystectomy: results from the International Robotic Cystectomy Consortium. Eur Urol. 2014;65:340–7.
23. Pagano F, Artibani W, Ligato P, Piazza R, Garbeglio A, Passerini G. Vescica Ileale Padovana: A technique for total bladder replacement. Eur Urol. 1990;17:149–54.
24. Fontana D, Destefanis P, Cugiani A. Evolution and progress in bladder replacement. Riv Urol. 2007;74:49–52.
25. Cacciamani GE, De Marco V, Sebben M, Rizzetto R, Cerruto MA, Porcaro AB, Gill IS, Artibani W. Robot-assisted vescica ileale padovana: a new technique for intracorporeal bladder replacement reproducing open surgical principles. Eur Urol. 2019;76:381–90.
26. Simone G, Papalia R, Misuraca L, Tuderti G, Minisola F, Ferriero M, Vallati G, Guaglianone S, Gallucci M. Robotic intracorporeal padua ileal bladder: surgical technique, perioperative, oncologic and functional outcomes. Eur Urol. 2018;73:934–40.
27. Minervini A, Vanacore D, Vittori G, Milanesi M, Tuccio A, Siena G, Campi R, Mari A, Gavazzi A, Carini M. Florence robotic intracorporeal neobladder (FloRIN): a new reconfiguration strategy developed following the IDEAL guidelines. BJU Int. 2018;121:313–7.
28. Minervini A, Vanacore D, Sforza S, et al. Florence robotic intracorporeal neobladder (FLORIN). What about following the IDEAL guidelines? Eur Urol 2018;Suppl 17:e2151.
29. Tasso G, Vanacore D, Mari A, Bossa R, Sforza S, Tellini R, Di Maida F, Bigazzi B, Carini M, Minervini A. Neo-bladder functional outcomes after radical cystectomy performed in a single center institution, description of results in traditional surgery Vescica Ileale Padovana (VIP) and Florence Robotic Intracorporeal Neo-Bladder (FloRIN). Eur Urol Suppl. 2018;17:227–8.
30. Tasso G, Di Maida F, Tuccio A, et al. Florin robot-assisted intracorporal neobladder reconstruction, oncologic outcomes three years after the introduction of the technique. Eur Urol Suppl. 2019;18:e3241–2.
31. Le Duc A, Camey M, Teillac P. [Antireflux uretero-ileal implantation via a mucosal sulcus]. Ann Urol (Paris). 1987;21:33–4.
32. Hautmann RE. Surgery illustrated—surgical atlas ileal neobladder. BJU Int. 2010;105:1024–35.
33. Dal Moro F, Zattoni F. Ves.Pa.-designing a novel robotic intracorporeal orthotopic ileal neobladder. Urology. 2016;91:99–103.
34. Hassan AA, Elgamal SA, Sabaa MA, Salem KA, Elmateet MS. Evaluation of direct versus non-refluxing technique and functional results in orthotopic Y-ileal neobladder after 12 years of follow up. Int J Urol. 2007;14:300–4.
35. Sim A, Todenhofer T, Mischinger J, et al. Y pouch neobladder—a simplified method of intracorporeal neobladder after robotic cystectomy. J Endourol. 2015;29:387–9.

Chapter 20
Stone Treatment: The Endoscopic Perspective

Eugenio Ventimiglia, Felipe Pauchard, Bhaskar K. Somani, and Olivier Traxer

20.1 Position and Operative Setup

The retrograde endoscopic treatment of urinary stones is usually performed in lithotomy position [1–6]. However, thanks to the introduction of flexible scopes it can be performed in supine position with the surgeon standing beside the patient. This alternative position is recommended especially in patients with cardiovascular comorbidities at the level iliac vessels such as vascular stents [7], in order to avoid serious adverse vascular events.

During standard procedures, the surgeon is usually standing, and it is recommended that he/she is not directly facing the patient, but rather implements a

E. Ventimiglia (✉)
GRC n°20, Groupe de Recherche Clinique sur la Lithiase Urinaire, Hôpital Tenon, Sorbonne Université, Paris, France

Service d'Urologie, Assistance-Publique Hôpitaux de Paris, Hôpital Tenon, Sorbonne Université, Paris, France

Division of Experimental Oncology/Unit of Urology, URI-Urological Research Institute IRCCS Ospedale San Raffaele, Milan, Italy

F. Pauchard
Department of Urology, Hospital Carlos Van Buren, Valparaiso, Chile

B. K. Somani
University Hospital Southampton NHS Trust, Southampton, UK

O. Traxer
GRC n°20, Groupe de Recherche Clinique sur la Lithiase Urinaire, Hôpital Tenon, Sorbonne Université, Paris, France

Service d'Urologie, Assistance-Publique Hôpitaux de Paris, Hôpital Tenon, Sorbonne Université, Paris, France
e-mail: olivier.traxer@aphp.fr

© Springer Nature Switzerland AG 2021
E. Huri, D. Veneziano (eds.), *Anatomy for Urologic Surgeons in the Digital Era*,
https://doi.org/10.1007/978-3-030-59479-4_20

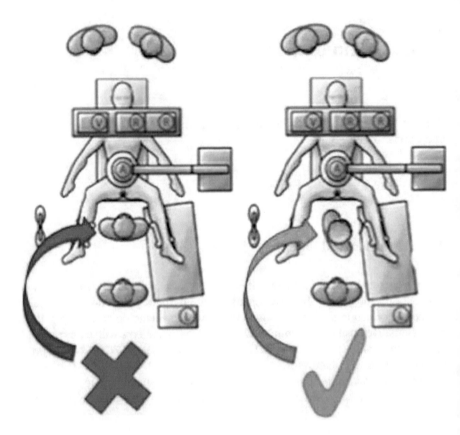

Fig. 20.1 A suggested operative setup for flexible ureteroscopy

90-degree rotation in a lateral position. This allows the operator to block and have a better control of the torque of the ureteroscope [8] (Fig. 20.1).

Although local, spinal anesthesia, and intravenous sedation are feasible options, general anesthesia is suggested because it offers some advantages: it eliminates possible unwanted movements and allows intervention in case of excessive renal movement during respiration [9]. It is possible either to induce temporary apnea [10] or to use low-volume ventilation protocols [11, 12] in order to avoid inconvenient kidney excursion interfering with renal endoscopy. A good collaboration and coordination with the anesthesiology team is fundamental at this regard, and the anesthesiologist should be aware before the beginning of the procedure that he/she might be asked to modify ventilation according to renal excursion.

20.2 Access to the Ureter

If the operative endoscopic access to the bladder performed by Jean Civiale almost 200 years ago gave birth to endourology [13], the endoscopic access to the ureter remains a much recent conquest [14]. It is fundamental to be aware of the urinary tract anatomy during this step, since a proper entry strategy is likely to determine the success of the procedure itself. The access to the ureter starts with the placement of a safety guidewire into the renal cavities. Our preference is to use a 0.035″ stiff hydrophilic guidewire. There are other options but a key point is that the guidewire has to be stiff in order to insert instruments and/or stents over it with ease and safety. It's a longstanding debate whether a safety guidewire should be in place, since it is feasible to perform fURS without it [15]. However, we suggest the use of a safety guidewire as it is still useful and does not add any relevant morbidity [16]. Moreover, the use of a safety guidewire ensures immediate access to the collecting system and facilitates the insertion of a stent in case of intraoperative complications [17, 18]. Before the introduction of the flexible ureteroscope in the ureter, a preliminary, although not mandatory, step is sometimes represented by a semirigid ureteroscopy [19]. When it comes to the access it is possible to choose at least among three different scenarios:

1. The flexible ureteroscope may be passed alongside the safety guidewire, i.e. using a modification of the so called "no-touch technique" [17, 20]
2. The flexible ureteroscope may be passed over a second stiff guidewire (e.g. inserted using a dual-lumen catheter) under fluoroscopic guidance
3. The flexible ureteroscope may be inserted through a ureteral access sheath (UAS)

These different options for endoscope insertion depend on stone burden, upper urinary tract anatomy, and surgeon's preference. The presence of a narrow ureteral orifice, a kinking ureter, or a stricture of the ureter will make it harder to achieve the access using the first option. Consider the use of a UAS in case of multiple passages for stone fragments removal and, most importantly, in order to provide irrigation with better fluid outflow, thereby decreasing the intrarenal pressure [21–24]. Again, it is key to keep into account the anatomy whenever a UAS is put in place, and in the choice of the UAS itself [25, 26] in term of size and functioning mechanism, in order to avoid possible adverse events such as ureteral wall lesions [27]. When using a 12-14 Fr UAS it is possible to observe ureteral wall injuries in up until 46% of patients [27] (Fig. 20.2), although most of them will not result in serious clinical sequelae after 3 years of follow-up [28].

In order to reduce the occurrence of ureteral lesions, we suggest the 10/12 Fr UAS as first-line choice as it is the best compromise in terms of intrarenal pressure and irrigation [21].

The use of this disposable is not mandatory since it has not been demonstrated to improve stone free rate [29] and is definitely not required in every case. Nowadays the use of UAS is reported in around a fifth of all cases in high volume centers [30]. The advantages related to UAS [31] are shown in Table 20.1. Always remember the importance of never forcing the UAS insertion and to position the tip of the UAS below the level of the uretero-pelvic junction (UPJ) in order not to traumatize this area.

Further factors related to anatomy have to be taken into account. Narrow ureteral orifices (UO) can be passed through by backloading the scope over the guidewire and rotating the scope 90°–180° over its main axis at the UO to help with access. Narrow and tortuous distal ureters have to be carefully managed, in order to avoid

UAS & URETERAL LESION

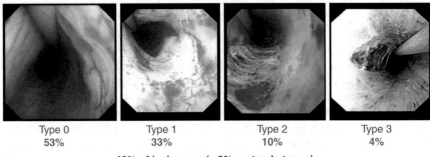

| Type 0 | Type 1 | Type 2 | Type 3 |
| 53% | 33% | 10% | 4% |

46% of lesions and >2% ureteral stenosis

Fig. 20.2 Incidence and classification of ureteral lesions following UAS placement. Type 0: No lesion found or only mucosal petechiae, Type 1: Ureteral mucosal erosion without smooth muscle injury, Type 2: Ureteral wall injury, including mucosa and smooth muscle, with adventitial preservation (periureteral fat not seen), Type 3: Ureteral wall injury, including mucosa and smooth muscle, with adventitial perforation (periureteral fat seen), Type 4: Ureteral avulsion. Adapted from Traxer et al. J Urol 2013

Table 20.1 Advantages related to the use of ureteral access sheaths

Advantage	Comment
Easier access for scopes and instruments	Theoretically some time is spared, but data is not conclusive
Better visualization	Irrigation can be increased with a safer control of renal pressure
Control of intrapelvic temperature	Higher irrigation flow can avoid temperature rise. This is a concern when high power lasers are used
Lower intrapelvic pressure	Outflow irrigation is increased if correct UAS is used in consideration of the scope

perforations at guidewire insertion. Anatomically difficult cases, such as following Cohen cross-trigonal ureteral reimplantation, can be managed with a 7 Fr angled orifice catheter used to direct a hydrophilic angled tip stiff guide-wire in the proper ureteral direction [32]. Once the scope is in the ureter, it can be advanced to the renal cavities. It is a key message never to force the access to the ureter, either with the scope or the UAS. In such challenging cases, it is imperative to stent and come back after a couple of weeks. Pre-stenting routinely may entail some advantages in terms of accessibility to the upper urinary tract and shorter operative time [33], although these benefits need to be weighed against the risk of overtreatment in patients not necessarily requiring presenting and the increased risk of post-operative sepsis [34].

20.3 Renal Exploration

An adequate knowledge of the collecting system anatomy is required in order to properly orientate during fURS. An anatomical study by the Brazilian endourologist Sampaio based on 140 polyester endocasts of the collecting system [35] originally identified four different types according to the drainage of the polar regions and of the mid (hilar) zone. The types described in the initial report as AI and AII (62% of the specimens) presented two major calyceal groups as a primary division of the renal pelvis and mid-zone drainage dependent on these two major groups. The types known as BI and BII (38% of the specimens) presented mid-zone drainage independent of the superior and inferior calyceal groups. This classification was further refined and developed by the same study group [36].

Once in the urinary tract, the manipulation of the scope is performed with the dominant hand movements of pronation and supination in order to obtain rotation (Fig. 20.3). Supination in a right-handed surgeon rotates the scope tip to the right of the patient, whereas pronation is the opposite. Therefore, pronation is the preferred movement in the left kidney, whereas supination allows for proper manipulation in the right one. The scope handle has a trigger for upper/lower deflection which is controlled with the thumb of the dominant hand as well. Two different systems are available for deflection: the European and the American type [37]. In the European system, the upwards deflection will deflect the tip of the scope downwards, and vice versa for the downwards deflection. In the American system, the direction of the trigger and tip of the scope are concordant. The non-dominant hand holds with the

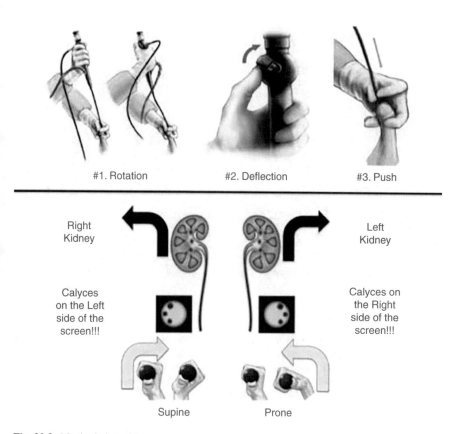

#1. Rotation   #2. Deflection   #3. Push

Right
Kidney

Left
Kidney

Calyces
on the Left
side of the
screen!!!

Calyces on
the Right
side of the
screen!!!

Supine   Prone

Fig. 20.3 Manipulation of the scope

thumb and the index finger the distal part of the ureteroscope near the patient urethral orifice or UAS. This hand helps with micro rotations and also pushing and
pulling the scope (Fig. 20.3).

The features of the ureteroscope should be further taken into account when planning an operative procedure. There are clinically relevant differences in terms of
quality of vision [38], deflectability, and scopes diameter [39] when analyzing available scopes [37]. More specifically, some peculiar situations are indicative for the
selection the most suitable ureteroscope. Fiberoptic ureteroscopes have shown better access to sharp angled calyces compared to digital ones, mainly because the tips
of the digital scope embed the digital chip, lowering its end tip deflection capabilities [39]. Fiberoptic scopes are also smaller in diameter [40], allowing for easier
access to thinner ureters. The working channel position is another major factor that
must be considered according to which kidney will be treated and where the stone
is located. It was recently shown in an in-vitro study that ureteroscopes with a 3
o'clock working channel position perform better for stones located in right posterior
calyces and left anterior cavities. Conversely, 9 o'clock working channel scopes are
better for stones located in the left posterior and right anterior calyces [41]
(Fig. 20.4).

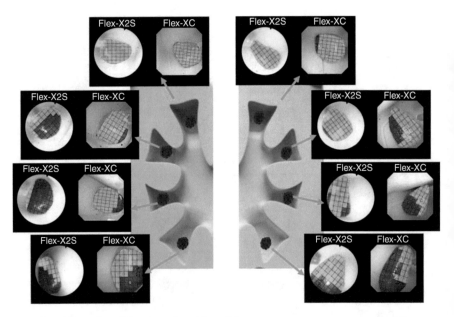

Fig. 20.4 Effect of working channel position of the ureteroscope on stone targeting. The green
surface of the stone represents the proportion targetable by the laser fiber. In the right posterior
renal cavities, the 3 o'clock position allows for better stone targeting, whereas in the left posterior
cavities the 9 o'clock position performs better. Flex-XC: ureteroscope with a 3 o'clock working
channel position. Flex-X2s: ureteroscope with a 9 o'clock working channel position

20.4 Laser Lithotripsy

After the stone is identified, the laser fiber is prepared, and laser parameters have to be properly set. Brand new laser fiber come with a stripped tip. Also, companies sell the stripping equipment and ceramic scissor to cut the fiber. However, this necessity has been challenged and demonstrated that coated laser fibers provide better lithotripsy performance and metal common scissors are as good as ceramic ones to cleave coated fibers [42]. Eyeglass protection can be potentially avoided if Ho:YAG laser tip of the fiber is more than 5 cm away from the eyes [43, 44]. It is now time for setting laser parameters. The surgeon has the possibility to choose between fragmentation or dusting settings (Table 20.2). However, different considerations need to be made according to stone location. In the ureter, the most important concept during laser lithotripsy is to avoid damaging the ureteral wall due to laser energy itself. Post-ureteroscopy ureteral stenosis is reported to be low. In limited series laser lithotripsy has shown higher rates of ureteral stenosis compared to pneumatic energy [45]. For this reason, we advocate to use low frequency in the ureter (max 5–6 Hz) irrespective of fragmentation or dusting technique. Another trick to avoid ureter laser injury is starting the lithotripsy in the center of the stone, avoiding the space between the stone and the mucosa.

It is recommended that at least one fragment of the stone should be removed and sent for stone analysis. Placement of a double j ureteral stent after the surgery is not mandatory. It depends on surgeon preferences, ureteral wall damage, risk of sepsis, residual fragments, need of second look and patient preference. If stent is placed, need for post-operative pain medication is supposed to be reduced. In uncomplicated procedures, there is no difference in terms of urinary tract infection compared to no stent, ureteral stricture may slightly be reduced, quality of life is lower and readmission rate slightly higher [46].

20.5 Anatomical and Functional Considerations for Treating Stones in the Renal Cavities

Irrigation in the renal cavity must be judicious trying not to overcome 40 cmH$_2$O, in order to avoid venous backflow and risk of post-operative sepsis [6]. Several irrigation systems are available in order to improve quality of vision during fURS, either automatic or manual such as handheld syringe or pumps [47]. However, few

Table 20.2 Laser settings during lithotripsy

	Fragmentation	Dusting
Pulse length	Short	Long
Energy (Joules)	High (0.8–1.2 J)	Low (<0.8 J)
Frequency (Hertz)	Low (≤5–6 Hz)	High (≥8–10 Hz)[a]

[a]Frequency during dusting should be as high as the surgeon can maintain a good vision and constant safe control laser activation, avoiding damage to the urothelium

comparative studies assessed both the efficacy and safety profile of these tools to date, leaving therefore little room for an evidence-based assessment of the best available irrigation system [48]. It is important to remark that many of the different commercially available systems increase intrarenal pressure up to risky values [49]. Our personal feeling is that handheld systems are preferred due to the possibility of prompt and direct control, provided that a well-trained assistant is in charge for the irrigation.

Lower pole stones represent a challenging scenario during flexible ureteroscopy [50], and both its clinical and economic efficiency are often questioned in this setting [51]. Moreover, treating lower pole stones can compromise the life span of the scope [52]. A possible recommendation when dealing with this kind of situations would be to relocate the stone in an upper calyx with the use of basket [53]. In case this is not possible, then the stone has to treated directly in the lower pole. It is usually not recommended to advance the laser fiber whenever the tip of the scope is deflected, in order to avoid possible working channel damage (e.g. perforation). However, there are at least three available options. First, to deflect the tip of the scope towards the lower pole with the laser fiber already in place; however, this is not always possible since the laser fiber per se will cause a loss of deflection [54]. Second, the use of ball-tip laser fibers [55], thus limiting the damage to the working channel when it is advanced inside a deflected scope. As a drawback, ball tip fibers will lose their safety profile after laser activation, limiting the possibility of multiple accesses through a deflected scope working channel. Third, it is possible to cut with regular scissors the laser fiber tip preserving the external coating and the advancing it through the working channel of the deflected scope. This practice was shown to be safe for the scope and its working channel [56]. Again, after a few minutes of laser activity, if the fiber has to be passed once more through the deflected scope, it has to be refreshed and cut again [56].

In contrast to the ureter, it is possible to use high and very-high frequencies when treating stones in the renal cavities, always paying close attention not to hit the mucosa with laser pulses. Whenever dusting in the renal cavities, the stone should be treated starting from the periphery towards the center, this way fragments detachment from the stone is avoided, ensuring better dusting and fewer residual fragments. The main factor for a good dusting technique is to keep proper control of the laser fiber, maintaining constant gentle of the fiber displacement over the stone as if painting the stone surface with the laser fiber. When high power laser are used, temperature rise in the renal cavity may be a concern, because it can produce parenchymal damage [57]. The common measures to avoid this rise in temperature are to increase irrigation and to pause during laser, or to switch to low power settings [58]. However, increasing the irrigation can also increase the intrarenal pressure with the subsequent rise in risk of sepsis. Pausing during lasering will translate into less efficient surgery. Lastly, high-power and high-frequency settings decreases considerably the quality of vision. This is why the role of high-power Ho:YAG lasers during laser lithotripsy is still controversial, despite interesting laboratory data [59–61]. The linear relationship between increasing power and decreasing lasering time observed during laboratory controlled lithotripsy is challenged in real life experience, and lasering with ordinary low power system might achieve similar results [62].

Renal movements due to ventilation can make the lithotripsy challenging. The use of apnea to facilitate the procedure has been shown to be a good option in these cases. Before initiation the apnea, the patient must be ventilated with 100% concentration of oxygen: this allows to maintain apnea for approximately five minutes [10].

After completion of lithotripsy, there is no available technology nowadays capable of measuring endoscopically remaining stone fragments size. The comparison between the fragment size and the laser fiber diameter is an easy way to infer the size. In particular, a commercially available 200 μm laser fiber has a real diameter of approximately 400 μm [63, 64] due to its external coating. Therefore, a fragment whose main axis is twice as wide as the laser fiber section, could be roughly considered as a 1 mm fragment. It is important to estimate the size of remaining fragment in order to achieve as much as possible the stone-free status. To date, there is no consensus definition for what real dust is in terms of size [65]. On the other hand, the extraction of very small fragments remains unpractical with the available baskets. If small fragments (less 2–3 mm) want to be extracted, the glue-clot technique can be used. This consist of injection of 10 mL of autologous venous blood into the renal cavity, then wait for 5–10 min for the clot to form and extract it with a basket [66].

A final anatomical challenging situation is represented by stones in calyceal diverticula. These stones can be reached and treated using the "Blue Spritz" technique, which consist of an injection of contrast medium mixed with methylene blue or indigo carmine. Fluoroscopy aids to identify the calyceal diverticulum. Then, with the ureteroscope irrigating normal saline the renal cavity, the blue dye is washed, whereas there is some persistence of contrast inside the diverticulum, as shown during fluoroscopy. Exploration of the cavities and identification of leakage of the blue dye from the diverticulum to the cavities reveals the neck that should be opened with laser [67] in order to access the diverticular stones.

References

1. Seklehner S, Laudano MA, Del Pizzo J, Chughtai B, Lee RK. Renal calculi: trends in the utilization of shockwave lithotripsy and ureteroscopy. Can J Urol. 2015;22:7627–34.
2. Dauw CA, Simeon L, Alruwaily AF. Contemporary practice patterns of flexible ureteroscopy for treating renal stones. J Endourol. 2015;29:1221–30. https://doi.org/10.1089/end.2015.0260.
3. Geraghty RM, Jones P, Herrmann TRW, Aboumarzouk O, Somani BK. Ureteroscopy is more cost effective than shock wave lithotripsy for stone treatment: systematic review and meta-analysis. World J Urol. 2018;36:1783–93. https://doi.org/10.1007/s00345-018-2320-9.
4. De Coninck V, Keller EX, Somani B, Giusti G, Proietti S, Rodriguez-Socarras M, et al. Complications of ureteroscopy: a complete overview. World J Urol. 2020;38(9):2147–66. https://doi.org/10.1007/s00345-019-03012-1.
5. Cindolo L, Castellan P, Scoffone CM, Cracco CM, Celia A, Paccaduscio A, et al. Mortality and flexible ureteroscopy: analysis of six cases. World J Urol. 2016;34:305–10. https://doi.org/10.1007/s00345-015-1642-0.

6. Doizi S, Traxer O. Flexible ureteroscopy: technique, tips and tricks. Urolithiasis. 2018;46:47–58. https://doi.org/10.1007/s00240-017-1030-x.

7. Emiliani E, Talso M, Beltran-Suarez E, Doizi S, Traxer O. Reperfusion and compartment syndrome after flexible ureteroscopy in a patient with an iliac vascular graft. J Endourol Case Rep. 2016;2:224–6. https://doi.org/10.1089/cren.2016.0108.

8. Somani BK, Ploumidis A, Pappas A, Doizi S, Babawale O, Dragos L, et al. Pictorial review of tips and tricks for ureteroscopy and stone treatment: an essential guide for urologists from PETRA research consortium. Transl Androl Urol 2019;8:S371–80. https://doi.org/10.21037/tau.2019.06.04.

9. Cybulski PA, Joo H, Honey RJD. Ureteroscopy: anesthetic considerations. Urol Clin North Am. 2004;31:43–7, viii. https://doi.org/10.1016/S0094-0143(03)00087-9.

10. Emiliani E, Talso M, Baghdadi M, Ghanem S, Golmard J, Pinheiro H, et al. The use of apnea during ureteroscopy. Urology. 2016;97:266–8. https://doi.org/10.1016/j.urology.2016.06.016.

11. Kourmpetis V, Dekalo S, Levy N, Nir T, Bar-Yosef Y, Beri A, et al. Toward respiratory-gated retrograde intrarenal surgery: a prospective controlled randomized study. J Endourol. 2018;32:812–7. https://doi.org/10.1089/end.2018.0231.

12. Gadzhiev N, Oibolatov U, Kolotilov L, Parvanyan S, Akopyan G, Petrov S, et al. Reducing kidney motion: optimizing anesthesia and combining respiratory support for retrograde intrarenal surgery: a pilot study. BMC Urol. 2019;19:61. https://doi.org/10.1186/s12894-019-0491-3.

13. Herr HW. Civiale, stones and statistics: the dawn of evidence-based medicine. BJU Int. 2009;104:300–2. https://doi.org/10.1111/j.1464-410X.2009.08529.x.

14. Somani BK, Aboumarzouk O, Srivastava A, Traxer O. Flexible ureterorenoscopy: Tips and tricks. Urol Ann. 2013;5:1–6. https://doi.org/10.4103/0974-7796.106869.

15. Rizkala ER, Monga M. Controversies in ureteroscopy: Wire, basket, and sheath. Indian J Urol. 2013;29:244–8. https://doi.org/10.4103/0970-1591.117287.

16. Doizi S, Herrmann T, Traxer O. Death of the safety guidewire. J Endourol. 2017;31:619–20. https://doi.org/10.1089/end.2016.0756.

17. Johnson GB, Portela D, Grasso M. Advanced ureteroscopy: wireless and sheathless. J Endourol. 2006;20:552–5. https://doi.org/10.1089/end.2006.20.552.

18. Patel SR, McLaren ID, Nakada SY. The ureteroscope as a safety wire for ureteronephroscopy. J Endourol. 2012;26:351–4. https://doi.org/10.1089/end.2011.0406.

19. Giusti G, Proietti S, Villa L, Cloutier J, Rosso M, Gadda GM, et al. Current standard technique for modern flexible ureteroscopy: tips and tricks. Eur Urol. 2016;70:188–94. https://doi.org/10.1016/j.eururo.2016.03.035.

20. Johnson GB, Grasso M. Ureteroscopic management of upper tract urothelial malignancies. Rev Urol. 2000;2:116–28. https://doi.org/10.1097/01.mou.0000160622.13366.a1.

21. Rehman J, Monga M, Landman J, Lee DI, Felfela T, Conradie MC, et al. Characterization of intrapelvic pressure during ureteropyeloscopy with ureteral access sheaths. Urology. 2003;61:713–8. https://doi.org/10.1016/s0090-4295(02)02440-8.

22. Auge BK, Pietrow PK, Lallas CD, Raj GV, Santa-Cruz RW, Preminger GM. Ureteral access sheath provides protection against elevated renal pressures during routine flexible ureteroscopic stone manipulation. J Endourol. 2004;18:33–6. https://doi.org/10.1089/089277904322836631.

23. Kaplan AG, Lipkin ME, Scales CDJ, Preminger GM. Use of ureteral access sheaths in ureteroscopy. Nat Rev Urol. 2016;13:135–40. https://doi.org/10.1038/nrurol.2015.271.

24. Newman RC, Hunter PT, Hawkins IF, Finlayson B. The ureteral access system: a review of the immediate results in 43 cases. J Urol. 1987;137:380–3. https://doi.org/10.1016/s0022-5347(17)44039-0.

25. Al-Qahtani SM, Letendre J, Thomas A, Natalin R, Saussez T, Traxer O. Which ureteral access sheath is compatible with your flexible ureteroscope? J Endourol. 2014;28:286–90. https://doi.org/10.1089/end.2013.0375.

26. Sener TE, Cloutier J, Villa L, Marson F, Butticè S, Doizi S, et al. Can we provide low intrarenal pressures with good irrigation flow by decreasing the size of ureteral access sheaths? J Endourol. 2016;30:49–55. https://doi.org/10.1089/end.2015.0387.

27. Traxer O, Thomas A. Prospective evaluation and classification of ureteral wall injuries result-ing from insertion of a ureteral access sheath during retrograde intrarenal surgery. J Urol. 2013;189:580–4. https://doi.org/10.1016/j.juro.2012.08.197.
28. Stern KL, Loftus CJ, Doizi S, Traxer O, Monga M. A prospective study analyzing the associa-tion between high-grade ureteral access sheath injuries and the formation of ureteral strictures. Urology. 2019;128:38–41. https://doi.org/10.1016/j.urology.2019.02.032.
29. Traxer O, Wendt-Nordahl G, Sodha H, Rassweiler J, Meretyk S, Tefekli A, et al. Differences in renal stone treatment and outcomes for patients treated either with or without the sup-port of a ureteral access sheath: The Clinical Research Office of the Endourological Society Ureteroscopy Global Study. World J Urol. 2015;33:2137–44. https://doi.org/10.1007/s00345-015-1582-8.
30. Tracey J, Gagin G, Morhardt D, Hollingsworth J, Ghani KR. Ureteroscopic high-frequency dusting utilizing a 120-W holmium laser. J Endourol. 2018;32:290–5. https://doi.org/10.1089/end.2017.0220.
31. De Coninck V, Keller EX, Rodriguez-Monsalve M, Audouin M, Doizi S, Traxer O. Systematic review of ureteral access sheaths: facts and myths. BJU Int. 2018;122:959–69. https://doi.org/10.1111/bju.14389.
32. Emiliani E, Talso M, Audouin M, Traxer O. Modern flexible ureteroscopy in Cohen cross-trigonal ureteral reimplantations. J Pediatr Urol. 2017;13:329–31. https://doi.org/10.1016/j.jpurol.2017.03.009.
33. Chu L, Sternberg KM, Averch TD. Preoperative stenting decreases operative time and reopera-tive rates of ureteroscopy. J Endourol. 2011;25:751–4. https://doi.org/10.1089/end.2010.0400.
34. Nevo A, Mano R, Baniel J, Lifshitz DA. Ureteric stent dwelling time: a risk factor for post-ureteroscopy sepsis. BJU Int. 2017;120:117–22. https://doi.org/10.1111/bju.13796.
35. José F, Sampaio B, Mandarim-de-lacerda CA. Anatomic classification of the kidney collecting system for endourologic procedures. J Endourol. 1988;2:247–51.
36. Sampaio FJ. Renal anatomy. Endourologic considerations. Urol Clin North Am. 2000;27:585–607, vii. https://doi.org/10.1016/s0094-0143(05)70109-9.
37. Dragos LB, Somani BK, Keller EX, De Coninck VMJ, Herrero MR-M, Kamphuis GM, et al. Characteristics of current digital single-use flexible ureteroscopes versus their reusable coun-terparts: an in-vitro comparative analysis. Transl Androl Urol 2019;8:S359–70. https://doi.org/10.21037/tau.2019.09.17.
38. Talso M, Proietti S, Emiliani E, Gallioli A, Dragos L, Orosa A, et al. Comparison of flexible ureterorenoscope quality of vision: an in vitro study. J Endourol. 2018;32:523–8. https://doi.org/10.1089/end.2017.0838.
39. Dragos LB, Somani BK, Sener ET, Buttice S, Proietti S, Ploumidis A, et al. Which flexible ureteroscopes (digital vs. fiber-optic) can easily reach the difficult lower pole calices and have better end-tip deflection: in vitro study on K-box. A PETRA evaluation. J Endourol. 2017;31:630–7. https://doi.org/10.1089/end.2017.0109.
40. Gridley CM, Knudsen BE. Digital ureteroscopes: technology update. Res Rep Urol. 2017;9:19–25. https://doi.org/10.2147/RRU.S104229.
41. Villa L, Ventimiglia E, Proietti S, Giusti G, Briganti A, Salonia A, et al. Does working channel position influence the effectiveness of flexible ureteroscopy? Results from an in vitro study. BJU Int. 2019. https://doi.org/10.1111/bju.14923.
42. Kronenberg P, Traxer O. Are we all doing it wrong? Influence of stripping and cleaving meth-ods of laser fibers on laser lithotripsy performance. J Urol. 2015;193:1030–5. https://doi.org/10.1016/j.juro.2014.07.110.
43. Villa L, Cloutier J, Comperat E, Kronemberg P, Charlotte F, Berthe L, et al. Do we really need to wear proper eye protection when using holmium:YAG laser during endourologic proce-dures? Results from an ex vivo animal model on pig eyes. J Endourol. 2016;30:332–7. https://doi.org/10.1089/end.2015.0232.
44. Doizi S, Audouin M, Villa L, Rodriguez-Monsalve Herrero M, De Coninck V, Keller EX, et al. The eye of the endourologist: what are the risks? A review of the literature. World J Urol. 2019;37:2639–47. https://doi.org/10.1007/s00345-019-02667-0.

45. Chen S, Zhou L, Wei T, Luo D, Jin T, Li H, et al. Comparison of holmium: YAG laser and pneumatic lithotripsy in the treatment of ureteral stones: an update meta-analysis. Urol Int. 2017;98:125–33. https://doi.org/10.1159/000448692.

46. Ordonez M, Hwang EC, Borofsky M, Bakker CJ, Gandhi S, Dahm P. Ureteral stent versus no ureteral stent for ureteroscopy in the management of renal and ureteral calculi. Cochrane Database Syst Rev. 2019. https://doi.org/10.1002/14651858.CD012703.pub2.

47. Doersch KM, Hart KD, Elmekresh A, Milburn PA, Machen GL, El Tayeb MM. Comparison of utilization of pressurized automated versus manual hand irrigation during ureteroscopy in the absence of ureteral access sheath. Proc (Bayl Univ Med Cent). 2018;31:432–5. https://doi.org/10.1080/08998280.2018.1482518.

48. Lama DJ, Owyong M, Parkhomenko E, Patel RM, Landman J, Clayman RV. Fluid dynamic analysis of hand-pump infuser and UROMAT endoscopic automatic system for irrigation through a flexible ureteroscope. J Endourol. 2018;32:431–6. https://doi.org/10.1089/end.2017.0811.

49. Proietti S, Dragos L, Somani BK, Buttice S, Talso M, Emiliani E, et al. In vitro comparison of maximum pressure developed by irrigation systems in a kidney model. J Endourol. 2017. https://doi.org/10.1089/end.2017.0005.

50. Dauw CA, Simeon L, Alruwaily AF, Sanguedolce F, Hollingsworth JM, Roberts WW, et al. Contemporary practice patterns of flexible ureteroscopy for treating renal stones: results of a worldwide survey. J Endourol. 2015;29:1221–30. https://doi.org/10.1089/end.2015.0260.

51. Koo V, Young M, Thompson T, Duggan B. Cost-effectiveness and efficiency of shockwave lithotripsy vs flexible ureteroscopic holmium:yttrium-aluminium-garnet laser lithotripsy in the treatment of lower pole renal calculi. BJU Int. 2011;108:1913–6. https://doi.org/10.1111/j.1464-410X.2011.10172.x.

52. Salvadó JA, Cabello JM, Moreno S, Cabello R, Olivares R, Velasco A. Endoscopic treatment of lower pole stones: is a disposable ureteroscope preferable? Results of a prospective case-control study. Cent Eur J Urol. 2019;72:280–4. https://doi.org/10.5173/ceju.2019.1962.

53. Moore SL, Bres-Niewada E, Cook P, Wells H, Somani BK. Optimal management of lower pole stones: the direction of future travel. Cent Eur J Urol. 2016;69:274–9. https://doi.org/10.5173/ceju.2016.819.

54. Pasqui F, Dubosq F, Tchala K, Tligui M, Gattegno B, Thibault P, et al. Impact on active scope deflection and irrigation flow of all endoscopic working tools during flexible ureteroscopy. Eur Urol. 2004;45:58–64. https://doi.org/10.1016/j.eururo.2003.08.013.

55. Carlos EC, Li J, Young BJ, Radvak D, Wollin DA, Winship BB, et al. Let's get to the point: comparing insertion characteristics and scope damage of flat-tip and ball-tip holmium laser fibers. J Endourol. 2019;33:22–6. https://doi.org/10.1089/end.2018.0229.

56. Baghdadi M, Emiliani E, Talso M, Servian P, Barreiro A, Orosa A, et al. Comparison of laser fiber passage in ureteroscopic maximum deflection and their influence on deflection and irrigation: Do we really need the ball tip concept? World J Urol. 2017;35:313–8. https://doi.org/10.1007/s00345-016-1873-8.

57. Aldoukhi AH, Hall TL, Ghani KR, Maxwell AD, MacConaghy B, Roberts WW. Caliceal fluid temperature during high-power holmium laser lithotripsy in an in vivo porcine model. J Endourol. 2018;32:724–9. https://doi.org/10.1089/end.2018.0395.

58. Winship B, Wollin DA, Carlos EC, Peters C, Li J, Terry R, et al. The rise and fall of high temperatures during ureteroscopic holmium laser lithotripsy. J Endourol. 2019. https://doi.org/10.1089/end.2019.0084.

59. Aldoukhi AH, Roberts WW, Hall TL, Teichman JMH, Ghani KR. Understanding the popcorn effect during holmium laser lithotripsy for dusting. Urology. 2018;122:52–7. https://doi.org/10.1016/j.urology.2018.08.031.

60. Pauchard F, Traxer O. RE: Winship et al., The rise and fall of high temperatures during ureteroscopic holmium laser lithotripsy (From: Winship B, Wollin D, Carlos E, et al. J Endourol 2019;33:794–799; DOI: 10.1089/end.2019.0084). J Endourol. 2019;33:801. https://doi.org/10.1089/end.2019.0363.

61. Ventimiglia E, Traxer O. Is very high power/frequency really necessary during laser lithotripsy? RE: understanding the popcorn effect during holmium laser lithotripsy for dusting (Aldoukhi et al, Urology. 2018 Dec;122:52–57). Urology. https://doi.org/10.1016/j.urology.2019.01.032.
62. Pauchard F, Ventimiglia E, Traxer O. Letter to the Editor RE: Mekayten et al., Will stone density stop being a key factor in endourology? The impact of stone density on laser time using lumenis laser p120w and standard 20w laser: a comparative study (from: Mekayten M, Lorber A, Katafigiotis, et al. J Endourol 2019;33:585–589; DOI: 10.1089/end.2019.0181). J Endourol. 2019. https://doi.org/10.1089/end.2019.0438.
63. Knudsen BE. Laser fibers for holmium:YAG lithotripsy: what is important and what is new. Urol Clin North Am. 2019;46:185–91. https://doi.org/10.1016/j.ucl.2018.12.004.
64. Kronenberg P, Traxer O. The truth about laser fiber diameters. Urology. 2014;84:1301–7. https://doi.org/10.1016/j.urology.2014.08.017.
65. Doizi S, Keller EX, de Coninck V, Traxer O. Dusting technique for lithotripsy: what does it mean? Nat Rev Urol. 2018;1–2. https://doi.org/10.1038/s41585-018-0042-9.
66. Cloutier J, Cordeiro ER, Kamphuis GM, Villa L, Letendre J, de la Rosette JJ, et al. The glue-clot technique: a new technique description for small calyceal stone fragments removal. Urolithiasis. 2014;42:441–4. https://doi.org/10.1007/s00240-014-0679-7.
67. Sejiny M, Al-Qahtani S, Elhaous A, Molimard B, Traxer O. Efficacy of flexible ureterorenoscopy with holmium laser in the management of stone-bearing caliceal diverticula. J Endourol. 2010;24:961–7. https://doi.org/10.1089/end.2009.0437.

Chapter 21
Stone Treatment: The Percutaneous Perspective

Panagiotis Kallidonis, Athanasios Vagionis, Evangelos Liatsikos, Cesare Marco Scoffone, and Cecilia Maria Cracco

21.1 The Case for Percutaneous Nephrolithotomy in Urolithiasis: Indications and Contraindications

According to EAU (European Association of Urology) guidelines percutaneous nephrolithotomy (PCNL) represents the gold standard for the treatment of staghorn renal calculi sized 20 mm or more. PCNL is also an option for the treatment of 15–20 mm lower pole stones when factors are unfavourable for SWL (Shock Wave Lithotripsy) [1], stone patients with renal fusion abnormalities such as horseshoe kidneys [2], symptomatic calculi in calyceal diverticula [3], or large impacted urolithiasis of the proximal ureter [4].

Absolute contraindications of PCNL include untreated urinary tract infection, potential malignant kidney tumor, tumor in the presumptive access tract area and pregnancy [1]. An ongoing anticoagulant therapy and problems in performing general anaesthesia are relative contraindications [5, 6].

21.2 Different Approaches to PCNL

PCNL is a complex surgery made up by several steps, each one susceptible to variations implying possible advantages and disadvantages. Technical modifications in the position of the patient, intraoperative imaging approaches, tract size, type of dilators and intracorporeallithotripsy devices have been reported [7].

P. Kallidonis · A. Vagionis · E. Liatsikos (✉)
Department of Urology, University of Patras, Patras, Greece

C. M. Scoffone · C. M. Cracco
Department of Urology, Cottolengo Hospital, Torino, Italy

© Springer Nature Switzerland AG 2021   305
E. Huri, D. Veneziano (eds.), *Anatomy for Urologic Surgeons in the Digital Era*,
https://doi.org/10.1007/978-3-030-59479-4_21

Several different positions for PCNL have been described [8, 9]. Among them the most common are the prone and the supine positions with their modifications, equivalent in terms of efficacy and safety but offering different advantages. Prone position is preferred in upper pole, multiple accesses and bilateral procedures, offering for sure more puncturing space and shorter distance between skin and kidney [5]. The supine access has undeniable anaesthesiological advantages, offering the possibility of simultaneous RIRS (Retrograde IntraRenal Surgery) [9–11].

Fluoroscopy, ultrasonography, or combination of ultrasound and fluoroscopy are currently used to gain access to the pelvicalyceal system and guide the PCNL procedure [12]. Fluoroscopy offers the advantages of a clear imaging of the collecting system anatomy depicted by retrograde contrast and a fast puncture; ultrasonography offers the advantages of X-ray-free puncture, the possibility to see surrounding organs and a significantly lower cost of the imaging device.

The standard size PCNL has been 30F for several years. Endoscopes and accessories with reduced diameter (midi- and mini-PCNL, microPerc, UMP) have been introduced along the years in an attempt to decrease the morbidity related to percutaneous tract creation [13].

Tract dilation can be performed with the use of polymeric semirigid Amplatz dilators, metal Alken dilators, or balloon dilators. Alken and Amplatz dilators are more economic, multiple and sequential, balloon ones perform a one-step dilation with less bleeding risk and are less efficient in case of previous surgery with perirenal and fascial scarring [14, 15].

The most common lithotripsy devices are ultrasonic, pneumatic, combined ultrasonic and pneumatic, and Holmium: YAG laser [16, 17]. Pneumatic and ultrasonic lithotripters offer the advantage of shorter operative times in staghorn stones, lower intrarenal temperatures and high efficacy. Lasers can be inserted through the working channel of miniaturized endoscopes.

21.3   Anatomy: Relationships with Neighboring Organs

Familiarity with basic renal anatomy is a necessity for achieving a successful percutaneous renal access and minimizing bleeding complications [18]. The kidneys have a definite inclination (with the upper poles nearer and more posterior than the lower poles, and the lateral margins more posterior than the medial margins) and lie in the intermediate perirenal space of the retroperitoneal cavity, which is created by the two layers of Gerota's fascia. The posterior layer is stronger and better defined than the anterior one, which is softer and usually adherent to the peritoneum. Posteriorly to kidneys, psoas and quadratus lumborum muscles can be found. Because of the shape of the psoas muscle, the kidney inclines dorsally following the muscles course. The left kidney borders with the 11th and the 12th rib, being its location usually 2–3 cm higher than the right kidney. The latter is located more caudally due to the presence of the liver. Pleuras extend inferiorly till the 12th rib. There is a possibility of traversing the pleura without symptoms when puncturing. It should be noted though that it is not recommended puncturing over the 11th rib because of the danger of injuring the ipsilateral lung. The diaphragm is attached on the 11th and the 12th ribs and attaches also over the posterior abdominal muscles. Therefore, traversing the diaphragm when puncturing to perform an access to the kidney is possible. An injury to the intercostal artery can lead to the potential complication of hemothorax, and can be avoided by staying in the middle of the intercostal space [19], or immediately above the upper border of the lower rib [20]. The risk for hydrothorax or hemothorax increases in the case of a right-sided procedure and non-obese patients [21]. The location of the posterior costophrenic sulcus should be identified both in inspiration and expiration by fluoroscopy for obtaining safe access via the tenth or 11th intercostal space, especially on the left side [22]. A short and viable trajectory to the posterior superior pole calyx that is not related to intrusion of the pleural space or injury of the lung can be achieved when accessing in expiration or mid-inspiration. The diaphragm can be displaced to a cephalad direction by intraperitoneal infusion of saline or pneumo-peritoneum. The retrorenal position of the left colon (10% of patients) or a large spleen may not allow an access either through the tenth or 11th intercostal space [22].

21.4   Anatomy: Vascularization of the Kidney

Knowing the basic vascular anatomy is also essential for accessing the kidney safely. The main renal artery divides into an anterior and a posterior branch, giving rise to the interlobar arteries, which course parallel to the calyceal infundibula. Most of the renal parenchymais densely vascularized by those branches apart from a relatively avascular zone, known also as Brödel's bloodless line. The Brödel's line was described in 1901 as an avascular plane allowing surgeons to perform a bloodless incision just posterior to the lateral convex border of the kidney during open anatrophic nephrolithotomy for the treatment of large staghorn stones, now of interest again not only for nephrostomy insertion and PCNL but also for laparoscopic and robotic anatrophic nephrolithotomies [23]. Of course, there are anatomical and radiological variations of the pattern of distribution of the Brödel's line, which might require preoperative investigation with dedicated imaging like an early arteriographic phase of the CT scan, and also a 3-D reconstruction [24], virtual reality models [25] and more advanced intraoperative tools [26, 27].

   Due to all these anatomic notions the least dangerous site for a percutaneous puncture from an hemorrhagic point of view is a posterior-inferior calyx [18, 28].

   Experiments on fresh human cadaveric kidneys [28, 29] investigated the probability of arterial and venous bleeding when puncturing different areas of the kidney, and of damaging an intrarenal vessel when puncturing a calyx in the upper, middle and lower pole. Puncturing the upper infundibulum resulted in vascular injury in 67% of the cases (26% arterial); similarly, an access through the mid-calyceal infundibulum was associated with an arterial injury in 23% of the investigated casts, access through the lower infundibulum resulted in13%of cases [30–32].

The area surrounding the infundibulum of each pole was divided into four quadrants, superior, anterior, inferior and posterior. The anterior pole was the most segmented by vessels, the inferior pole the least one. The anterior quadrant was the most dangerous site for puncturing as almost always neighboring with large vessels, so bleeding occurred in most cases in all lobes. Superior and inferior quadrants were found to be the safest place for puncturing the infundibulum; the posterior quadrant of the lower pole was also free of vessels and could be a possible target. Such results practically differ from the clinical practice, being the upper calyceal access commonly and safely performed for PCNL [20–22].

It is also relevant that the access to the chosen calyx follows a short and straight path to the renal pelvis, offering an easy access to the upper ureter and other calyces without significant angulation. When the Amplatz sheath is inserted along a straight path the possibility of injuring the peri-in fundibular venous plex us angulating the tract for approaching the stone-bearing area is reduced. To avoid torqueing and related bleeding risk the use of flexible scopes might also be of help [22].

21.5   The Papillary Puncture for PCNL

PCNL's success is heavily based on achieving a precise puncture of the desired calyx without causing significant bleeding, causing persistent hematuria, hemorrhage, parenchymal loss, and pseudo aneurysms requiring embolization to be controlled. As far as we know literature suggests that renal puncture for PCNL should be conducted through the papilla of the chosen renal calyx, the needle following the major axis of the infundibulum; on the contrary, a puncture crossing the infundibulum or blindly directed towards the renal pelvis/urolithiasis is not advisable because of the related increased risk of injury of infundibular vessels [29, 31–33].

For years PCNL has been made up by steps which were considered "dogmas", including the prone position (which was not a urological choice but simply an inheritance from the radiologists, directly puncturing hydronephrotic renal pelvis more than 40 years ago) [11] and the papillary puncture. Actually, the papillary puncture is not a tradition, or a blind adherence to a practice without the benefit of evidence [34], but is rather rooted in experience with variable levels of evidence, and additionally based on studies on cadaveric kidneys, evaluating the anatomic configuration of renal vascular supply in relation with the pelvicalyceal system. In fact, papillary punctures resulted in no discernable arterial injuries, venous injuries representing only 8% of cases. These are the anatomic basis of the papillary puncture: so why not?

Admittedly, these studies did not evaluate the occurrence of vascular injury in a clinical setting, after additional tract dilation and during/after PCNL, but under this respect there is ample evidence in the literature attesting the safety and efficacy of the papillary puncture for PCNL [34–38], with <7% transfusion rates (in case of single access, because multiple punctures have an increased risk of blood transfusions and angioembolization) [39]. Entry in the collecting system through the infundibulum might propagate a tear in the urothelium, increasing the like hood of secondary injury to underlying infundibular vessels secondary to nephroscope torqueing, possibly resulting in bleeding and/or pseudo aneurysm [34]. Moreover, since dilation of an access tract to a diameter of 24-30F might represent a higher degree of invasiveness to the renal tissue compared to needle punctures and miniaturized tracts it is clear that dilation will amplify the bleeding risk of a non-anatomic puncture, also depending upon the technique of dilation employed [13–15] possibly injuring vessels nearby. Therefore, before leaving established practice, further randomized clinical trials with significant sample sizes considering variables are warranted, also ruling out long-term development of infundibular stenosis due to scarring and possible parenchymal damage [40].

Both retrospective and prospective randomized trials supporting the performance of a nonpapillary puncture [41–43] report no increased blood loss or higher incidence of bleeding complications, but the results might be biased by the fact the endourologic team performing them is a referral group of endourologists with well-known surgical skills, (and this puncture should be safe also for inexperienced young urologists during their learning curve), and additionally do not report in detail all the pre-, intra- and postoperative measures applied in order to minimize hemorrhagic complications, interfering with the supposed mini-invasiveness of the procedure. Non-dilated systems.

21.6 Non-Papillary Puncture for PCNL

PCNL is constantly undergoing improvements in terms of efficacy and safety. Different approaches have been described regarding patients positioning, tract dilation methods and imaging techniques. Nonetheless, the target area on the kidney for the percutaneous access has not been studied adequately. The currently available concept on the percutaneous access is based on the anatomical studies which took place in cadaveric kidneys. The possibility of a non-papillary (non-forniceal) puncture has never been studied since the common clinical practice is to access the fornices of the papillae of the pelvicalyceal system. There is no current evidence that a non-papillary puncture is not safe in the clinical practice, while the available evidence on the incidence of injury of the renal vasculature is based on needle punctures of cadaveric kidneys, lacking any evidence on vascular trauma related to 30F dilation of the access tract. Moreover, the anatomical correlation of the kidney to the surrounding organs or the presence of dilation of the pelvicalyceal system, which highly common in the cases of PCNL, have never be considered in the available anatomical studies [20, 28, 29, 32].

Non-papillary punctures have been performed in our Department for more than ten years. The clinical experience gained by performing such an approach showed that the non-papillary approach is safe, could be related to technical advantages such as the higher degree of instrument movement or the direct pass of a guidewire into the ureter with a reduced risk for guidewire dislodgment.

Evidence on the safety of the non-papillary approach includes three published studies.

1. A retrospective clinical study examining safety and efficacy of non-papillary punctures in unselected cases over a 1-year period [41]. Hemoglobin loss and complication rates were comparable to the literature.

2. A prospective randomized trial comparing papillary and non-papillary percutaneous access in terms of operative time, hemoglobin drop and complication rate [42]. No statistical significance was found between the two groups in terms of complication rats sand the hemoglobin drop.

3. A prospective clinical study examining safety of puncturing and dilating the infundibulum of the middle renal calyx [43]. Single-photon emission computed tomography/computed tomography scintigraphies with Dimercaptosuccinic acid (SPECT-CT DMSA) and computed tomography perfusion were used as imaging tools to measure the angle of approach (AoA) for infundibular, pelvic and papillary accesses, comparing the vascularization of the areas related to dilation of the percutaneous tract. The AoA represented possible puncture tracts for the respective sites, both in prone supine positions. The comparison of the AoA's for infundibular and pelvic access did not show statistically significant differences, neither in dilated nor in non-dilated systems. The sites of the dilation tracts were overlapping for infundibular, pelvic and papillary accesses, and the vascularization was found no different. The above evidence practically show that the infundibular punctures are safe despite the current belief for the opposite. Thus, the performance of a non-papillary puncture could be advocated as any safe alternative to any practicing endourologist.

21.7 Conclusions

PCNL is a complex surgery made up by several steps, each one susceptible to variation simplying possible advantages and disadvantages, and always dealing with the anatomy of the patient and of the collecting system.

Familiarity with basic renal and vascular anatomy is a necessity for achieving a successful percutaneous renal access (which is the core step of PCNL) and minimizing bleeding complications (which are the most common and potentially dangerous ones).

You might believe or not in the existence of the Brödel's bloodless line, as well as decide between the traditional papillary puncture and the non-papillary one. In any case anatomy of the collecting system has to be taken into account and thoroughly evaluated pre- and intraoperatively with adequate imaging tools.

References

1. Turk C, Petrik A, Sarica K, Seitz C, Skolarikos A, Straub M, et al. EAU guidelines on interventionaltreatment for urolithiasis. Eur Urol. 2016;69(3):475–82.
2. Purkait B, Sankhwar SN, Kumar M, Patodia M, Bansal A, Bhaskar V. Do outcomes of percutaneous nephrolithotomy in horseshoe kidney in children differ from adults? A single-center experience. J Endourol. 2016;30(5):497–503.

3. Srivastava A, Chipde SS, Mandhani A, Kapoor R, Ansari MS. Percutaneous management of renal caliceal diverticular stones: ten-year experience of a tertiary care center with different techniques to deal with diverticula after stone extraction. Indian J Urol. 2013;29(4):273–6.
4. Goel R, Aron M, Kesarwani PK, Dogra PN, Hemal AK, Gupta NP, Gupta NP. Percutaneous antegrade removal of impacted upper-ureteral calculi: still the treatment of choice in developing countries. J Endourol. 2005;19(1):54–7.
5. Ecke TH, Barski D, Weingart G, Lange C, Hallmann S, Ruttloff J, et al. Presentation of a method at the Exploration Stage according to IDEAL: Percutaneous nephrolithotomy (PCNL) under local infiltrative anesthesia is a feasible and effective method - retrospective analysis of 439 patients. Int J Med Sci. 2017;14(4):302–9.
6. Solakhan M, Bulut E, Erturhan MS. Comparison of two different anesthesia methods in patients undergoing percutaneous nephrolithotomy. Urol J. 2019;16(3):246–50.
7. Ghani KR, Andonian S, Bultitude M, Desai M, Giusti G, Okhunov Z, et al. Percutaneousnephrolithotomy: update, trends, and future directions. Eur Urol. 2016;70(2):382–96.
8. De la Rosette JJ, Tsakiris P, Ferrandino MN, Elsakka AM, Rioja J, Preminger GM. Beyond prone position in percutaneous nephrolithotomy: a comprehensive review. Eur Urol. 2008;54(6):1262–9.
9. Cracco CM, Scoffone CM. ECIRS (Endoscopic Combined Intrarenal Surgery) in the Galdakao-modified supine Valdivia position: a new life for percutaneous surgery? World J Urol. 2011;29(6):821–7.
10. Cracco CM, Alken P, Scoffone CM. Positioning for percutaneous nephrolithotomy. Curr Opin Urol. 2016;26(1):81–7.
11. Scoffone CM, Cracco CM. Invited review: the tale of ECIRS (Endoscopic Combined IntraRenal Surgery) in the Galdakao-modified supine Valdivia position. Urolithiasis. 2018;46(1):115–23.
12. Zhang W, Zhou T, Wu T, Gao X, Peng Y, Xu C, et al. Retrograde intrarenal surgery versus percutaneous nephrolithotomy versus extracorporealshockwave lithotripsy for treatment of lower pole renal stones: a meta-analysis and systematic review. J Endourol. 2015;29(7):745–59.
13. Gao XS, Liao BH, Chen YT, Feng SJ, Gao R, Luo DY, et al. Different tract sizes of miniaturized percutaneous nephrolithotomy versus retrograde intrarenal surgery: asystematic review and meta-analysis. J Endourol. 2017;31(11):1101–11.
14. Tomaszewski JJ, Smaldone MC, Schuster T, Jackman SV, Averch TD. Factors affecting blood loss during percutaneous nephrolithotomy using balloon dilation in a large contemporary series. J Endourol. 2010;24(2):207–11.
15. Aminsharifi A, Alavi M, Sadeghi G, Shakeri S, Afsar F. Renal parenchymal damageafter percutaneous nephrolithotomy with one-stage tract dilation technique: a randomized clinical trial. J Endourol. 2011;25(6):927–31.
16. Wollin DA, Lipkin ME. Emerging technologies in ultrasonic and pneumatic lithotripsy. Urol Clin North Am. 2019;46(2):207–13.
17. Liu C, Zhou H, Jia W, Hu H, Zhang H, Li L. The efficacy of percutaneous nephrolithotomy using pneumatic lithotripsy vs. the holmium laser: a randomized study. Indian J Surg. 2017;79(4):294–8.
18. Cracco CM, Vercelli AE. Anatomy for PNL. In: Scoffone CM, Hoznek A, Cracco CM, editors. Supine percutaneous nephrolithotomy and ECIRS. Paris: Springer; 2014. p. 41–55.
19. Netto NR Jr, Ikonomidis J, Ikari O, Claro JA. Comparative study of percutaneous access for staghorn calculi. Urology 2005;65(4):659–662; discussion 62–3.
20. Aron M, Goel R, Kesarwani PK, Seth A, Gupta NP. Upper pole access for complex lower pole renal calculi. BJU Int. 2004;94(6):849–52.
21. Soares RMO, Zhu A, Talati VM, Nadler RB. Upper pole access for prone percutaneous nephrolithotomy: advantage or risk? Urology. 2019, pii: S0090–4295(19)30753–8. https://doi.org/10.1016/j.urology.2019.08.031.
22. Lang E, Thomas R, Davis R, Colon I, Allaf M, Hanano A, et al. Risks, advantages, and complications of intercostal vs subcostal approach for percutaneous nephrolithotripsy. Urology. 2009;74(4):751–5.

23. Macchi V, Picardi E, Inferrera A, Porzionato A, Crestani A, Novara G, et al. Anatomic and radiologic study of renal avascular plane (Brödel's line) and its potential relevance on percutaneous and surgical approaches to the kidney. J Endourol. 2018;32(2):154–9.

24. Cacciamani GE, Okhunov Z, Meneses AD, Rodriguez-Socarras ME, Rivas JG, Porpiglia F, et al. Impact of three-dimensional printing in urology: state of the art and future perspectives. A systematic review by ESUT-YAUWP Group. Eur Urol. 2019;76(2):209–21.

25. Parkhomenko E, O'Leary M, Safiullah S, Walia S, Owyong M, Lin C, et al. Pilot assessment of immersive virtual reality renal models as an educational and preoperative planning tool for percutaneous nephrolithotomy. J Endourol. 2019;33(4):283–8.

26. Sood A, Hemal AK, Assimos DG, Peabody JO, Menon M, Ghani KR. Robotic anatrophic nephrolithotomy utilizing near-infrared fluorescence image-guidance: Idea, Development, Exploration, Assessment, and Long-term Monitoring (IDEAL) Stage 0 Animal Model Study. Urology. 2016;94:117–22.

27. Xu C, Feng S, Lin C, Zheng Y. Reducing postoperative morbidity of mini-invasive percutaneous nephrolithotomy: would it help if blood vessels are left unharmed during puncture? A CONSORT-prospective randomized trial. Medicine (Baltimore). 2018 Nov;97(47):e13314.

28. Sampaio FJ. Renal anatomy. Endourologic considerations. Urol Clin North Am 2000;27(4):585–607, vii.

29. Sampaio FJ, Zanier JF, Aragao AH, Favorito LA. Intrarenal access: 3-dimensional anatomical study. J Urol. 1992;148(6):1769–73.

30. Sampaio FJ, Passos MA. Renal arteries: anatomic study for surgical and radiological practice. Surg Radiol Anat. 1992;14(2):113–7.

31. Sampaio FJ, Aragao AH. Anatomical relationship between the intrarenal arteries and the kidney collecting system. J Urol. 1992;148:1769–73.

32. Sampaio FJ. Renal collecting system anatomy: its possible role in the effectiveness of renal stone treatment. Curr Opin Urol. 2001;11:359–66.

33. Kallidonis P, Liatsikos E. Puncture for percutaneous surgery; is papillary puncture a dogma? Yes! Curr Opin Urol. 2019;29(4):470–1.

34. Pearle MS. Puncture for percutaneous surgery: is papillary puncture a dogma? No! Curr Opin Urol. 2019;29(4):472–3.

35. Olvera-Posada D, Tailly T, Alenezi H, et al. Risk factors for postoperative complications of percutaneous nephrolithotomy in a tertiary referral center. J Urol. 2015;194:1646–51.

36. Seitz C, Desai M, Häcker A, et al. Incidence, prevention, and management of complications following percutaneous nephrolitholapaxy. Eur Urol. 2012;61:146–58.

37. Kallidonis P, Panagopoulos V, Kyriazis I, Liatsikos E. Complications of the percutaneous nephrolithotomy: classification, management and prevention. Curr Opin Urol. 2016;26:88–94.

38. Single M, Srivastava A, Kapoor R, Gupta N, Ansari MS, Dubey D, Kumar A. Aggressive approach to staghorn calculi – safety and efficacy of multiple tracts percutaneous nephrolithotomy. Urology. 2008;71(6):1039–42.

39. Campobasso D, Ferretti S, Frattini A. Papillary puncture: still a good practice. World J Urol. 2019;37:573–4.

40. Scoffone CM, Cracco CM. ECIRS (Endoscopic Combined IntraRenal Surgery) in the Galdakao-modified supine Valdivia position. J Urol. 2017;197(4):E440–1.

41. Kyriazis IA, Kallidonis P, Vasilas M, Panagopoulos V, Kamal W, Liatsikos E. Challenging the wisdom of puncture at the calyceal fornix in percutaneous nephrolithotripsy: feasibility and safety study with 137 patients operated via a non-calyceal percutaneous track. World J Urol. 2017;35(5):795–801.

42. Kallidonis P, Kyriazis I, Kotsiris D, Koutava A, Kamal W, Liatsikos E. Papillary vs nonpapillary puncture in percutaneous nephrolithotomy: a prospective randomized trial. J Endourol. 2017;31(S1):S4–9.

43. Kallidonis P, Kalogeropoulou C, Kyriazis I, Apostolopoulos D, Kitrou P, Kotsiris D, et al. Percutaneous nephrolithotomy puncture and tract dilation: evidence on the safety of approaches to the infundibulum of the middle renal calyx. Urology. 2017;107:43–8.

Chapter 22
Benign Prostatic Hyperplasia: Elements of Embryology and Surgical Anatomy

Aldo Brassetti, Flavia Proietti, and Vito Pansadoro

The term "prostate" was first used in 335 B.C. by Herophilus of Alexandria to refer to the organ situated bellow the bladder. However, it was not until 1649 A.C. that the French physician and anatomist Jean Riolan speculated that enlargement of this organ could result in bladder outlet obstruction (BOO) [1]. He wrote in his *Opera Anatomica*:

"When, therefore, there is pain accompanied with a desire to urinate, but the urine is retained, one may suspect that (…) the prostate glands have become swollen or are indurated, all of which I have observed in various bodies"

22.1   Elements of Embryology

The Wolffian (mesonephric) ducts start to develop approximately 20–30 days after conception: these initially act as excretory canals for the mesonephros, which performs the renal function in the early embryo. The Müllerian (paramesonephric) ducts develop later and, by the eighth week, they extend between the mesonephric ducts reaching (but not breaking into) the urogenital sinus (UGS) which is produced by the septation of the cloaca by the uro-rectal septum [2].

Under the influence of Anti-Müllerian hormone (secreted by the Sertoli cells of the fetal testicles) the paramesonephric system regresses. Meanwhile, testosterone (produced by the Leydig cells) stabilizes the mesonephric ducts and stimulates the

A. Brassetti (✉)
Laparoscopic and Oncological Urology Center, Fondazione Vincenzo Pansadoro, Rome, Italy

Department of Urology, IRCCS Regina Elena National Cancer Institute, Rome, Italy

F. Proietti · V. Pansadoro
Laparoscopic and Oncological Urology Center, Fondazione Vincenzo Pansadoro, Rome, Italy
e-mail: vito@pansadoro.it

© Springer Nature Switzerland AG 2021
E. Huri, D. Veneziano (eds.), *Anatomy for Urologic Surgeons in the Digital Era*,
https://doi.org/10.1007/978-3-030-59479-4_22

Fig. 22.1 Development of the reproductive system. (**a**) Bisexual stage: the Wolffian ducts (light blue), which act as excretory canals for the mesonephros, coexist with the Müllerian ducts (purple). (**b**) At approximately 8 weeks of fetal development, in the male embryo, the anti-Müllerian hormone causes the paramesonephric ducts to degenerate; their cranial remnants become the hydatids of Morgagni while the caudal ends persist as the prostatic utricle. The mesonephric ducts will develop into the epididymides, the vasa deferentia, the seminal vesicles and the ejaculatory ducts

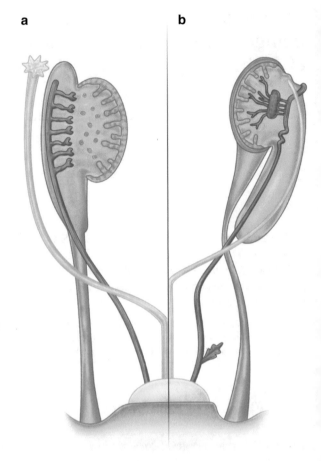

a   b

development of the vasa efferentia, the formation of the epididymal duct and the maturation of the vasa deferentia (Fig. 22.1). The androgenic stimulus also promotes the masculinization of the UGS leading to the formation of the prostate and the external genitalia [2].

Morphogenesis of the prostate begins at about 9–10 weeks of gestation with the appearance of solid epithelial buds that emerge from different quadrants of the prostatic urethra, over a considerable cranial-to-caudal distance, in the region of the verumontanum, which can be identified by the presence of the prostatic utricle (remnant of the Müllerian system) flanked by the paired ejaculatory ducts (derived from the Wolffian ducts) (Fig. 22.2) [3].

Under local mesenchymal control [2–4], buds elongation and branching occurs, via cell proliferation, at the solid cords tips [3]: the particular spatial arrangement is lobe-specific and defines the lobar division of the prostate [5–8]. From 12th week onward, canalization of these solid cords occurs, in a proximal to distal direction, and cell polarization is further observed [2, 3]. The relationship of the ductal

Fig. 22.2 Morphogenesis of the prostate. It begins at about 9–10 weeks of gestation with the appearance of solid epithelial buds that emerge from different quadrants of the prostatic urethra, in the region of the verumontanum, which can be identified by the presence of the prostatic utricle flanked by the paired ejaculatory ducts (*VD* vas deferens, *SV* seminal vesicle, *PU* prostatic utricle, *U* urethra)

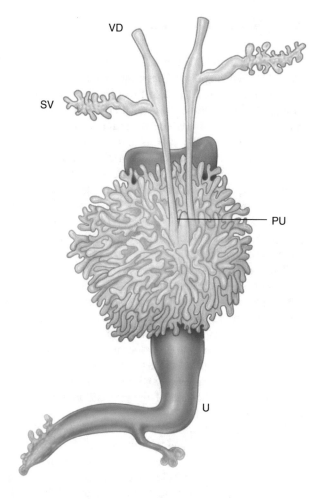

openings into the prostatic urethra remains identical through the entire fetal development and into adulthood [9]. Concurrent with epithelial maturation, the urogenital sinus mesenchyme proliferates and differentiates into interfascicular fibroblasts and prostatic smooth muscle cells [10]. Growth and development of the prostate is only completed at sexual maturity when, under the influence of androgens, epithelial cells begin to synthetize secretory products [11].

The human prostate does not grow significantly between birth and puberty, when growth commences in response to rising androgen levels. Its doubling time is 4.5 years between the ages of 31–50 and 10 years between 51–70 [12]. Sexual hormones, in fact, not only drive the development of the gland but also play a role in maintaining it quiescent in adulthood as young adult males, in whom androgen levels are at their peak, do not suffer from prostatic enlargement, which is associated with aging and decreased serum testosterone titers [13].

22.2   Surgical Anatomy

The prostate gland is a walnut-shaped organ located in the subperitoneal compartment, between the pelvic diaphragm and the peritoneal cavity. It sits posterior to the symphysis pubis, anterior to the rectum, and inferior to the urinary bladder. Conical in shape, it is referred as having anterior, posterior and lateral surfaces, with a narrowed apex inferiorly (which is continuous with the striated urethral sphincter) and a broad base superiorly (that is attached to the bladder neck and is pierced by the urethra and the internal urinary sphincter) [2, 14].

A sheet composed of collagen, elastin and smooth muscle cells covers the entire gland; being largely homogeneous in its muscle content and density with the prostate stroma, it is defined as 'pseudocapsule' [14]. On the anterior and anterolateral surfaces, this capsule fuses with the visceral continuation of the endopelvic fascia whose ventral condensations compose the puboprostatic ligaments that fix the gland to the posterior aspect of the pubic bone [15, 16].

The urethra runs through the prostate from the base to the apex. Along its course, it presents an anterior angulation of 30°-40° at the level of the seminal colliculus which divides the hollow organ into proximal ('preprostatic') and distal ('prostatic') segments that are functionally and anatomically discrete [17–19]. This angulation tends to be greater that 35° in men with nodular hyperplasia but it can also increase in those with an 'elevated bladder neck' in the absence of prostatic adenoma. By applying fluid dynamics to the process of micturition, it has been proven that energy loss increases proportionally with angulation, thus providing a theoretical basis for the transurethral incision of the prostate in symptomatic patients with a normal prostate volume [20].

The prostatic urethra is lined by transitional epithelium, surrounded by an inner longitudinal and an outer circular layer of smooth muscles. Actually, its entire length is encircled by sphincteric muscles (Fig. 22.3) [21, 22]. The *musculus sphincter trigonalis*, (best known as 'preprostatic' or "internal' urinary sphincter - IUS) is composed of smooth cells, originates at the level of the bladder trigone and inserts at the seminal colliculus; it is elliptic in shape and separates the urinary tract from the sexual tract [21, 22]. Any damage to this sphincter during transurethral resection of the prostate or treatment with alpha-blockers may cause retrograde ejaculation but do not affect continence. The *striated musculus sphincter urethrae* and *smooth musculus sphincter urethrae* are located below the verumontanum. The former (also known as 'external' urinary sphincter - EUS) is an horseshoe-shaped muscle that can trigger a voluntary micturition stoppage and avoids stress incontinence. The latter is a strongly developed circular involuntary muscle capable of producing long-term continence [21, 22]. Iatrogenic injuries to these distal sphincters during benign prostatic hyperplasia (BPH) surgery or radical prostatectomy may cause urinary incontinence.

The prostate is composed of approximately 70% tubuloalveolar glandular elements encircled with 30% fibromuscular stroma which contracts during ejaculation to express prostatic secretion into the urethra. All its major glandular elements open

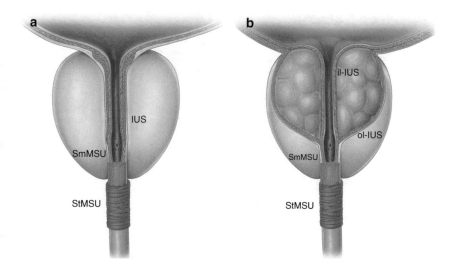

Fig. 22.3 Sphincteric muscles of the urethra. The *musculus sphincter trigonalis* (best known as 'preprostatic' or "internal' urinary sphincter-IUS) is composed of two layers of smooth cells, which originate at the level of the bladder trigone and insert at the seminal colliculus. It separates the urinary tract from the sexual tract (**a, b**). The cells composing the inner layer (il-IUS) are disposed longitudinally while the outer layer (ol-IUS) is elliptic in shape. The adenoma (only shown in (**b**) develops between the two layers of the IUS. The *striated musculus sphincter urethrae* (StMSU) and *smooth musculus sphincter urethrae* (SmMSU) are located below the verumontanum. The former (also known as 'external' urinary sphincter) is an horseshoe-shaped muscle that can trigger a voluntary micturition stoppage and avoids stress incontinence; the latter is a strongly developed circular involuntary muscle capable of producing long-term continence

into the distal urethra, to either side of a crest that projects inward from the posterior midline, widens and protrude as the verumontanum and disappears at the striated muscle [4, 6, 8, 9, 11, 14, 17–19]. The orifice of the prostatic utricle (müllerian remnant) is located at the apex of the seminal colliculus, while to either side the openings of the ejaculatory ducts are observed [14, 17–19].

As said above, the adult human prostate is a compact gland that does not exhibit distinct lobes seen in other mammals [8]; however, the focal nature of its diseases has suggested a similar but less conspicuous lobular design (Fig. 22.4) [4–6, 8, 11, 14, 17–19]. Up to one third of the organ mass may be attributed to the nonglandular anterior fibromascular stroma (AFMS) that extends as a shield from the bladder neck to the EUS [14, 17–19]. The central zone (CZ), which is only rarely affected by adenocarcinomas (<5%), is a wedge of glandular tissue surrounding the ejaculatory ducts and composing most of the prostate base; its ducts are structurally and immunohistochemically peculiar leading to the hypothesis that they are of wolffian origin [14, 17–19]. The bulk of the prostatic glandular tissue is made up by the peripheral zone (PZ) (which harbors the vast majority of the cancers but rarely becomes hyperplastic), composed of ducts that emanate from the postero-lateral recesses of the distal urethra and extend cranially to surround most of the CZ. It

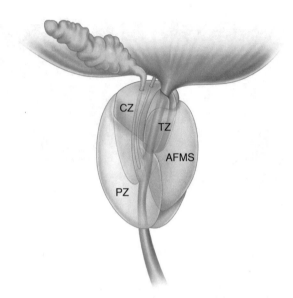

Fig. 22.4 Zonal anatomy of the prostate according to McNeal. The anterior fibromascular stroma (AFMS) extends as a shield from the bladder neck to the EUS (not shown) and composes up to one third of the organ mass. The central zone (CZ) is a wedge of glandular tissue surrounding the ejaculatory ducts and composing most of the prostate base. The peripheral zone (PZ) is composed of ducts that emanate from the postero-lateral recesses of the distal urethra and extend cranially to surround most of the CZ. The transition zone (TZ) encircles the proximal urethra and is surrounded by the circular smooth fibers of the IUS (not shown)

consists of small, simple round to oval acini emptying into long narrow ducts, lined with simple columnar epithelium, surrounded by a stroma of loosely arranged and randomly interwoven muscle bundles [14, 17–19]. The transition zone (TZ) encircles the proximal urethra and is surrounded by the circular smooth fibers of the IUS. It normally accounts for 5% of the glandular tissue but it commonly give rise to BPH [14, 17–19]. Being this zone surrounded by the musculus sphincter trigonalis, *the adenoma develops between the mucosa and inner longitudinal smooth muscle layer in front and the outer circular smooth muscle layer behind* (Fig. 22.3B and 22.5). Therefore, during BPH surgery, the surgeon should avoid entering the so called "false surgical capsule" (that represents the interface between the adenoma and the compressed PZ) and aim at *the proper enucleation plane* which *lies between the adenomatous tissue and the circular smooth muscle fibers of the proximal urethral sphincter* [23].

While the middle hemorrhoidals usually send a few small branches to the apex, the main source of arterial blood supply to the prostate gland comes from the prostatic branches of the inferior vesical artery (IVA) [24–27] (Fig. 22.6), which in turns may originate from the anterior division of the internal iliac artery (44% of cases), the internal pudendal artery (31% of cases) or the obturator artery (19% of cases)

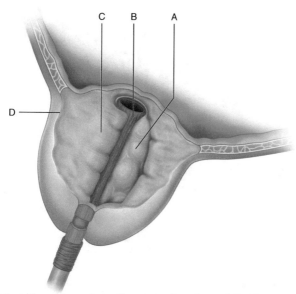

Fig. 22.5 The transition zone encircles the proximal urethra and lays between the two smooth muscle layers composing the internal urinary sphincter. Thus the adenoma (**a**) develops between the mucosa and inner longitudinal smooth muscle layer (**b**) in front and the outer circular smooth muscle layer (**c**) behind. During BPH surgery, the surgeon should avoid entering the so called "false surgical capsule" (**d**) that represents the interface between the adenoma and the compressed peripheral zone and aim at the proper enucleation plane which lies between the adenomatous tissue and the circular smooth muscle fibers of the proximal urethral sphincter

[25]. Actually there is no single prostatic artery, but there are about four or five twigs coursing more or less parallel to each other which can be divided into two groups: the 'urethral' (or 'penetrating') one immediately enters the tissue at the prostatic-vesical junction and travels inward, approaches the bladder neck in the 1- to 5-o'clock and 7- to 11-o'clock positions and then turns caudally, parallel to the urethra, to supply it and the TZ (thus providing the principal blood supply to the adenoma, in case BPH occurs. When these glands are resected/enucleated, *the most significant bleeding is encountered at the bladder neck at the 4- and 8- o'clock positions*) [24, 27]. The 'capsular' ('non-penetrating') group runs posterolateral to the prostate with the cavernous nerves and ends at the pelvic diaphragm; it gives off small twigs that pierce the prostate at right angle and follow the reticular bands of stroma to feed the outer glandular tissues [24, 27].

Venous drainage is abundant through the periprostatic plexus.

Innervation from the pelvic plexus travels to the prostate through the cavernous nerves: the parasympathetic system promotes secretion while the sympathetic one causes contraction of the smooth muscle of the capsule and stroma. The mnemonic "point (parasympathetic/erection and secretion) and shoot (sympathetic/ejaculation)" allows recall of vegetative innervation of the prostate gland [28].

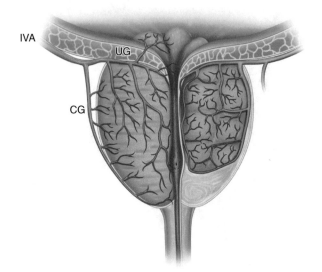

Fig. 22.6 Prostatic vasculature. The prostatic branches of the inferior vesical artery (IVA) provide the main source of arterial blood supply. There are about four or five twigs coursing more or less parallel to each other which can be divided into two groups: the 'urethral' (or 'penetrating') group (UG) immediately enters the tissue at the prostatic-vesical junction and travels inward, approaches the bladder neck and then turns caudally, parallel to the urethra, to supply it and the transition zone. The 'capsular' ('non-penetrating') group (CG) runs posterolateral to the prostate with the cavernous nerves and ends at the pelvic diaphragm; it gives off small twigs that pierce the prostate at right angle and follow the reticular bands of stroma to feed the outer glandular tissues

References

1. Oesterling JE. The origin and development of benign prostatic hyperplasia. An age-dependent process. J Androl [Internet]. 1991 [cited 2019 Nov 2];12(6):348–55. Available from: http://www.ncbi.nlm.nih.gov/pubmed/1722790.
2. Aaron L, Franco OE, Hayward SW. Review of prostate anatomy and embryology and the etiology of benign prostatic hyperplasia. Urol Clin North Am [Internet]. 2016 Aug [cited 2019 Jul 29];43(3):279–88. Available from: http://www.ncbi.nlm.nih.gov/pubmed/27476121.
3. Cunha GR, Vezina CM, Isaacson D, Ricke WA, Timms BG, Cao M, et al. Development of the human prostate. Differentiation [Internet]. 2018 Sep [cited 2019 Nov 2];103:24–45. Available from: http://www.ncbi.nlm.nih.gov/pubmed/30224091.
4. Timms BG, Hofkamp LE. Prostate development and growth in benign prostatic hyperplasia. Differentiation [Internet]. 2011 Nov [cited 2019 Nov 2];82(4–5):173–83. Available from: http://www.ncbi.nlm.nih.gov/pubmed/21939815.
5. Lowsley OS. The development of the human prostate gland with reference to the development of other structures at the neck of the urinary bladder. Am J Anat [Internet]. 1912 Jul 1 [cited 2019 Nov 3];13(3):299–349. Available from: http://doi.wiley.com/10.1002/aja.1000130303
6. Tisell LE, Salander H. The lobes of the human prostate. Scand J Urol Nephrol [Internet]. 1975 Jan 21 [cited 2019 Nov 3];9(3):185–91. Available from: http://www.tandfonline.com/doi/full/10.3109/00365597509134209

7. Cunha GR, Donjacour AA, Cooke PS, Mee H, Bigsby RM, Higgins SJ, et al. The endocrinology and developmental biology of the prostate*. Endocr Rev [Internet]. 1987 Aug [cited 2019 Nov 3];8(3):338–62. Available from: http://www.ncbi.nlm.nih.gov/pubmed/3308446.

8. Timms BG, Mohs TJ, Didio LJ. Ductal budding and branching patterns in the developing prostate. J Urol [Internet]. 1994 May [cited 2019 Nov 3];151(5):1427–32. Available from: http://www.ncbi.nlm.nih.gov/pubmed/8158800.

9. Price D. Comparative aspects of development and structure in the prostate. Natl Cancer Inst Monogr [Internet]. 1963 Oct [cited 2019 Nov 4];12:1–27. Available from: http://www.ncbi.nlm.nih.gov/pubmed/14072991.

10. Hayward SW, Baskin LS, Haughney PC, Cunha AR, Foster BA, Dahiya R, et al. Stromal development in the ventral prostate, anterior prostate and seminal vesicle of the rat. Cells Tissues Organs [Internet]. 1996 [cited 2019 Nov 3];155(2):94–103. Available from: http://www.ncbi.nlm.nih.gov/pubmed/8828707.

11. Timms BG. Prostate development: a historical perspective. Differentiation [Internet]. 2008 Jul [cited 2019 Nov 3];76(6):565–77. Available from: http://www.ncbi.nlm.nih.gov/pubmed/18462432.

12. Berry SJ, Coffey DS, Walsh PC, Ewing LL. The development of human benign prostatic hyperplasia with age. J Urol [Internet]. 1984 Sep [cited 2019 Nov 2];132(3):474–9. Available from: http://www.ncbi.nlm.nih.gov/pubmed/6206240.

13. Ho CKM, Habib FK. Estrogen and androgen signaling in the pathogenesis of BPH. Nat Rev Urol [Internet]. 2011 Jan 13 [cited 2019 Nov 3];8(1):29–41. Available from: http://www.nature.com/articles/nrurol.2010.207

14. Lee CH, Akin-Olugbade O, Kirschenbaum A. Overview of prostate anatomy, histology, and pathology. Endocrinol Metab Clin North Am [Internet]. 2011 Sep [cited 2019 Nov 6];40(3):565–75. Available from: http://www.ncbi.nlm.nih.gov/pubmed/21889721.

15. Raychaudhuri B, Cahill D. Pelvic fasciae in urology. Ann R Coll Surg Engl [Internet]. 2008 Nov [cited 2017 Feb 7];90(8):633–7. Available from.: http://www.ncbi.nlm.nih.gov/pubmed/18828961.

16. Cornu J-N, Phé V, Fournier G, Delmas V, Sèbe P. Fascia surrounding the prostate: clinical and anatomical basis of the nerve-sparing radical prostatectomy. Surg Radiol Anat [Internet]. 2010 Aug 29 [cited 2017 Feb 7];32(7):663–7. Available from.: http://www.ncbi.nlm.nih.gov/pubmed/20429006.

17. McNeal JE. Regional morphology and pathology of the prostate. Am J Clin Pathol [Internet]. 1968 Mar 1 [cited 2019 Nov 6];49(3):347–57. Available from: https://academic.oup.com/ajcp/article-lookup/doi/10.1093/ajcp/49.3.347

18. McNeal JE. Origin and evolution of benign prostatic enlargement. Invest Urol [Internet]. 1978 Jan [cited 2019 Nov 6];15(4):340–5. Available from.: http://www.ncbi.nlm.nih.gov/pubmed/75197.

19. McNeal JE. Anatomy of the prostate and morphogenesis of BPH. Prog Clin Biol Res [Internet]. 1984 [cited 2019 Jul 29];145:27–53. Available from.: http://www.ncbi.nlm.nih.gov/pubmed/6201879.

20. Cho KS, Kim J, Choi YD, Kim JH, Hong SJ. The overlooked cause of benign prostatic hyperplasia: prostatic urethral angulation. Med Hypotheses [Internet]. 2008 Jan [cited 2019 Nov 6];70(3):532–5. Available from.: http://www.ncbi.nlm.nih.gov/pubmed/17761390.

21. Brassetti A, Bollens R. Laparoscopic radical prostatectomy in 2018: 20 years of worldwide experiences, experimentations, researches and refinements. Minerva Chir [Internet]. 2019 Jan [cited 2019 Nov 8];74(1):37–53. Available from.: http://www.ncbi.nlm.nih.gov/pubmed/29658681.

22. Dorschner W, Stolzenburg JU. A new theory of micturition and urinary continence based on histomorphological studies. 3. The two parts of the musculus sphincter urethrae: physiological importance for continence in rest and stress. Urol Int [Internet]. 1994 [cited 2017 Oct 11];52(4):185–8. Available from.: http://www.ncbi.nlm.nih.gov/pubmed/8030163.

23. Hutch JA, Rambo ON. A Study of the Anatomy of the Prostate, Prostatic Urethra and the Urinary Sphincter System. J Urol [Internet]. 1970 Sep [cited 2019 Nov 6];104(3):443–52. Available from: http://www.jurology.com/doi/10.1016/S0022-5347%2817%2961756-7

24. Garcia-Monaco RD, Garategui LG, Onorati MV, Rosasco NM, Peralta OA. Cadaveric specimen study of prostate microvasculature: implications for arterial embolization. J Vasc Interv Radiol [Internet]. 2019 Sep [cited 2019 Nov 7];30(9):1471-1479.e3. Available from. http://www.ncbi.nlm.nih.gov/pubmed/31371136

25. de Assis AM, Moreira AM, de Paula Rodrigues VC, Harward SH, Antunes AA, Srougi M, et al. Pelvic arterial anatomy relevant to prostatic artery embolisation and proposal for angiographic classification. Cardiovasc Intervent Radiol [Internet]. 2015 Aug 12 [cited 2019 Nov 7];38(4):855–61. Available from.: http://www.ncbi.nlm.nih.gov/pubmed/25962991.

26. Clegg EJ. The arterial supply of the human prostate and seminal vesicles. J Anat [Internet]. 1955 Apr [cited 2019 Nov 7];89(2):209–16. Available from.: http://www.ncbi.nlm.nih.gov/pubmed/14367216.

27. Flocks RH. The arterial distribution within the prostate gland: its rôle in transurethral prostatic resection. J Urol [Internet]. 1937 Apr 1 [cited 2019 Nov 7];37(4):524–48. Available from: https://www.sciencedirect.com/science/article/abs/pii/S0022534717720526

28. McLaughlin PW, Troyer S, Berri S, Narayana V, Meirowitz A, Roberson PL, et al. Functional anatomy of the prostate: implications for treatment planning. Int J Radiat Oncol Biol Phys [Internet]. 2005 Oct 1 [cited 2019 Nov 7];63(2):479–91. Available from: https://linkinghub.elsevier.com/retrieve/pii/S0360301605002981

Chapter 23
Lymph Node Dissection Patterns

Bernardo Rocco, James Porter, Ahmed Eissa, Salvatore Micali, Stefano Puliatti, Luca Sarchi, Giulia Bonfante, and Maria Chiara Sighinolfi

23.1 Introduction

In clinical oncology, lymph nodes dissection (LND) represents an integral part of the diagnosis, staging and management of any solid tumor. A large autopsy study including 3827 autopsies with 9484 metastases from 41 primary neoplasms, demonstrated that regional and distant LNs were the most common sites of metastasis accounting for 20.5% and 12.9% of all metastases, respectively [1]. This fact applies also to the field of urologic oncology, where another autopsy study including 1589 prostate cancer (PCa) patients reported that LNs represent the most frequent site of metastasis and it was found in 26.1% of the autopsies [2]. In this setting, LN metastases is among the most important prognostic factors in urologic oncology [3–5].

23.2 Mechanism of LN Metastasis

The mechanism of tumoral cells dissemination to the regional LNs is complex; however, it is important for better comprehension of the patterns and concepts of nodal metastasis. The lymphatic system is responsible for gathering the extra-vasated

B. Rocco · S. Micali · S. Puliatti · L. Sarchi · G. Bonfante · M. C. Sighinolfi (✉)
Urology Department, University of Modena & Reggio Emilia, Modena, Italy
e-mail: Salvatore.micali@unimore.it

J. Porter
Swedish Urology Group, Seattle, WA, USA
e-mail: Porter@swedishurology.com

A. Eissa
Urology Department, University of Modena & Reggio Emilia, Modena, Italy

Urology Department, Faculty of Medicine, Tanta University, Tanta, Egypt

© Springer Nature Switzerland AG 2021   323
E. Huri, D. Veneziano (eds.), *Anatomy for Urologic Surgeons in the Digital Era*,
https://doi.org/10.1007/978-3-030-59479-4_23

fluid, and cells of the immune system and returning it to the blood system, thus it plays an important role in maintaining the body's fluid balance [6]. Nodal metastasis may occur through hematogenous spread but this pathway is extremely rare. On the other hand, the process of nodal metastasis starts by the secretion of lymphangiogenic cytokines from the neoplastic cells or host cells and stroma. Subsequently, these cytokines stimulate lymphangiogensis (the formation of new lymphatic capillaries) towards the tumor margins; however, some malignancies may be associated with intratumoral lymphangiogensis [7]. The lymphatic network is formed of unidirectional and blind-ended capillaries that is formed of single-layered but overlapped endothelial cells with incomplete or no intracellular junction [8]. Furthermore, lymphatic capillaries are characterized by the presence of anchoring filaments, which is responsible for maintaining the patency of the lymphatic capillaries and opening the intercellular junctions with the increase of the interstitial fluid pressure (IFP) and the interstitial fluid volume [9]. The IFP plays an important role in the directional motility of the tumoral cells towards the peritumoral lymphatic capillaries [10]. Once the neoplastic cells reach the peritumoral lymphatic capillaries, they start invading in to the lumen of these capillaries and embolize. Several factors may contribute to the passage of tumoral cells into the lymphatic system including; the large caliber of the lymphatic vessels, the absence of the basement membrane in these vessels with the scarcity of intercellular junction, the slower flow inside the lymphatic system compared to the blood system, and the similarity between the lymphatic fluid and the interstitial fluid [11]. Consequently, the malignant cells enter in to the sub-capsular sinus of the LN through the afferent lymphatic, followed by invasion of LN cortex [7].

23.3 Lymph Node Dissection in Urology

LNs dissection represent an important step in urologic oncology, where pelvic LNs dissection (PLND) provides staging information and potential therapeutic advantages in patients suffering from PCa and bladder cancer (BCa). Similarly, inguinal LN dissection is of pivot importance during penile and urethral carcinoma. On the same hand, retroperitoneal LNs dissection (RPLND) is an integral and critical part of the management of the testicular neoplasms. In this chapter we will discuss LND of inguinal and retroperitoneal LNs.

23.4 LND & Penile Cancer

23.4.1 Introduction

Penile carcinoma is a rare malignancy that accounts for approximately 0.2% of all the newly diagnosed cancer and 0.2% of all cancer deaths in the world in 2018 [12]. However, its incidence seems to be higher (3.7 per 100,000 men) in the developing countries, especially Brazil, where it is the fourth most common (2.8–6.8 per

100,000) malignancy in men [13, 14]. Interestingly, cancer statistics in United Kingdom (UK) show a 13% increase in the incidence of penile cancer over the last decade [15]. Several risk factors have been associated with the development of penile carcinoma including phimosis, lack of circumcision, lichen sclerosis, smoking, socioeconomic status, and human papilloma virus (HPV) [14]. Pathologically, squamous cell carcinoma is most common histologic subtype of penile carcinoma accounting for 95% of all cases [14]. The management of penile carcinoma consists of the radical excision of the primary tumor while preserving as much as possible of the penis with regional LN staging either through inguinal lymphadenectomy or dynamic sentinel node biopsy (DSNB) for patients with >T1G2 [16].

23.4.2 Pattern of LN Metastasis in Penile Carcinoma

The pattern of lymphatic drainage from primary penile neoplasm follows a well-known pathway, where it initially passes to the superficial inguinal LNs then to the deep inguinal LNs prior to reaching the pelvic LNs [17]. The superficial inguinal LNs lie between the fascia lata inferiorly and the subcutaneous fascia superiorly and it consists of approximately 8–25 nodes representing the first regional LNs to be affected by metastasis in penile carcinoma [18]. It is divided according to the work of Daseler et al. [19], into five anatomical zones with the central zone (zone V) located at the junction between the femoral vein and the saphenous vein. The remaining four zones are the superomedial (zone I), superolateral (zone II), inferolateral (zone III), and inferomedial (zone IV) [19]. Leijte et al. [20], analyzed the lymphatic drainage of 50 patients with penile carcinoma using a hybrid single-photon-emission-computed-tomography (SPECT-CT) imaging showing that 73%, 8.7%, and 18.3% of the sentinel LNs (SLNs) were located in the superomedial, superolateral, and central zones with no drainage to the inferior quadrants. In this setting, the authors suggested that inguinal LN dissection (ILND) can be limited to the superior and central zones in patients with cN0 to decrease the associated morbidity [20]. On the same hand, Omorphos et al. [17], confirmed that most of the SLNs were located in the superomedial (38.2%), superolateral (45%) and central zones (13%). Interestingly, they reported that SLNs were found in the inferolateral (3%), and inferomedial (0.8%) regardless the boundaries used for defining zone V (uroradiological classification, 5 mm radius, or 10 mm radius) [17].

Following the superficial inguinal LNs, metastasis can proceed to the deep inguinal lymph nodes that is situated medial to the femoral vein below the fascia lata in the region of the fossa ovalis and consists of approximately 5 nodes [21, 22]. The largest inguinal LN is called the Cloquet's (or Rosenmüller's) node and it lies at the transition between inguinal and pelvic regions [22]. Subsequently, nodal metastasis can progress to the pelvic LNs including the obturator, external iliac, and internal iliac and it may occur in 15–32% of patients [21, 23]. The lymphatic drainage of the penis occurs to the inguinal LNs on both sides in the majority of the patients [18].

23.4.3 Incidence of LN Metastasis in Penile Cancer

Approximately, 85% of patients with palpable inguinal LNs and 28% of those with impalpable nodes will have micometastasis [24]. The 5-years cancer specific survival of penile carcinoma has improved over time in cN0 patients (85% between 1956 and 1987, 78% from 1988 to 1993, 89% from 1994 to 2000, and 92% between 2001 and 2012) with significant improvement starting by the introduction of SNDB in 1994, this improvement reflects the prognostic value of LN metastasis [25]. Furthermore, the overall survival of penile carcinoma patients at 5-years is significantly affected by the absence or presence of LN metastasis (>90% vs 29–51%, respectively) [26]. Similarly, Zhu et al. [27], demonstrated that penile cancer specific survival at 3 years was 92.2%, 80.4%, 58.8%, and 49.7% for penile cancer patients with pN0, pN1, pN2, and pN3, respectively. Pelvic LN involvement in penile carcinoma is a sign of poor prognosis with a 3-years overall survival of 12.1% [23].

Other prognostic variables have been reported in the literature. Ball et al. [28], demonstrated that LN density (ratio of positive nodes to total nodes retrieved) of >15% resulted in a decrease in the recurrence free survival and the overall survival of penile carcinoma. Likewise, a recent meta-analysis of 1001 patients with penile cancer showed that perineural invasion was associated with higher risk of inguinal LN metastasis, worse cancer specific survival, and higher cancer specific mortality; however, it had no effect on overall survival [29]. Extranodal extension (ENE), which is the extension of the tumor beyond the nodal capsule to the perinodal fibrous tissue, was associated with worse prognosis and higher risk of pelvic LN metastasis [30]. Other prognostic variables include tumor stage, grade, depth of invasion, and histologic subtype; however, the data about all these variables remains a matter of debate. In these settings, the presence and the extent of LN metastasis in penile cancer patients remains among the most critical prognostic factors for survival [22].

23.4.4 Sentinel Lymph Node Biopsy & Imaging

Conventional imaging modalities (computed tomography [CT] and magnetic resonance imaging [MRI]) are characterized by low sensitivity and variable specificity for detection of micometastatic disease in inguinal LNs as the LNs' size represents the main parameter for assessment resulting in increased false negative and false positive rates [31]. Thus, dynamic sentinel LN biopsy (DSNB) was developed to overcome the drawbacks of the imaging modalities.

In 1960, Gould et al. [32], described the concept of SLNs in parotid carcinomas. It was not late until this concept was introduced in the management of penile carcinoma, where, Cabanas et al. [33], showed that this concept is applicable also for penile cancer. The concept of SLNs is based on the fact that lymph node metastasis in penile cancer follows the normal anatomical pathway of lymphatic drainage and that skip lesions do not occur [22]. However, the early experience with SLNs in penile cancer was associated with inconsistent negative false rate, which rendered it globally unacceptable. It was not until 1994, when this concept was brought back to life as the Amsterdam group performed the first DSNB, which consists of pre-operative lymphoscintigraphy after intradermal injection of colloid particles labeled with radioactive technetium-99 m close to the tumor followed by marking of the SLNs locations on the skin using a dual head gamma camera. Intra-operatively, a gamma probe was used for the localization of hot spots with the aid of patent blue dye. Yet, this technique was also associated with high false negative rates (17–22%) [34]. Leijte et al. [35], introduced several modifications to this technique including the use of preoperative ultrasound for all patients with non-palpable groin nodes with fine needle aspiration cytology (FNAC) of suspicious nodes. Furthermore, when the SLNs are not visualized on scintigraphy, surgical exploration and excision was performed with expanded serial sectioning of the SLNs for histopathological analysis. These modifications resulted in significant decrease in the rate of false negative biopsies down to 4.8% [35]. On the same hand, Naumann et al. [36], showed the use of SPECT-CT is superior to the planar scintigraphy and it is capable of reducing the number of false positive results and precisely localizing the SLNs. Furthermore, a novel hybrid radioactive and fluorescent tracer (indocyanine green (ICG)-^{99m} Technetium nanocolloid) was proposed as an alternative for patent blue. This novel tracer significantly increased the rate of the intra-operatively visualized SLNs compared to patent blue (96.8% vs 55.7%, respectively, $p < 0.0001$) [37]. Moreover, ICG and near infrared fluorescence imaging has been used to facilitate the detection of LNs during robotic inguinal lymphadenectomy for penile carcinoma [38, 39].

A recent meta-analysis assessing the DSNB in patients with non-palpable nodes in the groin showed a pooled sensitivity and negative predictive value (NPV) of 88% and 99%, respectively [34]. On the other hand, several authors showed DSNB alone is reliable in patients with palpable groin LNs; however, it may be associated with high false negative rates (11.9–13.9%), thus they suggested that adding ultrasound examination of the inguinal LNs with surgical excision of suspicious nodes may improve the sensitivity and specificity of DSNB in these group of patients [40, 41]. Non-visualization on the pre-operative lymphoscintigraphy is not rare event and it may occur either unilaterally (19%) or bilaterally (2%). These patients are usually subjected to more aggressive procedure (superficial modified inguinal lymphadenectomy) or extensive ultrasonographic follow up. Sahdev et al. [42], tried to develop a treatment algorithm for patients with non-visualized SLNs, where they demonstrated that re-DSNB will result in successful visualization in 86% of patients. If the SLN can not be visualized after re-biopsy patient should be referred to inguinal lymphadenectomy. Furthermore, they suggested that low risk patients with no-visualization of SLNs may be offered clinical and ultrasonographic surveillance of the groins [42]. Interestingly, several authors suggested that frozen section can be used for the intraoperative evaluation of SLNs with a specificity, sensitivity, positive predictive value (PPV) and NPV of 74%, 100%, 100%, and 72% [42, 43].

Recently, 18 Fluorodeoxyglucose positron emission tomography ([18F] FDG PET/CT) was suggested as a non-invasive alternative to DNSB. The sensitivity, specificity, PPV and NPV for [18F] FDG PET/CT ranges from 20–93%, 68–100%, 25–100%, and 89–96%, respectively [44].

23.4.5 Nomograms for Prediction of LN Involvement

Hence, radical inguinal lymphadenectomy is associated with high morbidity, the selection process for patients who will undergo inguinal lymphadenectomy should be optimal to avoid overtreatment and select only the patients who will benefit from this procedure [45]. In this setting, several authors have developed nomograms for prediction of LNI in patients with penile carcinoma. Ficarra et al. [45], used variables like tumor thickness, growth pattern, grade, presence of embolization, cavernosal or spongiosual infiltration, urethral infiltration and cN grouping to predict LN metastasis. Zhu et al. [46], developed a nomogram based on three simple variables (T stage, lymphovascular invasion, and p53 expression); however, on external validation this nomogram was not reliable [47]. Similarly, Peak et al. [48], used the same variables of Zhu's nomogram with only replacement of the p53 expression by the clinical nodal stage showing a high c-index for the new nomogram (0.880).

23.4.6 Management of Nodal Involvement

The European Association of Urology (EAU) guidelines recommends active surveillance for low grade tumors (Tis, TaG1, and T1G1), while patients with >T1G2 must undergo nodal staging through DSNB or bilateral modified lymphadenectomy. On the other hand, patients with cN1 or cN2 should be referred for radical lymphadenectomy, and patients with fixed inguinal lymph nodes (cN3) should start neoadjuvant chemotherapy before the lymphadenectomy. Finally, pelvic lymphadenectomy is recommended in patients with pN2 and pN3, followed by adjuvant chemotherapy [16].

Radical inguinal lymphadenectomy is defined as the excision of the LNs that are situated in the region bounded by the adductor longus on the medial side, the Sartorius muscle on the lateral side, and the inguinal ligament and the spermatic cord superiorly. The pectineus muscle forms the floor of dissection [21]. In the femoral triangle, the long saphenous vein is ligated and divided at its junction with the femoral vein and the anterior surface of the femoral vessels and nerves are dissected. Subsequently, the Sartorius muscle is used as a rotational flap to cover the femoral vessels. In this setting, all the superficial and deep inguinal LNs will be dissected [22]. However, this approach is associated with overall complication rate of 80% and a major complication rates of 20% [21]. Common complications of these approach includes wound infection, skin necrosis, lymphedema, and lymphocele [24].

In 1988, Catalona et al. [49], proposed the modified inguinal lymphadenectomy technique in order to decrease the inguinal lymphadenectomy associated morbidity without compromising its therapeutic benefits. The main proposed modifications included shorter skin incision, limiting the caudal and the lateral nodal dissection, avoiding the ligation and division of saphenous vein, and eluding the Sartorius transposition. These modification was associated with reduction of the rate of early and late complications of inguinal lymphadenectomy from 41.1% to 6.8% and from 43.1% to 3.4%, respectively [50].

Video endoscopic inguinal lymph node dissection (VE-IND), which resembles the open approach but performed using laparoscopic instruments, was proposed in 2003. A recent meta-analysis demonstrated that the VE-IND was associated with significantly less estimated blood less (EBL), shorter drainage time, and hospitalization period; however, the operative time was significantly longer when compared to open approach. Furthermore, VE-IND is associated with less minor and major complications but the LN yield was higher in the open approach [24]. The VE-IND can be performed through either a leg sub-cutaneous approach (port placement on leg) or a hypogastric subcutaneous approach (port placement on the lower abdomen). The hypogastric VE-IND allows bilateral inguinal LND through the abdomen rather than both legs in the leg subcutaneous approach. Furthermore, the hypogastric VE-IND can be used in case PLND is required [51]. Coping with the introduction of robotic technology in the urologic field, Josephson et al. [52], proposed robotic-assisted surgery for inguinal LNs dissection and it was associated with significantly lower morbidity compared to the open approach [53]. A recent systematic review showed that the most common reported complications of robotic inguinal LND are lymphocele (13.7%), lymphedema (7.8%), cellulitis (7.8%), seroma (3.9%), abscess (3.9%), wound infection or dehiscence (3.9%), and sepsis, lymphorrhea, and skin necrosis (1.9% each). Furthermore, the conversion rate was as low as 1.9% [54].

23.4.7 Salvage Inguinal LN Dissection

Inguinal recurrence may occur within a median 6 months after primary treatment of penile carcinoma. Neoadjuvant systemic chemotherapy followed by salvage inguinal LN dissection can be considered for management of delayed inguinal recurrence (>1 year after treatment). The dissection template is similar to that of the radical inguinal LN dissection with excision of all nodal metastasis even if outside the template of dissection. The morbidity of this approach is still considerably high with approximately 50% of patients experiencing lymphedema [21].

23.4.8   Role of PLND in Penile Carcinoma

PLND is indicated in patients with metastasis to two or more inguinal LNs on the same side or patients with pathologically confirmed ENE. However, different extents of PLND have been proposed including a limited PLND (external iliac and obturator LNs only) and extended PLND (extended to the bifurcation of the aorta) [55]. Since the pelvic LNs involvement is a rare event, there is scarce data in the literature to guide its management. Zargar-Shoshtari et al. [55], suggested that patients with pelvic LN involvement may have some survival benefit from bilateral PLND than unilateral dissection (estimated median overall survival 21.7 months vs 13.1 months, respectively, p = 0.051). On the contrary, Li et al. [56], demonstrated that only patients with pN2 may have survival benefit from bilateral PLND, while patients with pN3 showed no survival benefit when compared with patients with no-PLND. Several factors have been associated with increased risk of pelvic LNs involvement including strong p53 expression, vascular or lymphatic invasion, LN density greater than 30% and involvement of more than two inguinal LNs on the same side [23].

23.5   LND & Testicular Cancer

23.5.1   Introduction

However, testicular cancer is a rare neoplasm accounting for 0.4% of all malignancies and 0.1% of cancer-specific mortality [12], it is considered the most common solid tumor in young men between 15 and 34 years old [57]. Its incidence has shown steady increase over the last three decades but fortunately this was associated with improvement of the therapeutic approaches resulting in an overall 5-years survival of 97% [58]. Testicular cancer can be divided in two categories including; germ cell tumors, which is more common accounting for 90–95% of cases, and stromal tumors [59]. RPLND plays an important role in the multimodal treatment of testicular cancer [5]. According to the EAU guidelines on testicular cancer, primary RPLND may be offered for patients with high risk stage I and stage IIA non-seminomatous germ cell tumors (NSGCT) [60]. Furthermore, RPLND has been used for the management of stage IIB NSGCT; however, it was associated with high relapse rates. It has been also used in post-chemotherapy settings, when there is a residual mass of ≥1 cm. On the other hand, in seminomas, RPLND has been used in the management of post-chemotherapy residual masses >3 cm [61]. Moreover, RPLND is an essential part of the management of other malignancies including gynecological neoplasms [62], mesothelioma of the tunica vaginalis [63], and paratesticular rhabdomyosarcoma [64].

23.5.2   Patterns of LN Metastasis in Testicular Cancer

The lymphatic drainage of the testis is simple and predictable unless the lymphatics of the testis have been disrupted by a previous surgery [59]. The lymphatic drainage of the testis follows the paraaortic pathway and consists of two sets of vessels; the superficial vessels that drains the surface of the tunica vaginalis; and the deep vessels, which, carries the lymph from the epididymis and the body of the testis [65]. The lymphatic vessels of the testis ascend through the spermatic cord along the sides of the gonadal blood vessels. At the level of the inguinal ring, the lymphatic vessels passes anterior to the psoas muscle and proceed to end in the paraaortic and paracaval nodes at the level of the renal hilum [66]. Particularly, the primary landing sites differ between the right and the left testis, where on the right side they are located in the aortocaval chain opposite to the body of the second lumber vertebrae, and on the left side they are located in the left paraaortic nodes just inferior to the left renal vein [59]. Furthermore, right-to-left and left-to-right crossover of lymphatic drainage may occur in 13% and 20%, respectively [66]. Metastasis from the paraaortic LNs can pass in a retrograde fashion to reach the LNs at the level of the aortic bifurcation. Rarely, the external iliac LNs may drain the testis [65].

23.5.3   Indications for RPLND

Historically, surgical treatment (with RPLND) was the standard of care for the management of patients with germ cell tumors (GCTs); however, the introduction of cisplatin in 1965 as a part of the multimodal treatment of GCTs has revolutionized the treatment options resulting in great controversies about the role of primary RPLND in the management of testicular cancer [5].

23.5.3.1   Clinical Stage I NSGCT

Clinical stage I testicular carcinoma defines a group of patients with the tumor confined to the testis in the absence of clinical, serological, or radiological evidence of metastasis [67]. Several treatment options are available for the management of clinical stage I NSGCT including active surveillance, adjuvant chemotherapy (bleomycin etoposide cisplatin [BEP]), and RPLND, all of which, are associated with very high cure rates approaching 99% [68]. Mazzone et al. [69], retrospectively analyzed the data of 5034 patients with clinical stage I NSGCT between 1988 and 2015, demonstrating that active surveillance, chemotherapy, and RPLND were the treatment of choice in 61.2%, 24.9%, and 13.9% of patients, respectively. Further analysis showed that there was 1.1% and 2.3% annual increase in the use of active surveillance and chemotherapy, respectively, while, RPLND rates decreased by

5.7% over the study period (from 1988 to 2015). Furthermore, there was no statistical significant difference between active treatment (chemotherapy and RPLND) and surveillance as regards the 10-years cancer-specific mortality (2.1% Vs 1.8%, $p = 0.2$, respectively), while, on sub group analysis RPLND was associated with significantly lower 10-years cancer-specific mortality compared to chemotherapy (0.6% Vs 3.2%, $p = 0.002$, respectively) [69]. In this setting, the long-term side effects and the treatment-associated toxicities remains the driving factors in the decision-making strategy [70].

Risk-adapted management for this group of patients is important to identify patients who might benefit from adjuvant therapy following orchiectomy, hence the risk of relapse after orchiectomy alone was 42.4% for high-risk NSGCT and 17.3% for low-risk NSGCT [71]. Particularly, patients showing dominant embryonal carcinoma in the pathological analysis of the orchiectomy specimen (analyzed by experienced uropathologists) or those with lymphovascular invasion are at high risk of distant metastasis (up to 50%) [70]. Thus, primary nerve-sparing RPLND may be considered as an alternative treatment option to one cycle BEP only in high volume centers with experienced surgeons to ensure good therapeutic outcomes [71].

23.5.3.2   Clinical Stage IIA & IIB NSGCT

The American urological association (AUA) and the NCCN guidelines recommend either chemotherapy or primary RPLND for patients with clinical stage IIA NSGCT with negative serum tumor markers (STM); however, in case of clinical stage IIB NSGCT with negative STM, chemotherapy is the recommended treatment option and primary RPLND can be used as an alternative option in only highly selected patients. On the other hand, clinical stage IIC should always be treated with primary chemotherapy [72, 73]. Stephenson et al. [74], reported that clinical stage II NSGCT patients receiving primary chemotherapy with post-chemotherapy RPLND had a significantly higher 5-years relapse free survival compared to those receiving primary RPLND alone (98% Vs 79%, $p < 0.001$); however, the 5-years specific survival between both groups was not different (100% Vs 98%, $p = 0.3$). Furthermore, the authors illustrated that patients treated with primary RPLND either received fewer cycles of chemotherapy (1.4 Vs 4.2 cycles, $p < 0.001$) or avoided the need for chemotherapy (51%) [74]. On the same hand, a recent study demonstrated that 83% and 17% of the clinically stage II NSGCT patients received primary chemotherapy and primary RPLND, respectively, with decreasing trends in the use of primary RPLND specially among stage IIA and IIC patients from 2004 to 2014. Furthermore, the authors reported that intermediate- to high-volume centers more commonly offers RPLND as primary treatment to their patients [75].

Primary RPLND is considered an attractive treatment option for those patients for many reasons including; (1) avoidance of overtreatment with systematic chemotherapy (with its associated short- and long-term side effects) in approximately 13–35% of patients, whose enlarged nodes (1–2 cm) are due to reactive lymphoid hyperplasia exhibiting radiological false-positive results [5]; (2) approximately,

30% of clinical stage II NSGCT will require RPLND for residual or recurrent disease after primary treatment with chemotherapy [70]; (3) treatment of teratoma, which is found in approximately 20% of patients and is characterized by being resistant to chemotherapy [76]. On the other hand, bulky tumors (>5 cm) are ideal candidates for primary chemotherapy as the probability of relapse (requiring chemotherapy) after primary RPLND in those patients reaches up to 50–70% [70].

23.5.3.3 Seminomas

Unlike the NSGCT, the main treatment options of seminomas include surveillance, chemotherapy or radiotherapy and the role of RPLND is limited to patients with clinical stage II or III seminomas with persistent residual mass (>3 cm), positive PET scan and normal STM after primary chemotherapy, according to the NCCN guidelines [73]. However, both chemotherapy and radiotherapy are associated with high morbidity like cardiovascular disease, insulin resistance and secondary malignancies, which resulted in increasing interest in the use of primary RPLND in the management of early stage seminomas [5]. A recent review article by Hu et al. [77], summarized the results of four retrospective studies concerned with the use of primary RPLND for the management of seminoma, showing promising results with recurrence rate of 14% (14/92) at a median follow up ranging from 18–79 months. Currently, there are two ongoing trials for evaluation of primary RPLND in the management of patients with seminomas; the SEMS trial and the PRIMETEST trial, which will give better insights about this treatment strategy in the management of seminomas [68].

23.5.3.4 Post-Chemotherapy RPLND & Desperation RPLND

Approximately, 70% of patients receiving primary cisplatin-based chemotherapy for management of advanced testicular carcinoma will show complete response on radiography and normal post-orchiectomy STM; however, for the remaining 30% of patients, post-chemotherapy RPLND (PC-RPLND) or resection of the residual tumor are considered as the standard of care, when there is a persisting radiographic disease with negative STMs [70, 78]. Woldu et al. [78], used a propensity score matched cohorts demonstrating that patients who underwent PC-RPLND had a higher 5-years overall survival compared to those who did not (77% Vs 72%, $p = 0.007$, respectively) and thus highlighting the importance of PC-RPLND in highly selected patients.

Alpha fetoprotein (AFP) and beta-human chorionic gonadotropin (β-HCG) play an important role in the diagnosis, staging, and prognosis of testicular cancer [70]. In this setting, salvage surgery (also known as desperation RPLND) may be indicated in patients with elevated STM following second-line chemotherapy [79]. A recent study showed that salvage RPLND accounted for 6.8% of the RPLND performed in the UK between 2012 and 2013 [80]. Beck and colleagues presented a series of 114 patients who underwent PC-RPLND for elevated STM after first-line chemotherapy in 43.9% and desperation RPLND after second-line chemotherapy in 56.1% of patients, between 1977 and 2000. Pathological analysis revealed GCT, teratoma, and fibrosis in 53.5%, 34.2%, and 12.3% of patients, respectively. Germ cell tumor was found in 28% of patients after first-line chemotherapy and 75.8% of patients after second-line chemotherapy. Preoperative predictors of the presence of GCT in the surgical specimen included elevated β-HCG >100 ng/ml, increasing STM, second-line chemotherapy, and redo RPLND. The 5-years survival differed based on the pathology of the surgical specimen (31.4% for GCT, 77.5% for teratoma, and 85.7% for fibrosis) and the indication of RPLND (81.1% in the first-line chemotherapy group and 33.3% in the second-line chemotherapy group [81]. Interestingly, a highly selected group of patients may benefit from immediate PC-RPLND following first-line chemotherapy including patients with elevated STM without any tumoral cause of STM elevation. This group defines patients with stable and low-level increase of the STM and patients with cystic teratoma, which, may enclose large amount of tumor markers that leaks slowly in to the serum resulting in low elevations of STMs [82].

Generally, PC-RPLND (following first-line chemotherapy) is indicated in patients with NSGCT with tumor residuals in order to render the patient tumor free and excise any residual retroperitoneal masses. Size of the residual tumor is an important determinant of the type of intervention, where PC-RPLND is indicated for residual masses >1 cm as it may harbor teratoma in 40–45% of patients and viable GCT in 10–15% of patients. However, a residual mass following second-line chemotherapy may harbor viable GCT in approximately 50% of cases rendering desperation RPLND an imperative procedure [83]. On the other hand, the use of PC-RPLND for small residual masses ≤1 cm is still a matter of debate. A recent systematic review and meta-analysis reported that the pooled estimates of necrosis, teratoma and viable GCT in 588 men who underwent post-chemotherapy RPLND for residual masses ≤1 cm were 71%, 24%, and 4%, respectively. This meta-analysis highlighted that surveillance is considered a good option for men with subcentimeter residuals following primary chemotherapy and it avoids RPLND in approximately 97% of patients [84].

23.5.3.5 Late Relapse

Furthermore, late relapse defined as the recurrence occurring two or more years following primary curative treatment, is another indication for RPLND as the most common pathology reported in late relapses is teratoma [83].

23.5.4 Templates of RPLND

The RPLND for testicular cancer include the region of the embryologic origin close to the great vessels. The templates of RPLND has evolved and changed over time in order to decrease the associated morbidity, while maintaining the staging and therapeutic accuracy [85].

23.5.4.1 Extended (Supra-hilar) RPLND

Extended RPLND includes extensive bilateral dissection of the supra-hilar zones including the diaphragmatic crura and the region inferior to the renal hilum bounded laterally by both ureters. Furthermore, this template included the dissection of both iliac zones down to the bifurcation of the hypogastric and external iliac arteries. However, further pathological analysis of specimens from this template showed that supra-hilar zones are uncommon sites for nodal involvement in low stage diseases [86]. Furthermore, it is associated with increased pancreatic, lymphatic and vascular complications, thus, it has been limited to patients with hilar or supra-hilar masses [87].

23.5.4.2 Bilateral Infra-hilar RPLND (Standard Template)

The first modification of the RPLND template was the exclusion of the supra-hilar zones based on the scarcity of nodal metastasis to these zones, thus the boundaries of the infra-hilar template included the renal vessels superiorly, the ureters laterally, and the bifurcation of the common iliac vessels caudally [88]. This modification resulted in reduction of the operative time and the associated morbidity; however, one of the major concerns of this procedure was the loss of ante-grade ejaculation as a result of injury of the sympathetic nerves in this region [87].

23.5.4.3 Modified Template RPLND

The high rates or retrograde ejaculation (65–90%) with bilateral infra-hilar RPLND represented one of the major drawbacks of this procedure, which, was the main rationale for the modifications of the RPLND templates. The main modifications included; dissection of all the ipsilateral LNs between the renal vessels and the bifurcation of the common iliac; omitting the areas with known low risk of metastatic spread; and omitting the dissection in the area of the contralateral sympathetic trunk, especially below the inferior mesenteric artery [88]. The modified right RPLND included the dissection of the paracaval, precaval, intraaortocaval, preaortic, right iliac and right gonadal zones, while, the modified left RPLND included the dissection of para-aortic, preaortic, intraaortocaval, left iliac and left gonadal areas. This modification resulted in preservation of the antegrade ejaculation in approximately 90% of patients without affecting the oncological outcomes [89].

23.5.4.4 Nerve-Sparing RPLND

In 1988, Jewett et al. [90], presented the nerve-sparing approach to RPLND, which consisted of the identification and preservation of the sympathetic chain on both sides, the preservation of the post-ganglionic sympathetic nerves at vertebral levels of L1–L3, and the preservation of the branches of the hypogastric plexus. This nerve sparing approach preserved ejaculation in 90% (18/20) of patients, of which eight patients had bulky tumors (5 cm or more).

23.5.4.5 PC-RPLND Template

Commonly, PC-RPLND follow the full bilateral RPLND template; however, the use of modified templates for selected patients has been reported in the post-chemotherapy settings by some authors [91, 92]. Cho and colleagues used the modified template for post-chemotherapy RPLND in 100 patients with low-volume disease and normal STMs, reporting a 10-years survival of 99% [92].

23.5.5 Minimally Invasive RPLND

In 1992, the first minimally invasive RPLND was reported in the literature, when, Rukstalis et al. [93], performed the first laparoscopic bilateral RPLND in a patient with clinical stage I NSGCT. Since then and there was growing interest in laparoscopic RPLND as it was associated with shorter hospitalization and less complications compared to open surgery [94]; however, the main concerns to this approach were the lower lymph node yield, the steep learning curve and the difficult or absent dissection posterior to the great vessels, which limited the acceptance of this approach [68, 95]. In 2006, with the wide-spread of the robotic technology in the urological field, Davol et al. [96], were the first to report the feasibility of robotic assisted laparoscopic RPLND (RA-RPLND) in an 18 years old patient with mixed GCT. Stepanian et al. [97], reported their experience with RA-RPLND in 20 procedures (accounting for 19 patients as one patient underwent bilateral procedure). The median operative time was 293 min (IQR 257.3–317), EBL was 50 ml (IQR 50–100), and the hospitalization period was 1 day (IQR 1–2). Furthermore, the median LN yield was 19.5 (IQR 13.8–27.3). Only one patient suffered from ureteral transection that was repaired robotically and no patients required conversions or showed any sign of recurrence [97]. Likewise, Pearce et al. [98], presented one of the largest series (47 patients) for the use of the RA-RPLND in low stage patients (clinical stage I & IIA). The median operative time was 235 min, EBL was 50 ml, and the hospitalization period was 1 day. Furthermore, the authors reported a LN yield of 26. The authors reported a 2-years recurrence free survival rate of 97% [98]. A more recent and larger study including 58 patients with low stage (clinical stage I & IIA) reported a lower 2-years recurrence free survival (91%) after primary RA-RPLND; however, it is worth mentioning that all of the five reported recurrences were outside the template of dissection (one in the pelvis and four in the lung). Furthermore, the authors reported 3.3% intra-operative complications and 32.7% early post-operative complications; however, the majority of the post-operative complications were Clavien grade I & II [99]. RA-PLND has also been reported in post-chemotherapy setting by several authors [61, 100]. Noteworthy, RA-PLND is still considered an experimental approach and should be limited to high volume centers with highly experienced robotic surgeons.

23.5.6   Complications

The overall complication rate following primary RPLND may be as low as 1.3–24%; however, this rate is increased to 3.7–32% in the post-chemotherapy settings [101]. Approximately, 8.8% of patients with testicular cancer are infertile before starting any treatment, while, this percentage is increased up to 32.9%. Furthermore, erectile function is another concern of RPLND. However, the major andrological concern of RPLND is the retrograde ejaculation which ranged from 2–6.7% and 1.2–61% following primary RPLND in open and laparoscopic series, respectively [102]. A recent review article reported that the complications of primary RPLND can be divided to; (1) vascular complications (0–2.5%), which include venous thromboembolism, pulmonary embolism, and hemorrhage or vascular injury; (2) lymphatic complications that include symptomatic lymphocele (0–1.7%) and chylous ascites (0.2–2.1%); (3) other complications including neuropraxia, paralysis, pulmonary complications, ileus and small bowel obstruction; and 4-mortality, which should be nil following primary RPLND [101]. On the same hand, Gerdtsson et al. [103], demonstrated that the intra-operative complication rates was higher in bilateral PC-RPLND than in the unilateral approach (14% Vs 4.3%, $p = 0.003$) and the authors highlighted ureteral injury being the most common intra-operative complication (2%). Similarly, the authors reported that post-operative complications were more frequent in the bilateral post-chemotherapy RPLND compared to the unilateral approach (45% Vs 25%, $p = 0.001$) with lymphocele being the most frequent complication reported in 11% of patients [103].

23.6   Miscellaneous

23.6.1   LND and Renal Cell Carcinoma (RCC)

Renal cancers account for approximately, 2.2% and 1.8% of all newly diagnosed cancers and cancer-specific mortality, respectively [12]. The lymphatic drainage of the kidneys explains the unpredictable pattern of lymphatic spread in case of RCC. The efferent lymphatic vessels from the right kidney are divided into either anterior or posterior bundles; where, the anterior bundle runs anterior to the renal vein and drains into the paracaval, precaval, retrocaval (this nodes are connected to the thoracic duct), and interaortocaval nodes, while, the posterior bundle runs posterior to the renal artery and ends in the paracaval, retrocaval, and interaortocaval lymph nodes. Similarly, the anterior bundle of the left kidney drains into the para-aortic and preaortic nodes, while, the posterior bundle drains in the para-aortic and retroaortic lymph nodes. Furthermore, there is an extensive network of retroperitoneal lymphatic connections between the first and fifth lumber vertebrae [104].

Despite the essential diagnostic and prognostic value of LND in patients with RCC, the controversy and the lack of evidence about the therapeutic and survival benefit of such procedure [105] resulted in a significant drop in the rate of LND in patients with RCC overtime [106]. Where a recent systematic review and meta-analysis assessed the role of LND during the management of RCC demonstrating that LND was not associated with any survival benefit in patients with either non-metastatic or metastatic RCC; however, a survival benefit was reported in a small subset of patients with isolated lymph node metastasis [107].

According to the EAU guidelines on renal cell carcinoma, LND is indicated only in patients with clinically enlarged LNs [108]. Yet, there is no standardized template for LND in RCC patients. In this setting, Campi R et al. [109], performed a systematic review of literature to identify the most commonly used templates demonstrating that for the right kidney, most surgeons reported the dissection of the hilar, paracaval, and precaval lymph nodes between the crus of the diaphragm to the level of the bifurcation of the aorta. However, an extended dissection of the interaortocaval, retrocaval, common iliac, or preaortic and para-aortic nodes was also described. As regards the left kidney, the most commonly reported template includes the hilar, preaortic, and para-aortic lymph nodes between the crus of the diaphragm and the level of aortic bifurcation. Similarly, few authors reported an extended dissection that include the interaortocaval, retroaortic, common iliac, or paracaval lymph nodes [109]. Generally, LND in the setting of RCC represents a matter of debate and an area that requires further investigation.

23.6.2   LND and Upper Tract Urothelial Carcinoma (UTUC)

UTUCs are rare but aggressive urological malignancies that account for nearly 5% of all urothelial carcinomas. Regional lymph nodes are the most common site of metastasis of UTUCs, where, 30–40% of patients with muscle-invasive disease are expected to suffer of lymph node metastasis. Interestingly, several authors reported that LND in patients with UTUCs may be associated with survival benefits [110, 111]. Thus, LND is currently accepted as an important step of radical nephroureterectomy (RNU) with an increasing trend of LND rate overtime [112, 113]. Yet, LND is still not routinely performed during RNU due to the lack of standardized eligibility criteria for patients' selection, and the highly unpredictable lymphatic drainage of the UTUC [114]. Campi et al. [114], performed a systematic review in a trial to standardize the anatomical templates of LND during RNU. For right renal pelvis, upper, or middle ureteric tumors, the most commonly reported template included the right renal hilar, precaval, and paracaval LNs, which may be extended posterior to the inferior vena cava to include the retrocaval LNs, while, in case of left sided tumors (pelvis, upper, or middle ureteric), the dissection include the renal hilar, preaortic, and para-aortic LNs. On the contrary, in case of lower third ureteric tumors, most authors reported the dissection of the ipsilateral pelvic lymph nodes [114].

23.6.3 Robotic Approach for Inguinal and Pelvic LND in Case of Melanoma

Inguinal and pelvic LND is recommended also in case of high-risk lower limb cutaneous melanoma. Indications for superficial inguinal nodal dissection in melanoma include fine needle aspiration or clinically positive inguinal LN and sentinel LN [115]. Open inguinal LND may suffer from complications such as a poor wound healing, deep vein thrombosis, and lymphema. Robotically assisted dissection has been proposed; preliminary outcomes on small case series are encouraging, with minimal post-operative complications [115].

Pelvic LND for high-risk melanoma is recommended as well [116]: in these cases, the pelvic LND should include external iliac, internal iliac, common iliac and obturator nodes. As suggested from ASCO Guidelines on malignant melanoma 2012, the procedure could achieve a good regional disease control and, in most of the cases, it is followed by adjuvant oncological therapies [116].

Similar to what happens for the inguinal area, the open approach is well-established but traditionally impaired by a number of complications, often requiring medical and surgical management; adverse events could delay the initiation of adjuvant therapies. The most common side effect is the development of lymphocele, an event that—if symptomatic—may require drainage and prolonged antibiotic therapy [117]. The robotic approach provides several advantages including better visualization and a more precise dissection of nodes [118–120]; symptomatic lymphocele rate from a published series of more than 1300 robotic pelvic ND performed during prostatectomy was as low as 1.49% and 2.83% for the transperitoneal and extraperitoneal approach, respectively [121].

Overall, one of the main advantage of robotics over open surgery in the field of inguinal and pelvic ND for melanoma could be the faster recovery, advisable especially in the case of high-risk diseases requiring a prompt multimodal management.

References

1. Disibio G, French SW. Metastatic patterns of cancers: results from a large autopsy study. Arch Pathol Lab Med. 2008;132(6):931–9.
2. Bubendorf L, Schopfer A, Wagner U, Sauter G, Moch H, Willi N, et al. Metastatic patterns of prostate cancer: an autopsy study of 1,589 patients. Hum Pathol. 2000;31(5):578–83.
3. Svatek R, Zehnder P. Role and extent of lymphadenectomy during radical cystectomy for invasive bladder cancer. Curr Urol Rep. 2012;13(2):115–21.

4. Briganti A, Karnes JR, Da Pozzo LF, Cozzarini C, Gallina A, Suardi N, et al. Two positive nodes represent a significant cut-off value for cancer specific survival in patients with node positive prostate cancer. A new proposal based on a two-institution experience on 703 consecutive N+ patients treated with radical prostatectomy, extended pelvic lymph node dissection and adjuvant therapy. Eur Urol. 2009;55(2):261–70.

5. Mano R, Di Natale R, Sheinfeld J. Current controversies on the role of retroperitoneal lymphadenectomy for testicular cancer. Urol Oncol. 2019;37(3):209–18.

6. McMahon CJ, Rofsky NM, Pedrosa I. Lymphatic metastases from pelvic tumors: anatomic classification, characterization, and staging. Radiology. 2010;254(1):31–46.

7. Nathanson SD. Insights into the mechanisms of lymph node metastasis. Cancer. 2003;98(2):413–23.

8. Baluk P, Fuxe J, Hashizume H, Romano T, Lashnits E, Butz S, et al. Functionally specialized junctions between endothelial cells of lymphatic vessels. J Exp Med. 2007;204(10):2349–62.

9. Schmid-Schonbein GW. Microlymphatics and lymph flow. Physiol Rev. 1990;70(4):987–1028.

10. Jain RK, Munn LL, Fukumura D. Dissecting tumour pathophysiology using intravital microscopy. Nat Rev Cancer. 2002;2(4):266–76.

11. Weiss L, Schmid-Schonbein GW. Biomechanical interactions of cancer cells with the microvasculature during metastasis. Cell Biophys. 1989;14(2):187–215.

12. Bray F, Ferlay J, Soerjomataram I, Siegel RL, Torre LA, Jemal A. Global cancer statistics 2018: GLOBOCAN estimates of incidence and mortality worldwide for 36 cancers in 185 countries. CA Cancer J Clin. 2018;68(6):394–424.

13. Backes DM, Kurman RJ, Pimenta JM, Smith JS. Systematic review of human papillomavirus prevalence in invasive penile cancer. Cancer Causes Control. 2009;20(4):449–57.

14. Douglawi A, Masterson TA. Updates on the epidemiology and risk factors for penile cancer. Transl Androl Urol. 2017;6(5):785–90.

15. Cancer Research UK. Penile Cancer Statistics UK2019. Available from: https://www.cancerresearchuk.org/health-professional/cancer-statistics/statistics-by-cancer-type/penile-cancer/incidence-heading-Two#heading-Zero.

16. Hakenberg OW, Comperat EM, Minhas S, Necchi A, Protzel C, Watkin N. EAU guidelines on penile cancer: 2014 update. Eur Urol. 2015;67(1):142–50.

17. Omorphos S, Saad Z, Kirkham A, Nigam R, Malone P, Bomanji J, et al. Zonal mapping of sentinel lymph nodes in penile cancer patients using fused SPECT/CT imaging and lymphoscintigraphy. Urol Oncol. 2018;36(12):530.e1-.e6.

18. Horenblas S. Sentinel lymph node biopsy in penile carcinoma. Semin Diagn Pathol. 2012;29(2):90–5.

19. Daseler EH, Anson BJ, Reimann AF. Radical excision of the inguinal and iliac lymph glands; a study based upon 450 anatomical dissections and upon supportive clinical observations. Surg Gynecol Obstet. 1948;87(6):679–94.

20. Leijte JA, Valdes Olmos RA, Nieweg OE, Horenblas S. Anatomical mapping of lymphatic drainage in penile carcinoma with SPECT-CT: implications for the extent of inguinal lymph node dissection. Eur Urol. 2008;54(4):885–90.

21. Sharma P, Zargar H, Spiess PE. Surgical advances in inguinal lymph node dissection: optimizing treatment outcomes. Urol Clin North Am. 2016;43(4):457–68.

22. Protzel C, Alcaraz A, Horenblas S, Pizzocaro G, Zlotta A, Hakenberg OW. Lymphadenectomy in the surgical management of penile cancer. Eur Urol. 2009;55(5):1075–88.

23. Liu JY, Li YH, Zhang ZL, Yao K, Ye YL, Xie D, et al. The risk factors for the presence of pelvic lymph node metastasis in penile squamous cell carcinoma patients with inguinal lymph node dissection. World J Urol. 2013;31(6):1519–24.

24. Hu J, Li H, Cui Y, Liu P, Zhou X, Liu L, et al. Comparison of clinical feasibility and oncological outcomes between video endoscopic and open inguinal lymphadenectomy for penile cancer: A systematic review and meta-analysis. Medicine. 2019;98(22):e15862.

25. Djajadiningrat RS, Graafland NM, van Werkhoven E, Meinhardt W, Bex A, van der Poel HG, et al. Contemporary management of regional nodes in penile cancer-improvement of survival? J Urol. 2014;191(1):68–73.

26. Robinson R, Marconi L, MacPepple E, Hakenberg OW, Watkin N, Yuan Y, et al. Risks and benefits of adjuvant radiotherapy after inguinal lymphadenectomy in node-positive penile cancer: a systematic review by the european association of urology penile cancer guidelines panel. Eur Urol. 2018;74(1):76–83.

27. Zhu Y, Gu WJ, Xiao WJ, Wang BH, Azizi M, Spiess PE, et al. Important therapeutic considerations in T1b penile cancer: prognostic significance and adherence to treatment guidelines. Ann Surg Oncol. 2019;26(2):685–91.

28. Ball MW, Schwen ZR, Ko JS, Meyer A, Netto GJ, Burnett AL, et al. Lymph node density predicts recurrence and death after inguinal lymph node dissection for penile cancer. Invest Clin Urol. 2017;58(1):20–6.

29. Zhou X, Qi F, Zhou R, Wang S, Wang Y, Wang Y, et al. The role of perineural invasion in penile cancer: a meta-analysis and systematic review. Biosci Reports. 2018;38(5).

30. Zhang ZL, Yu CP, Liu ZW, Velet L, Li YH, Jiang LJ, et al. The importance of extranodal extension in penile cancer: a meta-analysis. BMC Cancer. 2015;15:815.

31. Gupta S, Rajesh A. Magnetic resonance imaging of penile cancer. Magn Reson Imaging Clin N Am 2014;22(2):191–199, vi.

32. Gould EA, Winship T, Philbin PH, Kerr HH. Observations on a "sentinel node" in cancer of the parotid. Cancer. 1960;13:77–8.

33. Cabanas RM. An approach for the treatment of penile carcinoma. Cancer. 1977;39(2):456–66.

34. Zou ZJ, Liu ZH, Tang LY, Wang YJ, Liang JY, Zhang RC, et al. Radiocolloid-based dynamic sentinel lymph node biopsy in penile cancer with clinically negative inguinal lymph node: an updated systematic review and meta-analysis. Int Urol Nephrol. 2016;48(12):2001–13.

35. Leijte JA, Kroon BK, Valdes Olmos RA, Nieweg OE, Horenblas S. Reliability and safety of current dynamic sentinel node biopsy for penile carcinoma. Eur Urol. 2007;52(1):170–7.

36. Naumann CM, Colberg C, Juptner M, Marx M, Zhao Y, Jiang P, et al. Evaluation of the diagnostic value of preoperative sentinel lymph node (SLN) imaging in penile carcinoma patients without palpable inguinal lymph nodes via single photon emission computed tomography/computed tomography (SPECT/CT) as compared to planar scintigraphy. Urologic oncology. 2018;36(3):92.e17–92.e24.

37. Brouwer OR, van den Berg NS, Matheron HM, van der Poel HG, van Rhijn BW, Bex A, et al. A hybrid radioactive and fluorescent tracer for sentinel node biopsy in penile carcinoma as a potential replacement for blue dye. Eur Urol. 2014;65(3):600–9.

38. Bjurlin MA, Zhao LC, Kenigsberg AP, Mass AY, Taneja SS, Huang WC. Novel use of fluorescence lymphangiography during robotic groin dissection for penile cancer. Urology. 2017;107:267.

39. Savio LF, Panizzutti Barboza M, Alameddine M, Ahdoot M, Alonzo D, Ritch CR. Combined partial penectomy with bilateral robotic inguinal lymphadenectomy using near-infrared fluorescence guidance. Urology. 2018;113:251.

40. Naumann CM, van der Horst S, van der Horst C, Kahler KC, Seeger M, Osmonov D, et al. Reliability of dynamic sentinel node biopsy combined with ultrasound-guided removal of sonographically suspicious lymph nodes as a diagnostic approach in patients with penile cancer with palpable inguinal lymph nodes. Urol Oncol. 2015;33(9):389.e9–14.

41. Lutzen U, Zuhayra M, Marx M, Zhao Y, Colberg C, Knupfer S, et al. Value and efficiency of sentinel lymph node diagnostics in patients with penile carcinoma with palpable inguinal lymph nodes as a new multimodal, minimally invasive approach. Eur J Nucl Med Mol Imaging. 2016;43(13):2313–23.

42. Sahdev V, Albersen M, Christodoulidou M, Parnham A, Malone P, Nigam R, et al. Management of non-visualization following dynamic sentinel lymph node biopsy for squamous cell carcinoma of the penis. BJU Int. 2017;119(4):573–8.

43. Chipollini J, Tang DH, Manimala N, Gilbert SM, Pow-Sang JM, Sexton WJ, et al. Evaluating the accuracy of intraoperative frozen section during inguinal lymph node dissection in penile cancer. Urol Oncol. 2018;36(1):14.e1–e5.

44. Drager DL, Heuschkel M, Protzel C, Erbersdobler A, Krause BJ, Hakenberg OW, et al. [18F]FDG PET/CT for assessing inguinal lymph nodes in patients with penile cancer – cor-

relation with histopathology after inguinal lymphadenectomy. Nuklearmedizin Nucl Med. 2018;57(1):26–30.

45. Ficarra V, Zattoni F, Artibani W, Fandella A, Martignoni G, Novara G, et al. Nomogram predictive of pathological inguinal lymph node involvement in patients with squamous cell carcinoma of the penis. J Urol 2006;175(5):1700–1704; discussion 4–5.

46. Zhu Y, Zhang HL, Yao XD, Zhang SL, Dai B, Shen YJ, et al. Development and evaluation of a nomogram to predict inguinal lymph node metastasis in patients with penile cancer and clinically negative lymph nodes. J Urol. 2010;184(2):539–45.

47. Maciel CVM, Machado RD, Morini MA, Mattos PAL, Dos Reis R, Dos Reis RB, et al. External validation of nomogram to predict inguinal lymph node metastasis in patients with penile cancer and clinically negative lymph nodes. International braz j urol. 2019;45(4):671–8.

48. Peak TC, Russell GB, Dutta R, Rothberg MB, Chapple AG, Hemal AK. A National Cancer Database-based nomogram to predict lymph node metastasis in penile cancer. BJU Int. 2019;123(6):1005–10.

49. Catalona WJ. Modified inguinal lymphadenectomy for carcinoma of the penis with preservation of saphenous veins: technique and preliminary results. J Urol. 1988;140(2):306–10.

50. Bouchot O, Rigaud J, Maillet F, Hetet JF, Karam G. Morbidity of inguinal lymphadenectomy for invasive penile carcinoma. Eur Urol 2004;45(6):761–765; discussion 5–6.

51. Yuan P, Zhao C, Liu Z, Ou Z, He W, Cai Y, et al. Comparative study of video endoscopic inguinal lymphadenectomy through a hypogastric vs leg subcutaneous approach for penile cancer. J Endourol. 2018;32(1):66–72.

52. Josephson DY, Jacobsohn KM, Link BA, Wilson TG. Robotic-assisted endoscopic inguinal lymphadenectomy. Urology 2009;73(1):167–170; discussion 70–1.

53. Singh A, Jaipuria J, Goel A, Shah S, Bhardwaj R, Baidya S, et al. Comparing outcomes of robotic and open inguinal lymph node dissection in patients with carcinoma of the penis. J Urol. 2018;199(6):1518–25.

54. Gkegkes ID, Minis EE, Iavazzo C. Robotic-assisted inguinal lymphadenectomy: a systematic review. J Robot Surg. 2019;13(1):1–8.

55. Zargar-Shoshtari K, Sharma P, Djajadiningrat R, Catanzaro M, Ye DW, Zhu Y, et al. Extent of pelvic lymph node dissection in penile cancer may impact survival. World J Urol. 2016;34(3):353–9.

56. Li ZS, Deng CZ, Yao K, Tang Y, Liu N, Chen P, et al. Bilateral pelvic lymph node dissection for Chinese patients with penile cancer: a multicenter collaboration study. J Cancer Res Clin Oncol. 2017;143(2):329–35.

57. Baird DC, Meyers GJ, Hu JS. Testicular cancer: diagnosis and treatment. Am Fam Physician. 2018;97(4):261–8.

58. Smith ZL, Werntz RP, Eggener SE. Testicular cancer: epidemiology, diagnosis, and management. Med Clin North Am. 2018;102(2):251–64.

59. Hale GR, Teplitsky S, Truong H, Gold SA, Bloom JB, Agarwal PK. Lymph node imaging in testicular cancer. Transl Androl Urol. 2018;7(5):864–74.

60. Albers P, Albrecht W, Algaba F, Bokemeyer C, Cohn-Cedermark G, Fizazi K, et al. EAU guidelines on testicular cancer: 2011 update. Eur Urol. 2011;60(2):304–19.

61. Klaassen Z, Hamilton RJ. The role of robotic retroperitoneal lymph node dissection for testis cancer. Urol Clin North Am. 2019;46(3):409–17.

62. Iavazzo C, Gkegkes ID. Robotic retroperitoneal lymph node dissection in gynaecological neoplasms: comparison of extraperitoneal and transperitoneal lymphadenectomy. Arch Gynecol Obstet. 2016;293(1):11–28.

63. Faraj KS, Abdul-Muhsin HM, Navaratnam AK, Rose KM, Stagg J, Ho TH, et al. Role of robot-assisted retroperitoneal lymph node dissection in malignant mesothelioma of the tunica vaginalis: case series and review of the literature. Can J Urol. 2019;26(3):9752–7.

64. Rague JT, Varda BK, Wagner AA, Lee RS. Delayed Return of ejaculatory function in adolescent males treated with retroperitoneal lymph node dissection and adjuvant therapy for paratesticular rhabdomyosarcoma. Urology. 2019;124:254–6.

65. Park JM, Charnsangavej C, Yoshimitsu K, Herron DH, Robinson TJ, Wallace S. Pathways of nodal metastasis from pelvic tumors: CT demonstration. Radiographics: a review publication of the Radiological Society of North America, Inc. 1994;14(6):1309–1321.
66. Pano B, Sebastia C, Bunesch L, Mestres J, Salvador R, Macias NG, et al. Pathways of lymphatic spread in male urogenital pelvic malignancies. Radiographics: a review publication of the Radiological Society of North America, Inc 2011;31(1):135–160.
67. Kollmannsberger C, Tandstad T, Bedard PL, Cohn-Cedermark G, Chung PW, Jewett MA, et al. Patterns of relapse in patients with clinical stage I testicular cancer managed with active surveillance. J Clin Oncol. 2015;33(1):51–7.
68. Werntz RP, Pearce SM, Eggener SE. Indications, evolving technique, and early outcomes with robotic retroperitoneal lymph node dissection. Curr Opin Urol. 2018;28(5):461–8.
69. Mazzone E, Mistretta FA, Knipper S, Tian Z, Palumbo C, Gandaglia G, et al. Contemporary assessment of long-term survival rates in patients with stage I nonseminoma germ-cell tumor of the testis: population-based comparison between surveillance and active treatment after initial orchiectomy. Clin Genitourin Cancer. 2019;
70. Masterson TA, Cary C, Foster RS. Current controversies on the role of lymphadenectomy for testicular cancer for the journal: urologic oncology: seminars and original investigations for the special seminars section on the role of lymphadenectomy for urologic cancers. Urol Oncol. 2019;
71. Heidenreich A, Paffenholz P, Nestler T, Pfister D. European association of urology guidelines on testis cancer: important take home messages. Eur Urol Focus. 2019;5(5):742–4.
72. Stephenson A, Eggener SE, Bass EB, Chelnick DM, Daneshmand S, Feldman D, et al. Diagnosis and treatment of early stage testicular cancer: AUA guideline. J Urol. 2019;202(2):272–81.
73. Motzer RJ, Jonasch E, Agarwal N, Beard C, Bhayani S, Bolger GB, et al. Testicular Cancer, Version 2.2015. J Natl Compr Cancer Netw JNCCN. 2015;13(6):772–99.
74. Stephenson AJ, Bosl GJ, Motzer RJ, Bajorin DF, Stasi JP, Sheinfeld J. Nonrandomized comparison of primary chemotherapy and retroperitoneal lymph node dissection for clinical stage IIA and IIB nonseminomatous germ cell testicular cancer. J Clin Oncol. 2007;25(35):5597–602.
75. Ghandour R, Ashbrook C, Freifeld Y, Singla N, El-Asmar JM, Lotan Y, et al. Nationwide patterns of care for stage II nonseminomatous germ cell tumor of the testicle. Eur Urol Oncol. 2019.
76. Ghandour RA, Singla N, Bagrodia A. Management of stage II germ cell tumors. Urol Clin North Am. 2019;46(3):363–76.
77. Hu B, Daneshmand S. Retroperitoneal lymph node dissection as primary treatment for metastatic seminoma. Adv Urol. 2018;2018:7978958.
78. Woldu SL, Moore JA, Ci B, Freifeld Y, Clinton TN, Aydin AM, et al. Practice patterns and impact of postchemotherapy retroperitoneal lymph node dissection on testicular cancer outcomes. Eur Urol Oncol. 2018;1(3):242–51.
79. Lakes J, Lusch A, Nini A, Albers P. Retroperitoneal lymph node dissection in the setting of elevated markers. Curr Opin Urol. 2018;28(5):435–9.
80. Wells H, Hayes MC, O'Brien T, Fowler S. Contemporary retroperitoneal lymph node dissection (RPLND) for testis cancer in the UK – a national study. BJU Int. 2017;119(1):91–9.
81. Beck SD, Foster RS, Bihrle R, Einhorn LH, Donohue JP. Outcome analysis for patients with elevated serum tumor markers at postchemotherapy retroperitoneal lymph node dissection. J Clin Oncol. 2005;23(25):6149–56.
82. Carver BS. Desperation postchemotherapy retroperitoneal lymph node dissection for metastatic germ cell tumors. Urol Clin North Am. 2015;42(3):343–6.
83. Ghodoussipour S, Daneshmand S. Postchemotherapy resection of residual mass in nonseminomatous germ cell tumor. Urol Clin North Am. 2019;46(3):389–98.
84. Ravi P, Gray KP, O'Donnell EK, Sweeney CJ. A meta-analysis of patient outcomes with subcentimeter disease after chemotherapy for metastatic non-seminomatous germ cell tumor. Ann Oncol. 2013;25(2):331–8.

85. Pearce S, Steinberg Z, Eggener S. Critical evaluation of modified templates and current trends in retroperitoneal lymph node dissection. Curr Urol Rep. 2013;14(5):511–7.
86. Donohue JP, Zachary JM, Maynard BR. Distribution of nodal metastases in nonseminomatous testis cancer. J Urol. 1982;128(2):315–20.
87. Jacobsen NE, Foster RS, Donohue JP. Retroperitoneal lymph node dissection in testicular cancer. Surg Oncol Clin N Am. 2007;16(1):199–220.
88. Yadav K. Retroperitoneal lymph node dissection: an update in testicular malignancies. Clin Transl Oncol. 2017;19(7):793–8.
89. Donohue JP, Thornhill JA, Foster RS, Rowland RG, Bihrle R. Retroperitoneal lymphadenectomy for clinical stage A testis cancer (1965 to 1989): modifications of technique and impact on ejaculation. J Urol. 1993;149(2):237–43.
90. Jewett MA, Kong YS, Goldberg SD, Sturgeon JF, Thomas GM, Alison RE, et al. Retroperitoneal lymphadenectomy for testis tumor with nerve sparing for ejaculation. J Urol. 1988;139(6):1220–4.
91. Beck SD, Foster RS, Bihrle R, Donohue JP, Einhorn LH. Is full bilateral retroperitoneal lymph node dissection always necessary for postchemotherapy residual tumor? Cancer. 2007;110(6):1235–40.
92. Cho JS, Kaimakliotis HZ, Cary C, Masterson TA, Beck S, Foster R. Modified retroperitoneal lymph node dissection for post-chemotherapy residual tumour: a long-term update. BJU Int. 2017;120(1):104–8.
93. Rukstalis DB, Chodak GW. Laparoscopic retroperitoneal lymph node dissection in a patient with stage 1 testicular carcinoma. J Urol 1992;148(6):1907–1909; discussion 9–10.
94. Porter JR. A Laparoscopic approach is best for retroperitoneal lymph node dissection: yes. J Urol. 2017;197(6):1384–6.
95. Abdul-Muhsin HM, L'Esperance JO, Fischer K, Woods ME, Porter JR, Castle EP. Robot-assisted retroperitoneal lymph node dissection in testicular cancer. J Surg Oncol. 2015;112(7):736–40.
96. Davol P, Sumfest J, Rukstalis D. Robotic-assisted laparoscopic retroperitoneal lymph node dissection. Urology. 2006;67(1):199.
97. Stepanian S, Patel M, Porter J. Robot-assisted laparoscopic retroperitoneal lymph node dissection for testicular cancer: evolution of the technique. Eur Urol. 2016;70(4):661–7.
98. Pearce SM, Golan S, Gorin MA, Luckenbaugh AN, Williams SB, Ward JF, et al. Safety and early oncologic effectiveness of primary robotic retroperitoneal lymph node dissection for nonseminomatous germ cell testicular cancer. Eur Urol. 2017;71(3):476–82.
99. Rocco NR, Stroup SP, Abdul-Muhsin HM, Marshall MT, Santomauro MG, Christman MS, et al. Primary robotic RLPND for nonseminomatous germ cell testicular cancer: a two-center analysis of intermediate oncologic and safety outcomes. World J Urol 2019.
100. Islamoglu E, Ozsoy C, Anil H, Aktas Y, Ates M, Savas M. Post-chemotherapy robot-assisted retroperitoneal lymph node dissection in non-seminomatous germ cell tumor of testis: Feasibility and outcomes of initial cases. Turk J Urol. 2018;45(2):113–7.
101. Cary C, Foster RS, Masterson TA. Complications of retroperitoneal lymph node dissection. Urol Clin North Am. 2019;46(3):429–37.
102. Crestani A, Esperto F, Rossanese M, Giannarini G, Nicolai N, Ficarra V. Andrological complications following retroperitoneal lymph node dissection for testicular cancer. Minerva urologica e nefrologica = The Italian journal of urology and nephrology. 2017;69(3):209–19.
103. Gerdtsson A, Hakansson U, Tornblom M, Jancke G, Negaard HFS, Glimelius I, et al. Surgical complications in postchemotherapy retroperitoneal lymph node dissection for nonseminoma germ cell tumour: a population-based study from the Swedish Norwegian Testicular Cancer Group. Eur Urol Oncol 2019.
104. John NT, Blum KA, Hakimi AA. Role of lymph node dissection in renal cell cancer. Urol Oncol. 2019;37(3):187–92.
105. Brito J 3rd, Gershman B. The role of lymph node dissection in the contemporary management of renal cell carcinoma: a critical appraisal of the evidence. Urol Oncol. 2017;35(11):623–6.

106. Capitanio U, Stewart GD, Larcher A, Ouzaid I, Akdogan B, Roscigno M, et al. European temporal trends in the use of lymph node dissection in patients with renal cancer. Eur J Surg Oncol. 2017;43(11):2184–92.
107. Bhindi B, Wallis CJD, Boorjian SA, Thompson RH, Farrell A, Kim SP, et al. The role of lymph node dissection in the management of renal cell carcinoma: a systematic review and meta-analysis. BJU Int. 2018;121(5):684–98.
108. European Association of Urology. EAU Guidelines on Renal Cell Carcinoma 2020 [Available from: https://uroweb.org/guideline/renal-cell-carcinoma/#7.
109. Campi R, Sessa F, Di Maida F, Greco I, Mari A, Takáčová T, et al. Templates of lymph node dissection for renal cell carcinoma: a systematic review of the literature. Front Surg. 2018;5:76.
110. Dominguez-Escrig JL, Peyronnet B, Seisen T, Bruins HM, Yuan CY, Babjuk M, et al. Potential benefit of lymph node dissection during radical nephroureterectomy for upper tract urothelial carcinoma: a systematic review by the european association of urology guidelines panel on non-muscle-invasive bladder cancer. Eur Urol Focus. 2019;5(2):224–41.
111. Dong F, Xu T, Wang X, Shen Y, Zhang X, Chen S, et al. Lymph node dissection could bring survival benefits to patients diagnosed with clinically node-negative upper urinary tract urothelial cancer: a population-based, propensity score-matched study. Int J Clin Oncol. 2019;24(3):296–305.
112. Duquesne I, Ouzaid I, Loriot Y, Moschini M, Xylinas E. Lymphadenectomy for upper tract urothelial carcinoma: a systematic review. J Clin Med. 2019;8(8).
113. Moschini M, Foerster B, Abufaraj M, Soria F, Seisen T, Roupret M, et al. Trends of lymphadenectomy in upper tract urothelial carcinoma (UTUC) patients treated with radical nephroureterectomy. World J Urol. 2017;35(10):1541–7.
114. Campi R, Minervini A, Mari A, Hatzichristodoulou G, Sessa F, Lapini A, et al. Anatomical templates of lymph node dissection for upper tract urothelial carcinoma: a systematic review of the literature. Expert Rev Anticancer Ther. 2017;17(3):235–46.
115. Hyde GA, Jung NL, Valle AA, Bhattacharya SD, Keel CE. Robotic inguinal lymph node dissection for melanoma: a novel approach to a complicated problem. J Robot Surg. 2018;12(4):745–8.
116. Wong SL, Balch CM, Hurley P, Agarwala SS, Akhurst TJ, Cochran A, et al. Sentinel lymph node biopsy for melanoma: American Society of Clinical Oncology and Society of Surgical Oncology joint clinical practice guideline. J Clin Oncol. 2012;30(23):2912–8.
117. Mall JW, Reetz C, Koplin G, Schafer-Hesterberg G, Voit C, Neuss H. Surgical technique and postoperative morbidity following radical inguinal/iliacal lymph node dissection – a prospective study in 67 patients with malignant melanoma metastatic to the groin. Zentralbl Chir. 2009;134(5):437–42.
118. Sohn W, Finley DS, Jakowatz J, Ornstein DK. Robot-assisted laparoscopic transperitoneal pelvic lymphadenectomy and metastasectomy for melanoma: initial report of two cases. J Robot Surg. 2010;4(2):129–32.
119. Pellegrino A, Damiani GR, Strippoli D, Fantini F. Robotic transperitoneal ilioinguinal pelvic lymphadenectomy for high-risk melanoma: an update of 18-month follow-up. J Robot Surg. 2014;8(2):189–91.
120. Ross AD, Kumar P, Challacombe BJ, Dasgupta P, Geh JL. The addition of the surgical robot to skin cancer management. Ann R Coll Surg Engl. 2013;95(1):70–2.
121. Horovitz D, Lu X, Feng C, Messing EM, Joseph JV. Rate of symptomatic lymphocele formation after extraperitoneal vs transperitoneal robot-assisted radical prostatectomy and bilateral pelvic lymphadenectomy. J Endourol. 2017;31(10):1037–43.

Chapter 24
Preventing Complications

Enanyeli Rangel, Jonathan Wingate, Robert Sweet, and Rene Sotelo

24.1 Error

To err is intrinsic to the human experience and our professional lives are not exempt. This is due to the imperfectness of human nature and of large, complex systems. The United States health care system first acknowledged error in medicine in the early 1990s by Leape and Gaba [1, 2]. This was brought to national attention in 1999 by the Institute of Medicine publication, "To Err is Human," which attributed between 44,000 to 98,000 deaths annually to medical error [3]. While most errors are not life threatening, they can significantly affect quality of care.

The predominant model of human error is that proposed by Reason: the person approach and the system approach [4]. The person approach focuses on unsafe acts and attributes them to forgetfulness, inattention, carelessness, etc. It attempts to mitigate error by reducing variability in human behavior. Conversely, the system approach concedes that humans are fallible and errors are unavoidable. By making these concessions, it attempts to reduce error by altering the system in which people work in order to create system defenses. Reason proposes a "Swiss cheese model" of system accidents where holes in the system defense are created by either active or latent failures. It is only when multiple layers align that the trajectory of the hazard opportunity is allowed to make contact with the patient, thus creating a demonstrable error or complication (Fig. 24.1).

E. Rangel · R. Sotelo (✉)
USC Institute of Urology and Catherine & Joseph Aresty Department of Urology, University of Southern California, Los Angeles, California, USA
e-mail: enanyeli.rangel@med.usc.edu; rene.sotelo@med.usc.edu

J. Wingate · R. Sweet
Department of Urology, University of Washington, Seattle, WA, USA
e-mail: jwingate@uw.edu; rsweet@uw.edu

© Springer Nature Switzerland AG 2021
E. Huri, D. Veneziano (eds.), *Anatomy for Urologic Surgeons in the Digital Era*,
https://doi.org/10.1007/978-3-030-59479-4_24

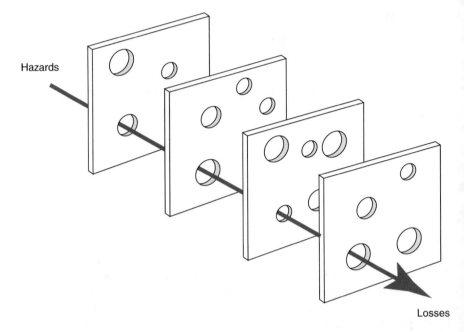

Hazards

Losses

Fig. 24.1 The Swiss cheese model of errors. Defenses, barriers, and safeguards may be penetrated by an accident and lead to error when certain conditions align. From James Reason, Human error: models and management, 2000

Achieving error-free medical care is a daunting, perhaps impossible, task; however, by implementing changes on both the personal and system level we can strive for perfection.

24.2 Preventing Complications

The art of preventing complications involves all series of actions that a surgeon and medical team do to prevent errors. This is a complex task as there are an infinite number of variables, many of which we cannot control.

24.2.1 Human Error

Although Reason argues that a person approach to error thwarts the development of safer healthcare institutions by ignoring or isolating it from their system context, we contend that these two approaches are not mutually exclusive and should be examined together [4]. A large study of operative error in an academic hospital found that the most common etiology of surgical errors was related to human factors (technique, judgment, inattention to detail, and incomplete understanding) rather than system factors [5].

Rasmussen's defines three types of operator performance and their associated errors: skill-based, rule-based, and knowledge-based. Surgeons operate at one of these three levels depending on the complexity of the task and the experience of the surgeon with the situation [6].

Skill-based tasks represent tasks that require the least experience and errors in this domain are largely errors of execution. To prevent skill-based errors, surgical and procedural simulators may play a critical role in teaching and remediation as it allows performers to practice tasks in a low risk environment [7].

Rule-based and knowledge-based tasks represent more advanced tasks than at the skill-based level. Errors at these levels are due to misclassification of the situation and applying improper rules/techniques or being unable to solve a problem due to lack of experience and knowledge. It is in this domain that surgical experience and formal residency education plays a vital role in error mitigation.

Sarker described surgical volume as an essential factor that will influence outcomes. The number of cases performed by a surgeon will affect the tactics used for challenges presented and experience is tightly bound to competence. Surgical competence, however, does not only involve technical abilities, but also communication and team-skills [7].

Case volume and time is also, closely related to the learning curve (LC) of every surgeon. The more the surgeon spends exercising their technique, the more dexterity they develop and obtain higher mastery of their craft; therefore, developing the skills needed to rectify complications or avoid them entirely [8].

The LC for a surgical procedure is related to the amount of time needed to gain competence [9]. This amount of time is variable and will depend on the procedure, previous experience, preparation intensity, as well as personal factors [10, 11].

There is no clear definition of how to measure a learning curve, however, most authors agree that increased volume is equated to increased competency, up to an asymptotic limit where increased case load start to have very marginal benefit [12]. Inexperienced surgeons have more complications in all three of Rasmussen's domains. Wang and Battista showed that surgical case volume was an independent predictor of outcomes with robotic prostatectomy with a substantial decrease in minor complications after the performance of 175 cases [13].

Volume, frequency, and variety of cases are other factors involved in the LC. It is difficult to compare a surgeon with 25 years of experience performing ten prostatectomies a year to a recent graduate performing ten prostatectomies per month. There will be different results for each case. However, data from Abboudi suggest that higher volume centers have better outcomes and superior long-term survival.

Effective risk management is also dependent on having a safe reporting culture [14]. This is not only to prevent error in real-time, but also to learn from mistakes to prevent the same errors from recurring. This has been adopted in the surgical community by allowing for anyone in the surgical team to speak-up against unsafe actions and with the non-attributional morbidity and mortality system to review complications [15].

24.2.2   System Error

The person-based approach to error views errors as a result of human fallacy and attempts to mitigate complications by increasing knowledge, technical skill, and allowing for a safe culture to explore one's errors. Conversely, the system approach views errors as consequences due to errors in the defense system.

High technology and reliable systems can help prevent error by creating barriers and defensive layers that serve as checks and balances. According to Reason, there are three main types of barriers:

1. Engineered, such as the use of medication dosage screens and allergy alerts in electronic medical record systems [16].
2. People, such as communication between the OR nursing team, surgical team, and anesthesia during a complex surgery.
3. Procedures and administrative controls, such as pre-operative time-outs and checklists.

These systems attempt to prevent hazards from ever reaching the patient by creating multiple barriers. For example, when a surgeon forgets a patient's penicillin allergy and orders a penicillin antibiotic, the electronic medical record should trigger an alert and the surgeon changes to a different medication. Although the surgeon made a mistake, the defenses prevented the mistake from causing any harm. However, complications can still occur when the holes in the defenses align. In the case previously mentioned, if the nurse or medical assistant does not update the patient's allergy in the computer system, the alert would not trigger.

24.3   Use of Novel Technology to Prevent Error

24.3.1   Simulation

Traditionally, the urologic training model has been one of apprenticeship. However, this experience is variable, and it does not provide an ethical means to practice complications. Due to these factors, surgical simulation provides a unique opportunity to practice procedural skills and complex decision-making in high fidelity, no-risk environment, thereby aiding in complication prevention and management. Multiple surgical disciplines have demonstrated a surgical learning curve with case volume and surgical proficiency being directly related [17–19]. Simulation training solutions have improved surgical skills acquisition and training, especially for imaging-based procedures [20].

Currently, simulation is predominately used to provide training in two domains: 1. Skills acquisition for commonly performed procedures and tasks, and 2. Training uncommon yet high-risk procedures and scenarios. By improving proficiency and

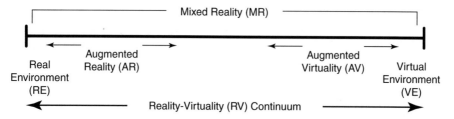

Fig. 24.2 Definition of mixed reality within the context of the RV continuum. From Milgram P, Colquhoun H., Jr. A taxonomy of real and virtual world display integration. Mixed reality: merging real and virtual worlds. Used with permission

aiding in skills acquisition, simulation can help play a role in a urologists' Dreyfus mastery of skills, thus decreasing their complication rate [21].

The simulation comprises of any technique to replace or amplify real experiences. Traditionally, they were live tissue training (LTT) with cadavers or animals. However, these are not only expensive, but social pressures have pushed for a move away from LTT. Simulators have progressed past the physical or "box" simulators and have entered the virtual reality domain [20]. We propose Milgram and Kishino's description of VR as a continuum between the real and virtual environments [22] (Fig. 24.2).

VR simulators have been shown to decrease operating time and improve performance in trainees with limited laparoscopic experience [9]. This improvement, however, is not limited to novice trainees as a randomized trial of a warm-up robotic curriculum on a VR simulator demonstrated a significant decrease in errors during the antecedent case [23]. VR is also being utilized as a pre-operative surgical planning tool for robotic partial nephrectomy and, in a randomized trial, demonstrated significant improvement in patient-centered outcomes [24].

Currently, simulators are utilized to prevent errors and complications by increasing proficiency and allowing for skills acquisition. As simulation sciences progress, we hope that there will be new curricula created that can also address how to respond to and fix surgical errors, that is, practice complications. The majority of the simulators currently available are limited to imaging-based surgeries, as current VR technology translates well to a screen-based simulated environment. With continued advances in technology, the future of simulation will be a virtual environment that can simulate open surgery in a high-fidelity manner.

24.3.2 Robotic Surgery

Robotic surgery was created in order to have more efficient and ergonomic laparoscopic platform. Robotics offered a solution to the limitations of operating in the confined space of the pelvis offering more degrees of articulation than a human wrist, 3-dimensional imaging, ergonomic operating environment, and a shorter LC for certain cases such as laparoscopic prostatectomy [25]. These factors help mitigate skill-based surgical errors [26].

24.3.3 Video Review

Skarecky proposed that observation is critical to error prevention. Taking time to view recordings of surgeries has been proven to be a valuable tool in pinpointing mistakes or revealing more efficient methods of performing a specific task [27].

The observation element in preventing complications represents a passive way of preventing mistakes and can be achieved by strict follow-up and documentation. With urologists eagerly adapting robotic technology, video recording is becoming more prevalent. With video recordings, surgeons are creating a log that can be reviewed many times over. Video recordings prove to be extremely useful to solve problems and hypothesize solutions for a specific setback [27]. Recent data also suggest that these videos can be graded by non-experts and provide objective feedback on surgical skills and areas of improvement [26].

The value of video review has been emphasized by Guerlain and Yang. Reviewing operative video can improve the understanding of surgical tasks and watching videos of errors could help learners avoid the same mistakes [28, 29].

24.3.4 Fluorescent Tracers

The use of fluorescent tracers, such as Indocyanine green, and complementary cameras allow for identification of specific anatomical geography and functional features. This dye was FDA approved in 1959, but it has started to gain popularity in 2011 [30, 31]. It is a water-soluble and anionic dye that bounds to protein getting confined to the vascular compartment allowing a rapid identification of blood vessels. It is often used in the reconstruction field for evaluation of flap perfusion [32]. By helping to identify perfusion and aberrant vascular anatomy, it attempts to decrease error by reducing rule- and knowledge-based deficits.

24.4 Conclusion

Error is intrinsic not only to the human condition, but also to large systems due to the complexity of medicine and the medical systems. Although perfection may be an impossible task, we should strive to provide error-free care. In order to do so, we should acknowledge the levels at which errors occurs, why they occur, and how we can learn and improve to mitigate both personal and system based errors.

The proliferation of technology in medicine and surgery also provide exciting opportunities to learn and reduce errors.

References

1. Leape LL, Brennan TA, Laird NAN, Anng L, et al. The nature of adverse events in hospitalized patients. N Engl J Med. 1991;324(6):377–84.
2. Gaba D. Human error in dynamic medical domains. NJ; 1994.
3. Linda T. Kohn, Janet M. Corrigan and MSD. To err is human. Building a safer health system, volume 6 [Internet]. Vol. 2, Int J Publ Health. 1999. 93–95 p. Available from: https://books.google.com/books?hl=en&lr=&id=Jj25GlLKXSgC&pgis=1
4. Reason J. Human error: models and management. Br Med J. 2000;320(7237):768–70.
5. Fabri PJ, Zayas-Castro JL. Human error, not communication and systems, underlies surgical complications. Surgery. 2008;144(4):557–65.
6. J R. Skills, Rules and Knowledge: signals, signs and symbols and other distintions in human perfomance models. 1983. 257–267 p.
7. Sarker SK, Vincent C. Errors in surgery. Int J Surg. 2005;3(1):75–81.
8. Doumas KAG. Surgical complications of laparoscopic urological surgery. Arch Esp Urol. 2002;56(6):730–6.
9. Nagendran M, Gurusamy KSAR, et al. Virtual reality training for surgical trainees in laparoscopic surgery. Cochrane Database Syst Rev. 2013:1–45.
10. Mazzon G, Sridhar A, Busuttil G, Thompson J, Nathan S, Briggs T, et al. Learning curves for robotic surgery: a review of the recent literature. Curr Urol Rep. 2017;18(11):1–6.
11. Wang L, Diaz M, Stricker H, Peabody JO, Menon M, Rogers CG. Adding a newly trained surgeon into a high-volume robotic prostatectomy group: are outcomes compromised? J Robot Surg. 2017;11(1):69–74.
12. Abboudi H, Khan MS, Guru KA, Froghi S, De Win G, Van Poppel H, et al. Learning curves for urological procedures: a systematic review. BJU Int. 2014;114(4):617–29.
13. Di Pierro GB, Wirth JG, Ferrari M, Danuser H, Mattei A. Impact of a single-surgeon learning curve on complications, positioning injuries, and renal function in patients undergoing robot-assisted radical prostatectomy and extended pelvic lymph node dissection. Urology. 2014;84(5):1106–11.
14. Reason J. Managing the risks of organizational accidents. Aldershot: Ashgate; 1997.
15. Tignanelli CJ, Embree GGR, Barzin A. House staff–led interdisciplinary morbidity and mortality conference promotes systematic improvement. J Surg Res [Internet]. 2017;214:124–30. Available from: doi:https://doi.org/10.1016/j.jss.2017.02.065.
16. Bates D, Cohen M, Leape LL, Overhage M, Shabot MST. Reducing the frequency of errors in medicine using information technology. JAMIA. 2001;8(4):299–308.
17. Lavery HJ, Samadi DB, Thaly R, Albala D, Ahlering T, Shalhav A, et al. The advanced learning curve in robotic prostatectomy: a multi-institutional survey. J Robot Surg. 2009;3(3):165–9.
18. Faris SF, Myers JB, Voelzke BB, Elliott SP, Breyer BN, Vanni AJ, Tam CAEB. Assessment of the male urethral reconstruction learning curve. Physiol Behav. 2017;176(5):139–48.
19. Maruthappu M, Duclos A, Lipsitz SR, Orgill D, Carty MJ. Surgical learning curves and operative efficiency: a cross-specialty observational study. BMJ Open. 2015;5(3):1–6.
20. Seymour NE, Gallagher AG, Roman SA, O'Brien MK, Bansal VK, Andersen DK, Richard MS. Virtual reality training improves operating room performance. results of a randomized, double blinded study. Ann Surg. 2002;236(4):458–64.
21. Dreyfus SE. The five-stage model of adult skill acquisition. Bull Sci Technol Soc. 2004;24(3):177–81.
22. Milgram P, Colquhoun H. A taxonomy of real and virtual world display integration. Mix Real 1999;5–30.

23. Lendvay TS, Brand TC, White L, Kowalewski T, Jonnadula S, Mercer L, Khorsand D, Andros JHB. Virtual reality robotic surgery warm-up improves task performance in a dry lab environment: a prospective randomized controlled study. J Am Coll Surg. 2013;216(6):1–25.

24. Shirk JD, Thiel DD, Wallen EM, Linehan JM, White WM, Badani KK, et al. Effect of 3-dimensional virtual reality models for surgical planning of robotic-assisted partial nephrectomy on surgical outcomes: a randomized clinical trial. JAMA Netw Open. 2019;2(9):e1911598.

25. Hussain A, Malik A, Halim MU, Ali AM. The use of robotics in surgery: a review. Int J Clin Pract. 2014;68(11):1376–82.

26. Ghani KR, Miller DC, Linsell S, Brachulis A, Lane B, Sarle R, et al. Measuring to improve: peer and crowd-sourced assessments of technical skill with robot-assisted radical prostatectomy. Eur Urol [Internet]. 2016;69(4):547–50. Available from: doi:https://doi.org/10.1016/j.eururo.2015.11.028.

27. Skarecky DW. Robotic-assisted radical prostatectomy after the first decade: surgical evolution or new paradigm. ISRN Urol. 2013;2013:1–22.

28. Yang K, Perez M, Hubert N, Hossu G, Perrenot C, Hubert J. Effectiveness of an integrated video recording and replaying system in robotic surgical training. Ann Surg. 2017;265(3):521–6.

29. Vaughn CJ, Kim E, O'Sullivan P, Huang E, Lin MYC, Wyles S, et al. Peer video review and feedback improve performance in basic surgical skills. Am J Surg [Internet]. 2016;211(2):355–60. https://doi.org/10.1016/j.amjsurg.2015.08.034.

30. Cacciamani GE, Shakir A, Tafuri A, Gill K, Han J, Ahmadi N, et al. Best practices in near-infrared fluorescence imaging with indocyanine green (NIRF/ICG)-guided robotic urologic surgery: a systematic review-based expert consensus. World J Urol [Internet]. 2019;(0123456789). https://doi.org/10.1007/s00345-019-02870-z.

31. van der Poel HG, Grivas N, van Leeuwen F. Comprehensive assessment of indocyanine green usage: one tracer, multiple urological applications. Eur Urol Focus [Internet]. 2018;4(5):665–8. https://doi.org/10.1016/j.euf.2018.08.017.

32. Kaplan-Marans E, Fulla J, Tomer N, Bilal K, Palese M. Indocyanine green (ICG) in urologic surgery. Urology. 2019;00(00):1–8.

Index

© Springer Nature Switzerland AG 2021
E. Huri, D. Veneziano (eds.), *Anatomy for Urologic Surgeons in the Digital Era*,
https://doi.org/10.1007/978-3-030-59479-4

Printed in the United States
by Baker & Taylor Publisher Services